O G P L

OXFORD GENERAL PRACTICE LIBRARY

Child Health

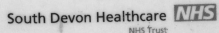

O G P L

OXFORD GENERAL PRACTICE LIBRARY

Child Health

Dr Francoise van Dorp

General Practitioner,
Laindon, UK

and

Dr Chantal Simon

MRC Research Fellow and
General Practitioner,
University of Southampton,
Southampton, UK

and Series Editor

OXFORD
UNIVERSITY PRESS

OXFORD
UNIVERSITY PRESS

Great Clarendon Street, Oxford OX2 6DP

Oxford University Press is a department of the University of Oxford.
It furthers the University's objective of excellence in research, scholarship,
and education by publishing worldwide in

Oxford New York

Auckland Cape Town Dar es Salaam Hong Kong Karachi
Kuala Lumpur Madrid Melbourne Mexico City Nairobi
New Delhi Shanghai Taipei Toronto

With offices in

Argentina Austria Brazil Chile Czech Republic France Greece
Guatemala Hungary Italy Japan Poland Portugal Singapore
South Korea Switzerland Thailand Turkey Ukraine Vietnam

Oxford is a registered trade mark of Oxford University Press
in the UK and in certain other countries

Published in the United States
by Oxford University Press Inc., New York

British Library Cataloguing in Publication Data

Data available

Library of Congress Cataloging in Publication Data

Data available

Typeset by Newgen Imaging Systems (P) Ltd., Chennai, India
Printed in Italy
on acid-free paper by
LegoPrint S.p.A.

ISBN 978–0–19–921568-3

10 9 8 7 6 5 4 3 2 1

Contents

Acknowledgements

We met on our first day at St. John's College in Cambridge as 18 year old medical students, when we discovered we were living next door to each other. This has not been an easy project as compressing the whole of child health for GPs into under 400 pages has been a real challenge. However, many years after our first encounter, and now both GPs, it has been a pleasure to work together after so long, and find that we still make such a good team.

This book would not have come into being without the support and drive of the editorial and production team at Oxford University Press and we would like to say a big thank you to all of you. We would also like to thank the authors of the Oxford Handbook of General Practice for allowing us to reproduce material, the authors and reviewers of many of the other books in the Oxford General Practice Library Series particularly Dr R. Davies, Dr A. Wilson, Dr N. Dunn, Dr H. Everitt, Mr R. Newsom, Mr D. Hargreaves, Prof. A. Kendrick, and Dr J. Lynch, and Theresa Gowing and Sandra Bryan for the information and advice they provided. Finally we would like to thank our major reviewer, Dr Judith Harvey, who, apart from correcting many minor typos, gave us a lot of helpful suggestions from her considerable experience of inner-city practice.

All those involved in writing while working clinically, will be very aware that the real cost of such work is borne by families, and our families in Brentwood and Hordle are no exception. We would particularly like to thank our children (Emma, Helena, Adam, Ben, Hannah and Kate) for the extensive first-hand experience of parenting they have given us, which has proved so valuable in writing this book. We would also like David and Peter, our ever-tolerant husbands, to know how much we both appreciate them for making this project possible through their never-ending patience, love and support.

FvD
CS

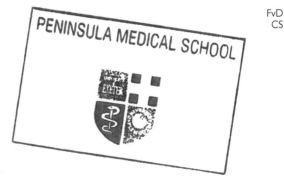

Symbols and abbreviations

⚠	Warning
❶	Important Note
💧	Controversial point
☎	Telephone number
💾	Website
📖	Cross reference to
±	With or without
↑	Increased/increasing
↓	Decreased/decreasing
→	Leading to
°	Degrees
1°	Primary
2°	Secondary
♂	Male
♀	Female
≈	Approximately equal
~	Approximately
%	Percent(age)
≥	Greater than or equal to
≤	Less than or equal to
>	Greater than
<	Less than
+ve	Positive
−ve	Negative
C	Cochrane review
G	Guideline from major guideline producing body
N	NICE guidance
R	Randomized controlled trial in major journal
S	Systematic review in major journal
ND	Notifiable disease

β	Beta
A&E	Accident and Emergency
ADHD	Attention deficit hyperactivity disorder
AED	Automated external defibrillator
AF	Atrial fibrillation
AIDS	Acquired immune deficiency syndrome
ALL	Acute lymphoblastic leukaemia
AML	Acute myeloid leukaemia
ASD	Atrial setal defect
ASO	Anti-strept.....
AV	Atrio-ventricular
A-V	Arterio-venous
bd	Twice daily
BCG	Bacillus Calmette-Guerin
BHF	British Heart Foundation
BM	Blood glucose using reagent strip
BMA	British Medical Association
BMI	Body mass index
BMJ	British Medical Journal
BNF	British National Formulary
BP	Blood pressure
bpm	Beats per minute
BTS	British Thoracic Society
C	Centigrade
Ca^{2+}	Calcium
CAH	Congenital adrenal hyperplasia
CDH	Congenital dislocation of the hip
CF	Cystic fibrosis
CHT	Congenital hypothyroidism
Cl^-	Chloride
cm	Centimetre(s)
CMV	Cytomegalovirus
CNS	Central nervous system
CO_2	Carbon dioxide
COC	Combined oral contraceptive
CPR	Cardiopulmonary resuscitation
Cr	Creatinine

CRP	C-reactive protein
CSF	Cerebrospinal fluid
CSM	Committee on Safety of Medicines
CT	Computerized tomography
CVD	Cardiovascular disease
CXR	Chest X-ray
d	Day(s)
DC	Direct current
DDH	Developmental dysplasaia of the hip
dL	Decilitre
DLA	Disability Living Allowance
DM	Diabetes mellitus
DNA	Deoxyribonucleic acid
DoH	Department of Health
DSH	Deliberate self-harm
DTaP	Diptheria, tetanus and pertussis vaccine
DTB	Drugs and Therapeutic Bulletin
DWP	Department of Work and Pensions
EBV	Epstein-Barr virus
Echo	Echocardiogram
ECG	Electrocardiograph
EEG	Electro-encephalogram
e.g.	For example
ENT	Ear, nose and throat
ESR	Erythrocyte sedimentation rate
ESRF	End-stage renal failure
etc.	Et cetera
F	Farenheit
FBC	Full blood count
FEV_1	Forced expiratory volume in one second
FH	Family history
FVC	Forced vital capacity
g	grams
G6PD	Glucose 6 phosphate dehydrogenase
GA	General anaesthetic
GBS	Group B streptococcus
GI	gastrointestinal

GMC	General Medical Council
GMS	General Medical Services
GnRH	Gonadotrophin releasing hormone
GORD	Gastro-oesophageal reflux disease
Gp.	Group
GP	General Practitioner
h	Hour(s)
Hb	Haemoglobin
HBeAg	Hepatitis e-antigen
HBeIg	Hepatitis B e-immunoglobulin
HBsAg	Hepatitis s-antigen
HBsIg	Hepatitis B s -immunoglobulin
HCV	Hepatitis C virus
Hib	Haemophilus influenza type b (vaccine)
HIV	Human immunodeficiency virus
HOCM	Hypertrophic obstructive cardiomyopathy
HSV	Herpes simplex virus
ICP	Intracranial pressure
Ig	Immunoglobulin
IM	Intramuscular
IO	Intraosseous
INR	International normalization ratio
IPV	Inactivated polio vaccine
IQ	Intelligence quotient
IRT	Immunoreactive trypsin
IS	Income support
IT	Information technology
IUCD	Intrauterine contraceptive device
IUGR	Intrauterine growth retardation
IV	Intravenous
IVF	In vitro fertilization
J	Joules
JCA	Juvenile chronic arthritis
JSA	JobSeekers Allowance
JVP	Jugular venous pressure
K^+	Potassium
kg	Kilogram(s)

l	Litre(s)
L	Left
LABA	Long acting beta agonist
LFT	Liver function test
LMWH	Low molecular weight heparin
LN	Lymph node
LOC	Loss of consciousness
LRTI	Lower respiratory tract infection
LSCS	Lower segment Caesarean Section
LTOT	Long term oxygen therapy
LVF	Left ventricular failure
m	Metres
M.	Mycobacterium
mcgm	Micrograms
M,C&S	Microscopy, culture and sensitivity
MCUG	Micturating cysto-urethrogram
MCV	Mean cell volume
MDI	Metered dose inhaler
Men C	Meningitis C vaccine
mg	Milligrams
MHRA	Medicines & Healthcare Products Regulatory Agency
MI	Myocardial infarct
min	Minutes
ml	Millilitres
mmHg	Millimetres of mercury
mmol	Millimole
MMR	Measles, mumps and rubella
mo	Month(s)
MRSA	Methicillin resistant Staphylococcus aureus
MSU	Mid-stream urine
Na^+	Sodium
NAI	Non-accidental injury
NHS	National Health Service
NICE	National Institute for Clinical Excellence
nmol	Nanomoles
NSAID	Non-steroidal anti-inflammatory drug
NSF	National Service Framework

O$_2$	Oxygen
od	Once daily
OM	Otitis media
OT	Occupational therapy/therapist
OTC	Over the counter
OUP	Oxford University Press
p.	Page number
P.	Plasmodium
PALS	Paediatric advanced life support
PBLS	Paediatric basic life support
PCO	Primary Care Organization
PDA	Patent ductus arteriosus
PE	Pulmonary embolus
PEFR	Peak expiratory flow rate
PFBAO	Paediatric foreign body airways obstruction
Physio	Physiotherapy
PIP	Proximal interphalangeal joint
PKU	Phenylketonuria
PMH	Past medical history
PMS	Personal Medical Services
po	Oral
prn	As needed
qds	Four times daily
QOF	Quality and outcomes framework
R	Right
RA	Rheumatoid arthritis
RCGP	Royal College of General Practitioners
RCN	Royal College of Nursing
RNA	Ribonucleaic acid
RSV	Respiratory syncitial virus
s or sec	Second (s)
S.	Streptococcus
SAH	Subarachnoid haemorrhage
SBE	Subacute bacterial endocarditis
s/cut	Subcutaneous
SIGN	Scottish Intercollegiate Guidelines Network
SOL	Space occupying lesion

SPF	Sun-protection factor
Staph.	Staphylococcus
STD	Sexually transmitted disease
Srep.	Streptococcus
SVT	Supraventricular tachycardia
TB	Tuberculosis
Td	Tetanus and low dose diphtheria vaccine
tds	Three times a day
TFTs	Thyroid function tests
TOF	Tracheo-oesophageal fistula
TSH	Thyroid stimulating hormone
u	units
U&E	Urea and electrolytes
UC	Ulcerative colitis
UK	United Kingdom
URTI	Upper respiratory tract infection
USS	Ultrasound scan
UTI	Urinary tract infection
VAT	Value added tax
VF	Ventricular fibrillation
VSD	Ventricular septal defect
VT	Ventricular tachycardia
VZ	Varicella zoster
WCC	White cell count
WHO	World Health Organization
wk	Week(s)
WPW	Wolff-Parkinson-White syndrome
y	Year(s)

Chapter 1

Assessing and screening children in primary care

1

Consultations with children

Child-friendly premises: Try to make the surgery, waiting room and consulting rooms child-friendly:
- Provide access for prams/pushchairs
- Have a few toys/books available
- Keep anything potentially dangerous (e.g. sharps box) well out of reach.

Aims: When assessing a child in primary care, objectives are to:
- Establish a constructive relationship with the child and carers to enable effective communication and serve as the basis for any subsequent therapeutic relationship. ❶ Be aware of cultural issues – if in doubt, ask.
- Determine whether the child has a physical or behavioural problem and, if so, what that is
- Find out (where possible) what caused that problem
- Assess the child's/family's emotions and attitudes towards the problem
- Establish how it might be treated.

History: Figure 1.1
- Check the relationship between the child and accompanying adult.
- Include the child and encourage him/her to contribute to the history when old enough to do so. For adolescents, consider seeing alone as well as with the carer.
- Use open questions at the start becoming directive when necessary – clarify, reflect, facilitate, listen.

Examination: Figure 1.1
- Young children may be best examined on the carer's lap.
- A minute or two playing (e.g. pretending to examine teddy, allowing the child to play with the stethoscope) may be well worth it to gain a child's cooperation.
- Some children are reluctant to be undressed – be flexible. Adequate examination is often possible without completely undressing the child.
- Leave any unpleasant parts of the examination (e.g. ENT or anything that is painful) until the end.

Investigation: Further investigations and interventions are guided by the findings on history and examination.

Assessment algorithm for sick infants: Figure 1.2 📖 p.4

Assessment of adolescents: 📖 p.6

Assessment of behaviour problems: 📖 p.8

Action:
- Summarize the history. Include children in discussion if old enough, and explain in terms the child and carer can understand. Give an opportunity for the child or carer to fill in any gaps.
- Attitudes and beliefs: how does the carer (and/or child) see the problem? What do they think is wrong? What does the family want you to do about it?
- Draw up a problem list and outline a management plan including review date if appropriate.

Figure 1.1 Paediatric assessment

ASK ABOUT

Presenting complaint
Chronological account of the presenting complaint
Past history of similar symptoms and previous treatments

Past medical history
Birth history – premature, significant birth injury, congenital disorder
Previous significant illnesses and chronic illness e.g. asthma
Current medication
Drug allergies/intolerances

Family history if relevant e.g. asthma if child has a chronic cough,
smoking history if child has asthma or recurrent otitis media

Social history
Housing
Social support
Family problems e.g. marriage breakdown, employment or
financial problems

EXAMINE

General examination: – Does the child look ill? General
appearance, alertness, hydration (skin turgor, mucus membranes,
fontanelle), colour, respiratory rate – temperature (if any suggestion
of infection)

Then tailor examination to confirm/refute suspected diagnosis.
Consider:
- Examination for meningitis – neck stiffness? Photophobia?
  Drowsiness? Non-blanching skin rash? Bulging fontanelle?
- Examination of the skin – colour (cyanosis, erythema), capillary
  refill time (≥3 seconds and/or cool peripheries – abnormal and
  suggests peipheral shutdown), rashes, scabies, scars, signs of NAI
- Examination of ears, nose and throat
- Examination of chest – heart sounds, murmurs/thrills, respiratory
  rate, intercostal/subcostal recession, crepitations, wheeze
- Check abdomen for hepatosplenomegaly, masses, tenderness
- Check neurology if history of visual/neurological deficit or fitting
- Check musculoskeletal system (look, feel, move) if history of
  bone, joint or limb pain
- Weigh/measure if failure to thrive, neurological deficit (head
  circumference), feeding problem or history of weight loss

GP Notes: Referring children

Remember: Parents know their children best – take any concerns
seriously. NICE recommends:
- Urgent referral when a child/young person presents several times
  (≥ 3x) with the same problem, but with no clear diagnosis.
- Persistent parental anxiety is sufficient reason for referral, even
  where a benign cause is considered most likely.

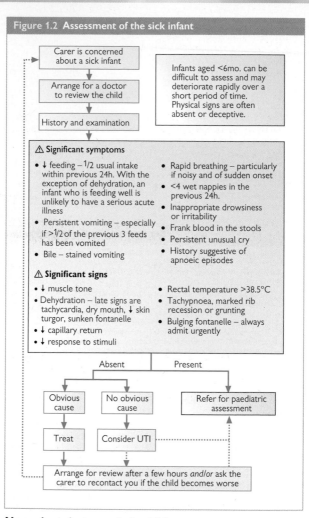

Figure 1.2 Assessment of the sick infant

```
Carer is concerned
about a sick infant
        ↓
Arrange for a doctor
to review the child
        ↓
History and examination
```

Infants aged <6mo. can be difficult to assess and may deteriorate rapidly over a short period of time. Physical signs are often absent or deceptive.

⚠ Significant symptoms

- ↓ feeding – ¹/2 usual intake within previous 24h. With the exception of dehydration, an infant who is feeding well is unlikely to have a serious acute illness
- Persistent vomiting – especially if >¹/2 of the previous 3 feeds has been vomited
- Bile – stained vomiting

- Rapid breathing – particularly if noisy and of sudden onset
- <4 wet nappies in the previous 24h.
- Inappropriate drowsiness or irritability
- Frank blood in the stools
- Persistent unusual cry
- History suggestive of apnoeic episodes

⚠ Significant signs

- ↓ muscle tone
- Dehydration – late signs are tachycardia, dry mouth, ↓ skin turgor, sunken fontanelle
- ↓ capillary return
- ↓ response to stimuli

- Rectal temperature >38.5°C
- Tachypnoea, marked rib recession or grunting
- Bulging fontanelle – always admit urgently

```
              Absent              Present
         ┌──────┴──────┐              │
    Obvious         No obvious    Refer for paediatric
    cause           cause         assessment
       │               │              ↑
    Treat         Consider UTI ········┘
       └───────────────┴──────────────────┐
  Arrange for review after a few hours and/or ask the
  carer to recontact you if the child becomes worse
```

Normal respiratory rate in children:

- *Neonate:* 30–60 breaths/min.
- *Infant:* 20–40 breaths/min.
- *1–3y.:* 20–30 breaths/min.
- *4–10y.:* 15–25 breaths/min.
- *>10y.:* 15–20 breaths/min.

Normal pulse rate in children:
- **≤1y.:** 110–160 beats/min.
- **2–5y.:** 95–140 beats/min.
- **5–12y.:** 80–120 beats/min.
- **>12y.:** 60–100 beats/min.

Normal temperature in children:
- *Oral:* 35.5–37.5°C (95.9–99.5°F)
- *Rectal:* 36.6–38.0°C (97.9–100.4°F)
- *Axillary:* 34.7–37.3°C (94.5–99.1°F)
- *Ear:* 35.8–38.0°C (96.4–100.4°F)

GP Notes: General rules for assessment of sick infants

- Always arrange for a sick baby who has not responded to simple measures (e.g. paracetamol and fluids) to be reviewed by a doctor.
- Always trust the mother's instinct.
- Always perform a full physical examination. Localizing signs might be absent (e.g. tonsillitis is a frequent cause of vomiting). Petechial rash under the nappy area can be easily missed.
- The younger the baby – the lower the threshold for seeking a paediatrician's opinion.

5

Advice for patients: Parents' and children's experiences of medical care

Putting children at ease

'They always used to sort of tickle his tummy while they were listening to him and say silly things. The doctor would be looking in his ears and they used to say, "Oh we've carrots growing today" or "Have you cleaned your ears?" They always used to play with him and ask him what he'd been doing either at nursery or at school, or about his home life and his food, and "Have you been to McDonald's?" and "Where are you going on holiday?" and "What are you doing today?" '

'They always had plenty of time for X which is, I think, really important to build a relationship, and it felt like we'd got a relationship with the doctors rather than just going to see a doctor.'

Children's experiences of communication with health professionals

'Most of the time it was really, really good. I found the nurses very easy to get on with, slightly easier than the doctors, they seemed to know a lot. Well they didn't know a lot more about it but they were a lot better at communicating it than the doctors were.'

'And when I woke up I was in the hospital with all my family around me and that was when I was told that I had a seizure. And this obviously meant absolutely nothing to me. I had absolutely no idea what a seizure was, I'd never been told or even heard about it before... I was just, I was just basically passed these pills and told that I was an epileptic and that's as far as it went.'

Consultations with adolescents

Adolescents visit their GPs on average 2–3x/y. but their needs are often poorly addressed. Aspects of general practice important to them include:

Confidentiality and consent: Posters/leaflets in the surgery about confidentiality help ↑ confidence. Usual principles of confidentiality and consent apply (📖 p.320). In particular, an adolescent judged competent:

- Can withhold permission for their parents to have access to medical information about them
- Can request to be seen alone without a parent.

🚫 Ensure confidentiality isn't breached when appointments are booked (e.g. for emergency contraception) and when telephoning about results, appointments or prescriptions.

Accessibility: Access to the primary care team can be a problem for teenagers, especially about issues they don't want to tell their parents about. To make services more accessible consider:

- *Timing and availability of appointments:* Special teenage clinics after school hours can help
- *Friendliness:* Ensure reception staff welcome teenagers when they come to the surgery without their parents. Listen to what teenagers say they want from the practice and try to be as accommodating as possible in providing those facilities/services
- *Information:* Provide leaflets and posters using language and presented in ways which are attractive for teenagers
- *Offer a choice of doctor:* Gender of the doctor is particularly important for sexual health matters. Often teenagers *don't* want to see the doctor they've always seen since being a small child or the doctor their mother always takes them to
- *Non-judgemental attitudes:* Teenagers often push the boundaries. They won't consult for help if they know they will be judged when they go too far or make mistakes. Listen and offer support, help, advice and treatment without being judgemental wherever possible.

Specific problems to look out for in teenagers:

- *Behavioural problems* – 📖 p.308
- *Psychiatric disease* – 📖 p.308
- *Eating disorders* – 📖 p.312
- *Drugs, solvent and/or alcohol abuse* – 📖 p.309
- *Sexual health problems* – > ½ have had sexual intercourse aged <16y. and so fear and risk of pregnancy are part of adolescent life. Those who have intercourse early are at greater risk of early pregnancy and health problems such as sexually transmitted disease and cervical cancer. Worries about sexuality for some can add to the pressure. Sensitive support, clear guidance and accurate information about contraception, sexuality and sexually transmitted disease is helpful.
- *Teenage pregnancy:* The UK has the highest teenage pregnancy rate in Western Europe. Not all are unplanned. Pregnant teenagers need information and non-judgemental support to help them reach a decision whether or not to continue with the pregnancy.

Cross-cultural issues: Adolescents can find themselves caught between the culture they were born and brought up in and their parents' culture. Be supportive.

GP Notes: Contraception and the under 16's

In England and Wales, a doctor is allowed to give advice to a girl aged <16y. without parental consent if:
- She has sufficient maturity to understand the moral, social and emotional implications of treatment
- She cannot be persuaded to inform (or allow the doctor to inform) her parents
- She is very likely to begin, or continue, sexual intercourse with or without contraception
- She is likely to suffer if no contraceptive advice or treatment is given
- It is in her best interest that contraceptive advice or treatment is given with or without parental consent.

Choice of contraceptive method:
- Condoms are adolescents' most commonly used form of contraception but have a relatively high failure rate. Suggesting their use in addition to another form of contraception will help prevent STDs.
- The low-dose combined oral contraceptive (COC) pill is the most suitable method of contraception for the under 16s. Poor compliance can be a problem and leads to a high failure rate.
- Progestogen implants/injectables are alternatives to the COC pill but the CSM advises that, in adolescents, medroxyprogesterone acetate (Depo-Provera®) should only be used when other methods of contraception are inappropriate. Can cause osteoporosis (use alternative if other risk factors and try not to use >2y.), menstrual irregularity and ↑ weight.
- The progestogen-containing intrauterine contraceptive device (IUCD) is less likely to cause pelvic inflammatory disease and ectopic pregnancy than other IUCDs but can be difficult to insert in a young woman.
- 'The morning after pill' (Levonelle) is not suitable as a regular method but valuable in preventing unwanted pregnancy. Information on availability and ability to make an urgent appointment is essential.

Do's and don'ts:
- **Don't** insist on vaginal examination or taking a smear unless there is a problem that necessitates it.
- **Do** discuss the merits of delaying sexual intercourse until older.
- **Do** stress the need for protection against sexually transmitted diseases.
- If prescribing the COC pill for dysmenorrhoea or cycle control in young women, **do** explain its use for contraception too.

Advice for patients: Information and support for teenagers

Childline 24h. confidential counselling ☎ 0800 1111 ▣ www.childline.org
Brook Advisory Service Contraceptive advice and counselling for teenagers ☎ 0800 0185 023 ▣ www.brook.org.uk
Sexwise For under 19s ☎ 0800 28 29 30
Teenage Health Freak ▣ www.teenagehealthfreak.org

Further information
BMJ McPherson *Adolescents in primary care* (2005) 330 pp.465–7
NICE Preventing sexually transmitted infections and reducing under 18 conceptions (2007). ▣ www.nice.org.uk

Child mental health assessment

2–5% of children are presented by their parents or carers with mental health or behaviour problems as the main complaint, often mixed with physical problems. GPs are commonly asked to 'sort out' behaviour problems of children by parents who are at their wit's end. 2–10% of all children are said to have behaviour problems depending on how the problems are defined and measured.

Differentiation between normal behaviour and behavioural problems can be difficult, especially if you don't know the child or family well. A significant problem is more likely:
• When the behaviour is frequent and chronic
• When >1 problem behaviour occurs *and*
• If behaviour interferes with social and/or cognitive functioning.

A feature of child psychiatry is that the child should be seen in the context of a family – any problems are an interaction between child, family and environment. The history is usually taken from the parents but it's helpful if the child can contribute. Older children may prefer to be seen alone.

Assessment: See Figure 1.3

Management: 📖 pp.289–315

Advice for patients

Information and support for parents:
Green *Toddler Taming*: a parent's guide to the first four years (2000) Vermilion ISBN 0091875285
Green *Beyond Toddlerdom*: every parent's guide to the 5–10s (2000) Vermilion ISBN 0091816246
Parentline ☎ 0808 800 2222 🖥 www.parentlineplus.org.uk

Information and support for children:
Childline 24h. confidential counselling service ☎ 0800 1111 🖥 www.childline.org

Figure 1.3 Assessment of childhood mental health problems

Start by gathering background information:
If the child is present, watch interactions between the child and parent/carer.

It is useful to interview parents both with and without the child and older children both with and without the parent.

Diaries can be helpful.

Consider:

Child:
Is the child acutely unwell?

Does the child have a chronic illness or disability?

Does the child have a physical deformity?

Does the child have any learning difficulty?

What is the child's normal temperament like?

Were there any problems in pregnancy or the neonatal period?

At what age did the child walk and talk?

Does the child have any feeding or sleeping difficulties?

Is the child clingy?

Does the child cry excessively?

Family:
What were the parents' childhoods like?

Is there family breakdown or marital stress?

Does either parent or a sibling have a chronic illness or disability? – depression, schizophrenia, cancer etc.

What were the circumstances of the child being born? – adoption, IVF, unwanted pregnancy etc.

Did the mother suffer from postnatal depression?

Is the child living in care or with short-term foster parents?

Have there been any major losses e.g. family death or parent leaving?

What are the parents' expectations of the child?

Environment:
Social deprivation?

Neighbourhood?

Frequent relocations?

How does the child integrate into play group, nursery or school?

Then:

Find out about the behavioural problems:
What does the child do?

When did it start?

When and where does that behaviour occur?

What seems to trigger it?

How do the parents and other carers/teachers react?

Child health promotion

Patients ≤15y. comprise 20% of the average practice list; schoolchildren visit the GP on average 2–3x/y. and the under-4s see their GP more often (average 6x/y.) and have more home visits than any other age group except the elderly.

The National Service Framework (NSF) for Children: Emphasizes child health promotion. It continues many elements of the previous child health surveillance programme but moves from rigid developmental screening to a more flexible assessment of the child within the family context. It includes:
* Immunization – 📖 p.84
* Childhood screening
* Holistic assessment of child and family followed by early intervention as required
* Health promotion, beginning antenatally and continuing to teenage years, covering the full range of child health issues e.g. diet, safety, substance abuse (drugs, smoking and alcohol), teenage sexual health.

Although most child health promotion is still carried out by the health visitor and other members of the primary health care team, the NSF stresses the need for partnership with parents and involvement of other care providers such as schools and nurseries.

Childhood screening: The aim of screening is to discover physical, developmental or behaviour problems as early as possible so that appropriate management can commence, preventing secondary complications. There has recently been a move away from set times for developmental screening but the neonatal (📖 p.14) and 6–8wk. check (with emphasis on checking the eyes, heart and hips as well as developmental milestones – 📖 p.12) are still recommended, as is a comprehensive assessment (usually by the health visitor) by 1y.

Beyond that assessments are carried out according to need. Any consultation can be used to check immunization status, monitor development and for health promotion. Expected developmental milestones are summarized in Table 1.1 (📖 pp.12–13). Liaise with the health visitor if:
* Immunizations are not up to date
* You have any worries regarding parenting abilities
* A child does not attend an appointment following referral
* You have concerns about neglect or abuse (but also see 📖 p.322).

Neonatal bloodspot screening: 📖 p.16

GP Notes: Diploma in Child Health

Designed to give recognition of competence in the care of children to GP vocational trainees, clinical medical officers and trainees in specialties allied to paediatrics. Administered by the Royal College of Paediatrics and Child Health (RCPCH). Further details are available at 🖥 www.rcpch.ac.uk

GMS contract

Child health surveillance 1	Child development checks are offered at intervals consistent with national guidelines and policy	6 points

GMS practices are expected to perform child health surveillance (excluding neonatal checks) for all children <5y. of age registered with the practice as an additional service. Opting out → a 0.7% ↓ in the global sum payment.

Neonatal checks can be provided by GMS GPs as a national enhanced service or by PMS GPs as part of their negotiated services.

Advice for patients: Information for new parents

Reducing the risk of cot death:
- Cut smoking in pregnancy and don't let anyone smoke in the same room as your baby.
- Place your baby on his back to sleep.
- Don't let your baby get too hot.
- Keep your baby's head uncovered – place your baby with his feet to the foot of the cot to prevent wriggling down under the covers.
- It's safest to sleep your baby in a cot in your bedroom for the first 6 months. It's dangerous to share a bed with your baby if either parent:
  - is a smoker – no matter where or when he/she smokes
  - has been drinking alcohol
  - feels, or has taken any drug which could make him/her, drowsy.
- It's very dangerous to sleep together with your baby on a sofa, armchair or settee.
- If your baby is unwell, seek medical advice promptly.

Protecting your baby from accidents and infections:
- Keep small objects out of your baby's reach.
- Stay with your baby when he is eating or drinking.
- Make sure your baby's cot and mattress are in good condition and that the mattress fits the cot properly.
- Install at least one smoke alarm and plan a way to escape a fire.
- Never leave your baby alone in a bath or near water.
- Make sure your baby can't reach hot drinks or the kettle or iron flex.
- Immunize your baby.
- Only use toys suitable for your baby's age.
- Never shake your baby – ask for help if crying gets too much.
- Use a properly fitted baby car seat that is the right size for your baby.
- Don't use a baby walker.
- Wash your hands before feeding your baby and make sure your baby's bottle and teats are properly sterilized.

Further information
Hall, Hill & Elliman *The child surveillance handbook* (1994) Radcliffe Medical Press ISBN: 1870905245
DoH Children's National Service Framework (2004) 🖳 www.dh.gov.uk

11

Table 1.1 Summary of developmental milestones

Development	6–week check	8 months
Gross motor	Controls head when pulled to sitting position (0–3mo.) Moro reflex (0–6mo.) – should be absent >6mo. Holds head in line/slightly higher than body with hips semi-extended during ventral suspension (0–10mo.) Lifts head momentarily when lying prone (from birth)	Bears weight on legs (3–7mo.) Can be pulled to sit (14wk.–6mo.) Sits with support (4–6mo.) Sits without support (5–8mo.) Crawls (6–9mo.)
Fine motor/ vision	Stares (from birth) – ▢ p.20 Follows horizontally to 90° (0–6wk.) – ▢ p.20	Reaches out to grasp (palmar grasp) (3–6mo.) Transfers and mouths (passes an object from 1 hand to the other and puts it in his mouth) (18wk.–8mo.) Fixes gaze on small objects (5–8mo.) Follows fallen toys (4–8mo.)
Hearing and speech	Responds to rattle or bell (from birth) Startle response (from birth)	Vocalizes (4–6mo.) Polysyllabic babbling (6–10mo.) Laughs (2–5mo.) Responds to own name (4–8mo.)
Social behaviour/play	Smiles (0–10wk. – mean 5wk.) Turns to look at observer's face (from birth)	Puts everything into mouth (4–8mo.) Hand and foot regard (4–8mo.) Plays peek-a-boo (5½–10mo.)
⚠ *Warning signs*	No red reflex No visual fixation or following Failure to respond to sound Asymmetrical neonatal reflexes Excessive head lag Failure to smile	Hand preference Fisting Squint Persistence of primitive reflexes – Moro response, stepping, asymmetrical tonic neck reflex

Table 1.1 (Contd.)		
18 months	**3 years**	**4 years**
Gets to sitting position (6–11mo.) Pulls to standing (6–10mo.) Walks holding onto furniture (7–13mo.) Walks alone (10–15mo.) Walks backwards (12–22mo.) Climbs stairs (14–22mo.)	Climbs and descends stairs Runs (~15mo.) Pedals tricycle (21mo.–3y.) Jumps in one place (21mo.–3y.) Kicks a ball (15–24mo.) Stands on 1 foot for 1sec. (22mo.–3¼ y.)	Hops forward on 1 foot for 2m (3–5y.) Stands on 1 foot for 5sec. (2¾ –4½ y.) Walks heel-to-toe (3½ –5¼ y. – backwards 4–6y.) Bounces and catches a ball (3¼ –5½ y.)
Points with index finger Casts (throws) (9–15mo.) Delicate pincer grasp (10–18mo.) Holds 2 bricks and bangs them together (7–13mo.) Scribbles (12–24mo.) Builds a tower of 3–4 bricks (16–24mo.)	Picks up 'hundreds and thousands' Imitates a vertical line (18mo.–33mo.) Copies a circle (2¼ –3½ y.) Threads beads Builds a tower of 8 bricks (21mo.–3½ y.) Matches 2 colours	Copies a cross (3–4½ y.) and square (4–5½ y.) Draws a man with 3 parts (with all features – 4½ –6y.) Recognizes colours (3–4¾ y.)
Turns to sound of name Jabbers continually Uses 'mama' & 'dada' (11–20mo.–½ by 15mo.) Can say ≥3 words other than 'mama' & 'dada' (10–21mo.) Points to eyes, nose & mouth (14–23mo.) Obeys simple instructions (15mo.–2½ y.)	Uses plurals (30mo.–3¼ y.) Uses prepositions (3–4½ y.) Joins words into sentences (50% by 23mo.; 97% by 3y.) Gives own name	Speaks grammatically (2½ y.–4¼ y.) Counts to 10
Holds spoon and gets food to mouth (14mo.–2½ y.) Explores environment (13–20mo.) Takes off shoes and socks (13–20mo.)	Plays alone Eats with spoon & fork Puts on clothes (2¼ –3½ y. – with supervision) Washes & dries hands Separates from mother easily (2–4y.) Dry in the day (2–4y.)	Shares toys Brushes teeth Dresses without supervision (3¼ –5½ y.) Comforts friends in distress (5y.)
Unable to sit, weight bear and/or stand without support Persistence of hand regard ± casting. No pincer grip Absence of babbling or cooing; inability to understand simple commands	Unable to speak in simple sentences Unable to understand speech	Speech difficult to understand due to poor articulation or because of omission or substitution of consonants (confusion of 's', 'f' and 'th' disappears by 6½ y.)

The neonatal check

It is essential that a full neonatal check is carried out <48h. after delivery. Most neonatal checks are carried out by paediatricians in maternity units before discharge. This does not happen if:
- The baby is discharged <24h. after delivery
- The birth occurs at home or in a GP unit or
- There is rapid discharge from an obstetric unit to a peripheral unit.

Parental concerns:
- Discuss any worries the parent(s) might have about the child.
- Review FH, pregnancy and birth.
- Arrange hepatitis B vaccination if mother is hepatitis B +ve (📖 p.75) or BCG vaccination if at high risk of TB (📖 p.161).

History: Check the baby has passed urine and meconium.
- *Has the baby passed urine?* If no urine in the 1st 24h., check if there is palpable bladder. If palpable bladder may be due to posterior urethral valves (📖 p.169). Otherwise suspect either that the baby has passed urine and it has been missed or that there is a renal abnormality. Check for low-set ears, beaked nose and possible limb abnormalities of Potter's syndrome and admit for further investigation.
- *Has the baby passed meconium?* If no meconium in the 1st 24h., suspect meconium ileus (CF), Hirschprung's or anorectal abnormality and admit for further investigation.

Examination: Check the baby systematically – Table 1.2.

Moro reflex: Support baby's head and shoulders about 15cm from the examination couch. Suddenly allow the baby's head to drop back slightly. The response – extension of the arms followed by adduction towards the chest should be brisk and symmetrical. This reflex disappears by 6mo.

Neonatal bloodspot screening: Discuss – 📖 p.16.

Check vitamin K has been given:
- Discuss any concerns with the parent(s).
- Deficiency of vitamin K can → *haemorrhagic disease of the newborn* with potentially serious effects including death.
- Vitamin K policies vary widely in the UK. Be aware of local policy.
- Babies at high risk of bleeding (premature, low birth weight, unwell babies and those who have undergone instrumental deliveries) – routine IM administration of vitamin K is the norm.
- Babies given oral vitamin K at birth – 1 dose doesn't confer full protection. Formula feeds contain vitamin K supplements but breast-fed babies require further doses – ensure they get them.

Health education: Discuss:
- Feeding and nutrition
- Sleeping position – 📖 p.11
- Baby care
- Sibling management
- Crying and sleep problems
- Transport in a car

Features of children with common chromosomal abnormalities: 📖 p.77

Table 1.2 Checklist for the neonatal examination

General appearance:

Syndrome? Clusters of features e.g. features of Downs/Turner's syndrome	Weight: small or large for gestation? Pallor, jaundice or cyanosis 🕛 slight peripheral cyanosis is normal	Skin: birth marks: meconium staining, purpura; lanugo or evidence of postmaturity

Head and facial features:

Head circumference Caput succedaneum or cephalhaematoma Fontanelles – number (if 3, ? Down's), size and tension Accessory auricles	Ptosis Subconjunctival haemorrhage, conjunctivitis or sticky eye? Cataract or red reflex?	Sternomastoid swelling Cleft lip Potter's facies Pierre Robin jaw (receding jaw with cleft palate)

Mouth:

Cleft palate? (📖 p.266)	Profuse saliva*	Epstein's pearls

Arms and hands:

Proportion of arms/fingers Oedema	Palmar creases Fingers – number, webbing, deformity	Normal movements Erb's palsy or Klumpke's palsy (📖 p.202)

Chest:

Distortion Breast enlargement	Respiratory rate** Added breath sounds	Air entry/added sounds Recession

Cardiovascular examination:

Pulses (femoral & brachial)	Heart sounds	Murmurs (📖 p.129)

Abdomen:

Umbilical infection/discharge or hernia	Anus: patency/position	Masses***

Genitalia:

♂ penis – size and shape; position of urethral orifice; testes (normal, undescended or maldescended), hernia or hydrocoele

♀ clitoromegaly; vaginal bleeding; posterior vaginal skin tag (common)

Back, legs and feet:

Sacral pit/spina bifida (📖 p.205) Scollosis (📖 p.26)	Hips (📖 p.24) Proportion of feet/legs/body	Club foot (📖 p.204) Toes – number, webbing, deformity

CNS:

Is the baby behaving normally?	Is the cry normal?	Are all 4 limbs moving equally and is the Moro reflex symmetrical?

* Profuse saliva is associated with oesophageal atresia.
** Respiratory rate <60 breaths/min is normal.
*** Liver is usually palpable as are the lower poles of the kidneys; the spleen and bladder are never palpable.

Neonatal bloodspot screening

Neonatal bloodspot screening involves taking a small blood sample obtained by pricking a baby's heel. The blood is placed on special filter paper (formerly called the Guthrie card) and sent for analysis. The test is usually carried out by the midwife when the baby is 5–8d. old.

Aim of bloodspot screening: To identify babies at high risk of having conditions for which early diagnosis and treatment improves outcome. Screening is not diagnostic and further tests are necessary to confirm diagnosis. When screening tests are positive it is essential that babies are referred quickly for further diagnostic tests/treatment.

Informed consent: As bloodspot screening is performed so soon after birth, it is important that parents have a chance to think about whether they wish their child to be screened for all or any of the conditions covered by the bloodspot screening programme, before the child is born. Where possible, ensure parents are given the national pre-screening leaflet during pregnancy at ~28wk. gestation.

Parents who decline screening: Parents are entitled to decline screening for all or any one of the conditions being screened for. Whilst screening is strongly recommended, parents' decisions must be respected. Discussions with parents and their consent (or decline) to screening should be recorded in the mother's health record. If a parent declines screening, explore the reasons why consent has not been given.

> ⚠ If screening is declined, it is important to flag in the child's notes that they have not been screened in case they become ill later on.

What conditions does bloodspot testing detect?
- Throughout the UK babies are screened for cystic fibrosis (CF), phenylketonuria (PKU) and congenital hypothyroidism (CHT).
- Throughout England, babies are screened for sickle cell disease.
- A pilot study of screening boys for Duchenne muscular dystrophy is underway in Wales and another pilot study of screening for medium chain acyl CoA dehydrogenase deficiency (MCADD) is underway in certain areas of England.

Phenylketonuria (PKU):
- In the UK 1:10,000 babies has PKU (autosomal recessive trait – higher incidence in Ireland).
- Children are unable to break down phenylalanine, an amino acid present in many foods. The baby appears normal at birth but develops severe developmental delay, learning difficulty and seizures in infancy.
- Prenatal diagnosis is possible if there is a FH and the bloodspot test is used to detect high levels of blood phenylalanine for all newborns in the UK.
- Treatment is with lifelong dietary restriction of phenylalanine. With treatment, growth and development are normal.

Advice for patients: Frequently asked questions about bloodspot screening

What are babies screened for?

Bloodspot screening identifies babies who may have rare but serious conditions. Please ask your midwife which conditions are screened for in your area.

Why should I have my baby screened?

Most babies screened will not have any of the conditions, but for the few who do, benefits of screening are enormous. Early treatment can improve health and prevent disability or even death.

What does screening involve?

When your baby is 5–8 days old, you will be offered a screening test for your baby. The midwife will prick your baby's heel using a special device and collect drops of blood onto a card. The test may be uncomfortable and your baby may cry.

Occasionally the midwife or health visitor will contact you to take another blood sample. This may be because there was not enough blood collected the first time or because the result was unclear. Usually repeat results are normal.

When will I get the result of the screening test?

Most babies will have normal results and you should know the result by the time your baby is 6–8 weeks old.

Will screening for these conditions show up anything else?

Screening for cystic fibrosis may identify some babies who are likely to be genetic carriers for cystic fibrosis. These babies may need further testing to find out if they are healthy carriers or have cystic fibrosis.

Screening for sickle cell disorders may also identify healthy genetic carriers of sickle cell or other unusual red blood cell disorders. Rarely, other red blood cell disorders are also detected. These disorders may not need treatment or benefit from early treatment too.

What if my baby has one of these conditions?

You will be told any abnormal results by the time your baby is 6 weeks old. Your baby will then be referred to a specialist for further tests to make sure the diagnosis is correct. If the diagnosis is confirmed the specialist will start treatment and provide you with information and support.

How accurate is screening?

Screening is not 100% accurate. Some babies will have a positive result and be referred for further testing and found not to have anything wrong. A few babies will not be detected by screening and their illness will be detected later when they get symptoms which need treatment.

Further information for parents

UK Newborn Screening Programme Centre leaflets about CF screening for parents ⊡ www.newbornscreening-bloodspot.org.uk
National Society for Phenylketonuria (NSPKU) ☎ 020 8364 3010
⊡ www.nspku.org

Congenital hypothyroidism:

- In the UK 1:4000 babies is born with congenital hypothyroidism ($♀>♂$).
- Untreated, children with abnormally low levels of thyroid hormone fail to grow properly and have mild to severe mental disability.
- The bloodspot is used to detect low levels of blood thyroxine.
- Treatment with thyroxine replacement results in normal growth and development. Usually thyroxine replacement is needed lifelong.

Cystic fibrosis (CF): 📖 p.162

- In the UK, 1:2500 babies is born with CF.
- Early treatment of cystic fibrosis improves outcome and prolongs both quality and quantity of life.
- Screening detects immunoreactive trypsin (IRT) which is ↑ in children with CF. If IRT is ↑, the blood is then DNA tested for the most common gene alterations (Figure 1.4).
- If a child tests positive, it is important that parents and siblings receive genetic counselling and are offered genetic testing for the condition. If both parents are carriers of a CF gene, there is a 1:4 chance of any subsequent children they have together being affected.
- Screening will also detect healthy carriers. This has implications not only for the child but also parents and other siblings. Ensure parents have a full explanation of results and understand their meaning.

⓵ As there are many more mutations described than tested for, not all gene mutations will be detected and some affected babies will be missed by newborn screening. Continue to watch for later presentations.

Sickle cell disease: 📖 p.114

- In the UK, 1:2400 babies is born with a sickle cell disorder (most common in people of Afro-Caribbean or sub-Saharan origin).
- Infants with sickle cell disease are at risk of presenting for the first time with severe overwhelming infections and splenic sequestration crises. Early diagnosis allows prophylaxis with penicillin and vaccines, and parent training to identify children with complications and to present early for treatment. This↓ complications and deaths in young infants.
- Abnormal haemoglobin is screened for using either high performance liquid chromatography (HPLC), or iso-electric focusing (IEF). If detected, a confirmatory test is performed on the original spot using a different technique from the initial screening test.
- If a child tests positive, it is important that parents and siblings receive genetic counselling, and are offered genetic testing for the condition.
- This test will detect babies with sickle cell trait or other heterozygous states as well as babies with sickle cell disease. It is important that parents understand the meaning and significance of results both for the child and other family members.
- The screening tests will also detect other haemoglobin abnormalities such as haemoglobin E and the thalassaemias. Even if these have no clinical consequences for the child the current policy is to inform parents of the results. It is essential that parents receive accurate information about what these results mean and the likely implications for the child and other family members.

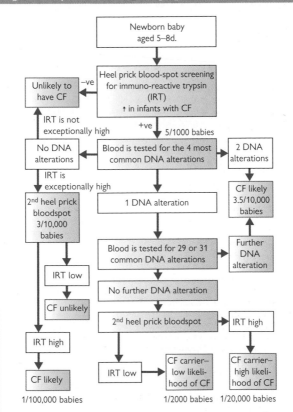

Figure 1.4 Cystic fibrosis screening algorithm

Newborn baby aged 5–8d.

Heel prick blood-spot screening for immuno-reactive trypsin (IRT) ↑ in infants with CF

Unlikely to have CF

–ve

+ve 5/1000 babies

IRT is not exceptionally high

No DNA alterations

Blood is tested for the 4 most common DNA alterations

2 DNA alterations

IRT is exceptionally high

CF likely 3.5/10,000 babies

2nd heel prick bloodspot 3/10,000 babies

1 DNA alteration

Further DNA alteration

Blood is tested for 29 or 31 common DNA alterations

IRT low

No further DNA alteration

CF unlikely

2nd heel prick bloodspot

IRT high

IRT high

CF likely

IRT low

CF carrier– low likeli-hood of CF

CF carrier– high likeli-hood of CF

1/100,000 babies

1/2000 babies

1/20,000 babies

Further information
UK Newborn Screening Programme Centre
⊞ www.newborn screening-bloodspot.org.uk

Vision and hearing screening tests for children

Operational senses are essential for normal development. Conditions which interfere with the normal senses, even if correctable, may lead to permanent impairment if not detected and treated early.

Routine developmental screening: Visual and hearing screening tests are carried out as part of routine child health surveillance at 6wk. and a year (Table 1.1, 📖 pp.12–13). Refer children for further assessment where there is any parental concern *or* concern about their vision or hearing as the result of screening.

Tests for vision at 6 weeks:

- *Stares (from birth):* Look at the baby's face – he will usually stare back. If not, ask the mother if the baby looks at her while feeding.
- *Follows horizontally to 90°:* Put the child on his back with head turned to 1 side. Move a bright coloured object 25cm from the child's face from 1 side to the other – the child should follow the object with his eyes ± head across the midline and through ≥90°. If the child's gaze wanders from one side to the other when happy, awake and >6wk. Old, suspect a visual problem.

Non-paralytic or congenital squint: Common abnormality of coordinated eye movement due to an imbalance of the muscles of the eye. 3% of children have a congenital squint – but only 1:3 squints are picked up by parents. There is a full range of eye movement in both eyes and no double vision. Squints may be convergent (esotropia) or divergent (exotropia). Convergent squint (Figure 1.5) is most common and often associated with long-sightedness. A and V syndromes are squints in which horizontal deviations are vertically inconstant (i.e. the squint is more pronounced on upward gaze – A pattern – or downward gaze – V pattern).

Predisposing factors: Family history of squint, high refractive errors, neurological disease (e.g. cerebral palsy), cataract, Down's syndrome, Turner's syndrome, retinoblastoma, optic atrophy, craniofacial anomalies, retinal disease

Testing for squint: Sit the child on the parent's lap. Stand in front of the child and shine a bright light (e.g. pen torch) at arm's length from the child. Fix the child's head in the midline and look for the reflection of the light on the child's corneas (Figure 1.5). The reflection should be symmetrical and near the centre of the pupil (usually slightly towards the nose). Turn the child's head to 1 side, keeping the eyes fixed on the light. The reflection should remain symmetrical. Repeat, turning the head to the other side. If reflections are not symmetrical perform a cover test.

Cover test: Sit the child comfortably on a parent's lap.
- Shine a bright light or place small bright object at arm's length from the child.
- Cover 1 eye with a card.
- Watch for any movement of the uncovered eye to fix on the object.
- Then remove the card and watch the covered eye to see if it moves to fix on the object.

- Repeat with the other eye. If either or both eyes move a squint is present – refer.

Management: Refer all non-paralytic squints as soon as recognized for ophthalmology assessment. Without treatment children with squint risk developing ambylopia, failure of binocular vision and long-term visual problems. Visual maturity occurs at 7–8y. Eye patching, correction of refractive errors (spectacles) and realignment surgery can improve sight up to this age.

> ### GP Notes:
>
> #### Conditions confused with squint (pseudosquint):
> - *Wide epicanthic folds:* Give the appearance of a squint but corneal reflections are symmetrical.
> - *Intermittent deviation of the eyes in neonates:* Common. Check red reflex is present. Normally settles by 3mo. – squint after this time is significant. Refer.
>
> #### ⚠ Warning signs for visual problems:
> - Lack of red reflex (Figure 1.6).
> - The child does not fix on the mother's face whilst feeding by 6wk.
> - In a child >6wk. old, the child's eye wanders about from one side of the eye socket to the other while the child is awake and happy.
> - A white spot is seen in the pupil at any age – could be cataract.
> - The child holds objects close to his face whilst trying to look at them.
> - A child >6mo. old has a squint in 1 or both eyes.

> ### Advice for patients: Information and support for parents and children
>
> **LOOK** Support for families of blind or visually impaired children
> ☎ 0121 428 5038 ▣ www.look-uk.org

Figure 1.5 Convergent squint

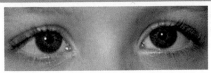

Figure 1.6 Loss of red reflex in a child with retinoblastoma

Figure 1.5 permission sought from Southampton University Hospital Trust.
Figure 1.6 is reproduced with permission from Childhood Eye Cancer Trust (CHECT)
▣ www.chect.org.uk

Hearing tests: Young babies have a startle response to loud sounds. There is a routine neonatal hearing screening programme (NHSP) in the UK and since December 2005 all newborn babies in the UK have been offered a routine hearing screen.

Neonatal screening: 2 types of screen are used by the NHSP:
- *Oto-acoustic emission (OAE) screen:* Involves placing a small soft-tipped earpiece in the outer part of the baby's ear and playing quiet clicking sounds. In a hearing ear, the cochlea produces sounds in response to the clicks which can be recorded and analysed by the computerized screening system. Screening takes a few minutes and can be done at the bedside when the baby is asleep, but it is not always possible to get clear responses, especially if the baby is <24h. old.
- *Automated auditory brainstem response (AABR) screen:* Involves placing small sensors on the baby's head and neck and then presenting quiet clicking sounds through tiny, soft headphones (muffs). A computer analyses the responses to sounds at and around the brainstem.

Tests for hearing at 6 weeks:
- *Rattle or bell 15cm away at ear level (from birth):* Ensure the baby cannot see the rattle or bell. The baby should quieten to the sound – other satisfactory responses are turning, widening eyes or change in breathing pattern. If the baby fails to respond, unless the parents are worried about the baby's hearing (when refer immediately), repeat in 2wk. and refer if the baby fails the test a second time.
- *Startle response (from birth):* Clap loudly close to the child – the child should make some response. If not, ask the parents if he reacts to loud noises at home.

The distraction hearing test: Can be used from 6mo. of age but is not very reliable. This test requires 2 testers and should be performed in a quiet room. Advise parents not to make any noise during the test.
- The child is placed on the parent's lap facing one of the testers.
- This tester attracts attention by moving a soundless toy just out of reach.
- The other tester makes a sound at ear level ~1m away from the child and slightly behind the child so that any movement cannot be seen.
- Both ears are tested.
- A positive test (implying the child can hear) occurs if the child localizes (searches for and finds) the sound.

Stimuli commonly used:
- Rattle – Manchester rattle (low-frequency sound); Nuffield rattle (high-frequency sounds).
- Cup and spoon – china cup and metal teaspoon. The spoon is run gently around the rim of the cup.
- Voice – high-pitched sound ('ss-ss'); low-pitched sound ('oo-oo'); speech including the child's name.

Pure tone audiometry: From 3y. pure tone audiometry is possible with a cooperative child.

GP Notes:

⚠ Warning signs for hearing problems:
- There is no startle response to loud noises at 6wk.
- The child does not respond to his name by 8mo.
- Absence of babbling or cooing by 1y.
- Inability to understand simple commands by 18mo.
- Inability to speak in short sentences by 2½ y.

Delayed speech development:
- If a child's speech is delayed always check his/her hearing.
- The range of normal for speech development is wide:
  - First words 11–20mo.
  - A 2y. old may use anything from a few words to 2000 words
  - Children start using prepositions at any time from 3–4½ y.
- Parents often compare their children's development to others, and this may lead to unnecessary anxiety.
- Check your local speech therapy department's referral guidelines.

When are further hearing tests necessary?
- If the newborn hearing test indicates a problem.
- If the newborn hearing test was missed or if the child is in a high-risk group for deafness e.g. cleft lip/palate, Down's syndrome, FH childhood deafness, congenital infection. Refer for screening at 8mo.
- If the child becomes at risk of developing deafness e.g. after bacterial meningitis, skull fracture or treatment with high doses of gentamicin.
- Parental or professional concern about a child's hearing.

Advice for patients: Helping your child's speech and language development
- Get your child's attention before you talk to him or her.
- Talk about what your child is doing.
- Play with your child – pretend play with dolls/teddies can be used to introduce common words and repeat them, for example 'Dolly has a cup. Give teddy a cup'.
- Speak clearly, not too fast, using short words and simple sentences.
- Ask questions that cannot be answered by just yes or no, for example 'Would you like ham or cheese on your bread?'
- Repeat and add to what your child says. For example, if your child says 'car', you say 'Yes, it's a red car'.
- If your child mispronounces words, repeat the correct word to your child without criticism. For example, if your child points at a cat and says 'dat', reply 'Yes, it's a cat'.

Further information
NHS Newborn hearing screening programme 🖳 www.nhsp.info

Information and support for parents and children
National Deaf Children's Society ☎ 0808 800 8880
🖳 www.ndcs.org.uk

Screening for childhood orthopaedic problems

Congenital dislocation of the hip (CDH) or developmental dysplasia of the hip (DDH): 3:2000 live births ($♀:♂≈6:1$) – though 10x that number have unstable hips and even more have 'clicks' detected on routine neonatal screening. Often there is a family history of CDH. Associated with breech presentation at term.

Encompasses varying degrees of instability, subluxation and dysplasia of the hip joint.

Presentation:
- Usually detected at routine screening. Screening should take place at birth, at the 6wk. check, at 6–8mo. and in the second year (15–21mo.).
- High-risk children (breech babies, family history, foot deformities, sternomastoid tumour) are routinely screened with USS.
- Screening tests should be taught *in vivo* by someone experienced in the technique.
- Despite screening some cases slip though the net. They present as toddlers with limp/waddling gait, frequent falls, asymmetric thigh creases or limited hip adduction noted at later developmental checks.
- Rarely some go unnoticed until adulthood when they present with premature osteoarthritis.

Screening a child <3mo.:
- In the newborn period limited abduction is uncommon as a sign of dislocation of the hip and more likely to be due to ↑ tone e.g. spina bifida. At this time the most important sign is instability of the hip.
- Screening tests should be performed in a warm room with the baby undressed and lying on a firm surface.
- Flex hips and knees to $90°$ using one hand for each leg with thumbs on the inner side of the baby's knee and ring and little fingers behind the greater trochanters (Figure 1.7).
- Each hip is tested separately. The examiner's hand on the opposite side from the hip being tested is used to stabilize the pelvis. Hold the thumb over the symphysis pubis and fingers under the sacrum.
- Only test once as repeated testing can damage the hips.

Ortolani manoeuvre: Each hip is gently abducted whilst lifting the greater trochanter forward. As a dislocated hip is abducted a clunk or jumping sensation is felt. It is difficult to tell the difference between a click of a normal hip and a clunk of an abnormal one, so refer any clicky or clunky hips for further investigation (usually USS or orthopaedic review).

Barlow manoeuvre: This establishes whether the hips are dislocatable. Holding the legs as described above, gently apply pressure along the line of the femur pushing it backwards out of the acetabulum. The judder of the femoral head slipping in and out of the acetabulum can be felt if the hip is dislocatable.

Figure 1.7 Screening for congenital dislocation of the hip (Ortolani test)

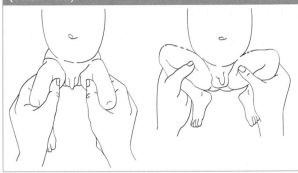

Screening a child >3mo.:

- After 3mo. of age, limited abduction is the most common finding in children with CDH. If the infant lies on his back with hips flexed at 90°, any hip which cannot abduct >75° should be viewed with suspicion.
- Perform the Ortolani and Barlow tests.
- *Other signs:*
  - Limb shortening on the affected side – compare knee levels.
  - Asymmetry of the thighs – particularly skin creases.
  - Flattening of the buttock – in a prone position, the affected side may look flatter.

Management: Refer to an orthopaedic surgeon specializing in paediatric problems. Treatment depends on when the condition is diagnosed:
- *Young babies:* Splinting in a pelvic harness to reduce and hold the hip – the hips are held in partial abduction using slings under each thigh attached to a body harness – e.g. von Rosen splint. Usually babies wear a splint for ~3mo.
- *Older babies, toddlers and adults:* Surgery is required.

Advice for patients: Support for parents and children

Steps Support for patients with lower limb conditions and their families ☎ 0871 717 0044 ▭ www.steps-charity.org.uk

Scoliosis: Lateral curvature of the spine. 2 types:
* **Structural (true) scoliosis:** Fixed deformity. Scoliosis is associated with rotation of the vertebrae ± ribs and wedging of the vertebrae. Causes – Box 1.1
* **Non-structural (mobile) scoliosis:** Curvature is 2° to another condition outside the spine and disappears when that is corrected – e.g. leg length disparity (disappears on sitting). No rotation of the vertebrae.

Presentation and management: Usually found incidentally or on screening. *Clinical features:*
* Difference in shoulder height
* Spinal curvature
* Difference in space between trunk and upper limbs.

🛈 Scoliosis which disappears on bending is postural and of no clinical significance.

Refer all children with suspected structural scoliosis to orthopaedics – urgently if painful. Complications include deformity, pain, limitation of activities and respiratory restriction.

Screening for childhood scoliosis: Early treatment of scoliosis prevents progression. Early-onset scoliosis (<8y.) is responsible for cosmetic problems, pain and cardiopulmonary disturbance. Late-onset scoliosis is less severe but also causes pain and significant deformity.

Screening tests:
* *<1y. old:* Place the child prone on his tummy and feel the shoulder and thoracic cage. There should be no rib hump or shoulder hump.
* *>1y. old:* Ask the child to bend forward whilst standing straight with both feet together and holding both hands straight. Look for a shoulder, thoracic or lumbar hump, difference in shoulder height and/or obvious spinal curvature (Figure 1.8). Check the gap between arm and waistline.

Idiopathic scoliosis: >10° of lateral curvature of the spine – thoracic curves tend to be more severe than lumbar. *Incidence:* 1–3%.

Infantile idiopathic scoliosis: ♂:♀≈6:4. 90% are left-sided convex scolioses. Associated with ipsilateral flattening of the skull. May resolve spontaneously (more likely if ♂, onset at <1y. of age and/or the rib – vertebral angle is <20°) or progress as the child grows. Progressive scoliosis is treated with braces and surgery. As a general rule, the younger the child and the higher the curve, the worse the prognosis.

Late-onset idiopathic scoliosis: Affects children aged 10–15y. ♀:♂≈9:1. Scoliosis is usually right-sided, convex and always gets worse without treatment as the child grows. Treatment is with observation (if scoliosis is mild and growth is nearly complete), braces and/or surgery.

Advice for patients: Information and support

Scoliosis Association (UK) ☎ 020 8964 1166 🖳 www.sauk.org.uk

Figure 1.8 Checking for scoliosis

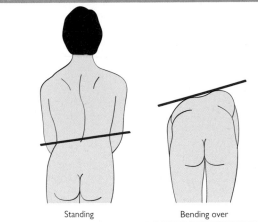

Standing   Bending over

Box 1.1 Causes of true scoliosis

- *Idiopathic*
- *Congenital:* Vertebral malformations produce severe scoliosis which is rapidly progressive. Major causes: hemivertebra; Klippel-Feil syndrome; congenital vertebral bar due to failure of segmentation
- *Neuromuscular imbalance* e.g. polio, cerebral palsy, muscular dystrophy, neurofibromatosis, syringomyelia
- *Trauma* → in damage to the vertebral growth plate and uneven growth
- *Neoplasm:*
  - 1°: Osteoid osteoma and osteoblastoma cause a painful scoliosis
  - 2°: Lytic metastases
  - Treatment of tumours e.g. radiotherapy can → scoliosis
- *Metabolic:* Osteoporosis and crush fracture
- *Infection:* TB of the spine (Pott's disease)

GP Notes: How can I detect scoliosis?

Look for:
- Difference in shoulder height
- Spinal curvature
- Difference in space between trunk and upper limbs

⓵ Structural scoliosis is often made more obvious by asking the child to bend forwards. Scoliosis which disappears on bending is postural and of no clinical significance.

⚠ If scoliosis is painful in a child or young person – especially at night – consider spinal tumour and refer for urgent orthopaedic assessment.

Figure 1.8 is reproduced with permission from the Merck Manual of Medical Information (2nd Home edition) (2003) by Merck & Co. Inc.

Chapter 2

Paediatric accidents and emergencies

Basic paediatric life support

Basic life support is a holding operation – sustaining life until help arrives.

Danger: Ensure safety of rescuer and child.

Response: Check the child for any response.
- Is he **A**lert?
- Does he respond to **V**ocal stimuli?
- Does he respond to **P**ainful stimuli (pinch lower part of nasal septum)?
- Is he **U**nconscious?

If he responds by answering or moving: Don't move the child unless in danger. Get help. Reassess regularly.

If he does not respond: Shout for help. Assess airway (below).

Airway: Open the airway. Don't move the child from the position in which you found him unless you have to:
- Gently tilt the head back with your hand on the child's forehead
- Lift the chin with your fingertips under the point of the child's chin.

If unsuccessful:
- Try jaw thrust – place the first 2 fingers of each hand behind each side of the child's jawbone and push the jaw forward.
- Try lifting the chin or jaw thrust after carefully turning the child onto his back.

⚠ Avoid head tilt as much as possible if trauma to the neck is suspected.

Breathing: Look, listen and feel for breathing (maximum 10sec.).

If breathing normally: Turn the child carefully into the recovery position (📖 p.33) if unconscious, and check for continued breathing.

If not breathing or making agonal gasps (infrequent irregular breaths):
- Carefully turn the child onto his back and remove any obvious airway obstruction.
- Give 5 initial rescue breaths – note any gag or cough response.

Technique for rescue breaths:
- Ensure head tilt (neutral position for children <1y.) and chin lift.
- If age ≥1y, pinch the soft part of the child's nose closed with the index finger and thumb of the hand which is on his forehead. Open the child's mouth a little, but maintain the chin upwards.
- Take a breath and place your lips around the child's mouth (mouth and nose if <1y.*), ensuring you have a good seal. Blow steadily into the child's airway over ~1–1.5 sec watching for chest rise.
- Maintaining head tilt and chin lift, take your mouth away and watch for the chest to fall as air comes out.
- Take another breath and repeat this sequence 5 times.

❶ If you have difficulty achieving an effective breath, consider airway obstruction – 📖 p.40.

---

* If the nose and mouth can't both be covered, place your lips around the mouth alone as for an older child, or nose alone (close the child's lips to prevent air escape).

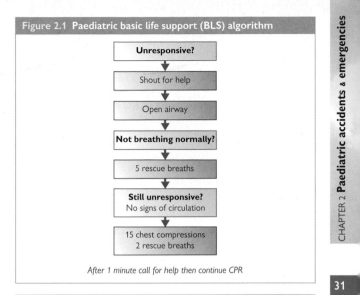

Figure 2.1 Paediatric basic life support (BLS) algorithm

Unresponsive?

↓

Shout for help

↓

Open airway

↓

Not breathing normally?

↓

5 rescue breaths

↓

Still unresponsive?
No signs of circulation

↓

15 chest compressions
2 rescue breaths

After 1 minute call for help then continue CPR

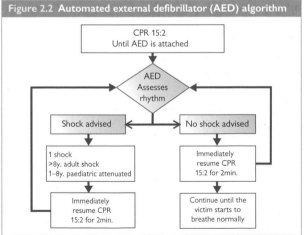

Figure 2.2 Automated external defibrillator (AED) algorithm

CPR 15:2
Until AED is attached

↓

AED
Assesses
rhythm

Shock advised ← → No shock advised

1 shock
>8y. adult shock
1–8y. paediatric attenuated

Immediately
resume CPR
15:2 for 2min.

Immediately
resume CPR
15:2 for 2min.

Continue until the
victim starts to
breathe normally

Circulation (signs of life): Check (maximum 10sec.) for:
- Any movement, coughing or normal breathing (not agonal gasps)
- Pulse – child ≥1y. carotid pulse; child <1y. brachial pulse.

If circulation is present: Continue rescue breathing until the child starts breathing effectively on his own. Turn the child into the recovery position (📖 p.33) if unconscious, and reassess frequently.

If circulation is absent, or slow pulse (<60 beats/min.) with poor perfusion, or you are not sure:
- Give 15 chest compressions. Then give 2 rescue breaths followed by 15 further chest compressions.
- Continue the cycle of 2 breaths followed by 15 chest compressions.
- ❶ Lone rescuers may use a ratio of 30 compressions: 2 rescue breaths.

Technique for chest compressions: Compress the sternum 1 finger's breadth above the xiphisternum by ~$^1/_3$ of the depth of the chest. Release the pressure then repeat at a rate of ~100 compressions/min.
- **Children <1y. with a lone rescuer:** Use the tips of 2 fingers.
- **Children <1y. with ≥2 rescuers:** Place both thumbs flat on the lower $^1/_3$ of the sternum with tips pointing towards the child's head and encircle the lower part of the child's ribcage with the tips of the fingers supporting the infant's back. Press down with both thumbs.
- **Children >1y.:** Place the heel of 1 hand over the lower $^1/_3$ of the sternum. Lift the fingers. Position yourself vertically above the chest with arm straight, and push downwards. For larger children use both hands with fingers interlocked to achieve satisfactory compressions.

⚠ Stop to recheck for signs of a circulation only if the child moves or takes a spontaneous breath – otherwise continue uninterrupted.

Use of automated external defibrillators (AEDs) in children
- **Children >8y.:** Use the standard adult AED.
- **Children aged 1–8y.:** Paediatric pads or a paediatric mode should be used if available; if not, use the adult AED as it is.
- **Children <1y.:** AED use is currently not advised.

If a patient arrests: Start CPR according to the guidelines for PBLS.

As soon as the AED arrives:
- Switch on the AED and attach the electrode pads. If >1 rescuer is present, continue CPR whilst this is done. (Some AEDs automatically switch on when the AED lid is opened.)
  - Place one AED pad to the right of the sternum, below the clavicle.
  - Place the other pad in the mid-axillary line with its long axis vertical.
- Follow the voice/visual prompts. Ensure nobody touches the victim whilst the AED is analysing the rhythm.

If a shock is indicated: Ensure nobody touches the victim. Push the shock button as directed (fully automatic AEDs deliver the shock automatically). Immediately resume CPR and continue to follow the prompts.
If no shock is indicated: Immediately resume CPR and continue to follow the prompts.

GP Notes: Emergency action

When to go for assistance: It is vital for rescuers to get assistance as quickly as possible when a child collapses.

When >1 rescuer is available: One should start resuscitation while another rescuer goes for assistance.

Lone rescuer: Perform resuscitation for *1 minute* before going for assistance (and consider taking a young child/infant with you to minimize interruption in CPR). The only exception to this is a *witnessed sudden* collapse, as in this case cardiac arrest is likely to be due to arrhythmia and the child may need defibrillation, so seek help immediately.

Duration of resuscitation: Continue resuscitation until:
- child shows signs of life (spontaneous respiration, pulse, movement)
- further qualified help arrives
- you become exhausted.

The recovery position: When circulation and breathing have been restored, it is important to:
- Maintain a good airway
- Ensure the tongue does not cause obstruction
- Minimize the risk of inhalation of gastric contents.

For this reason the victim should be placed in the recovery position. This allows the tongue to fall forward, keeping the airway clear:
- The child should be in as near a true lateral position as possible with his mouth dependant to allow free drainage of fluid
- The position should be stable. In an infant this may require the support of a small pillow or rolled-up blanket placed behind the infant's back to maintain the position.

Cervical spine injury:
- If spinal cord injury is suspected (e.g. if the victim has sustained a fall, been struck on the head or neck, or has been rescued after diving into shallow water), take particular care during handling and resuscitation to maintain alignment of the head, neck and chest in the neutral position.
- A spinal board and/or cervical collar should be used if available.

33

GMS contract

| Education 1 | There is a record of all practice-employed clinical staff having attended training/updating in basic life support skills in the preceding 18mo. | 4 points |
| Education 5 | There is a record of all practice-employed staff having attended training/updating in basic life support skills in the preceding 36mo. | 3 points |

Further information
Resuscitation Council (UK) Resuscitation guidelines (2005)
🖳 www.resus.org.uk

Advanced paediatric life support

Cardiac arrest in children is rare. Unless there is underlying heart disease, it is usually a consequence of respiratory arrest which results in asystole or pulseless electrical activity and has poor prognosis. Good airway management and providing high-flow oxygen for very sick children is therefore important in preventing cardiac arrest.

Basic paediatric life support: Follow the algorithm on 📖 p.31.

Unable to ventilate? Consider foreign body in the airway and initiate airway obstruction sequence – 📖 p.40.

Checking the pulse:
- Child – feel for the carotid pulse in the neck.
- Infant – feel for the brachial pulse on the inner aspect of the upper arm.

Once the airway is protected: If the airway is protected by tracheal intubation, continue chest compression without pausing for ventilation. Provide ventilation at a rate of 10/min. and compression at 100/min.

When circulation is restored, ventilate the child at a rate of 12–20 breaths/min.

Adrenaline (epinephrine) dose:
- Intravenous or interosseous (IO) access: 10mcgm/kg epinephrine/ adrenaline (0.1ml/kg of 1:10,000 solution)
- If circulatory access is not present and can't be quickly obtained, but the child has a tracheal tube in place, consider giving adrenaline/ epinephrine 100mcgm/kg via the tracheal tube (1ml/kg of 1:10,000 or 0.1ml/kg of 1:1,000 solution).This is the least satisfactory route of administration.

⚠ Don't give 1:1000 epinephrine/adrenaline IV or IO.

VF/Pulseless VT: Less common in paediatric life support.
- Defibrillation:
  - Give 1 shock of 4J/kg or
  - If using an AED for a child of 1–8y. deliver a paediatric attenuated adult shock energy
  - If using an AED for a child >8y. use the adult shock energy.
- For VF/pulseless VT persisting after the 3rd shock, try amiodarone 5mg/kg diluted in 5% dextrose.

Bradycardia: When bradycardia is unresponsive to improved ventilation and circulatory support, try atropine 20mcgm/kg (maximum dose 600mcgm; minimum dose 100mcgm).

Magnesium: Magnesium treatment is indicated in children with documented hypomagnesemia or with polymorphic VT ('torsade de pointes'), regardless of cause. Give IV magnesium sulphate over several minutes at a dose of 25–50mg/kg (to a maximum of 2g).

Intravenous fluids: In situations where the cardiac arrest has resulted from circulatory failure, a standard (20ml/kg) bolus of crystalloid fluid should be given if there is no response to the initial dose of epinephrine/adrenaline.

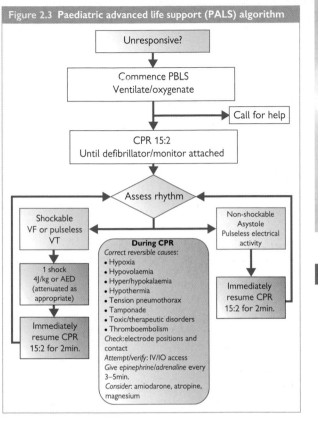

Figure 2.3 Paediatric advanced life support (PALS) algorithm

Unresponsive?

Commence PBLS
Ventilate/oxygenate

Call for help

CPR 15:2
Until defibrillator/monitor attached

Assess rhythm

Shockable
VF or pulseless
VT

Non-shockable
Asystole
Pulseless electrical
activity

1 shock
4J/kg or AED
(attenuated as
appropriate)

Immediately
resume CPR
15:2 for 2min.

During CPR
Correct reversible causes:
• Hypoxia
• Hypovolaemia
• Hyper/hypokalaemia
• Hypothermia
• Tension pneumothorax
• Tamponade
• Toxic/therapeutic disorders
• Thromboembolism
Check: electrode positions and
contact
Attempt/verify: IV/IO access
*Give epinephrine/adrenaline every
3–5min.*
Consider: amiodarone, atropine,
magnesium

Immediately
resume CPR
15:2 for 2min.

GP Notes: Estimating the weight of a child for drug/fluid doses

• May not be necessary – use a recent weight from the parent-held
  child record if available.
• Otherwise for children >1y., weight (in kg) ≈ 2 × (age + 4).

Resuscitation of the newborn

Follow the algorithm p.37 (Figure 2.4).

> **Rapid assessment of the infant at birth:**
> Start the clock. Assess colour, tone, breathing, heart rate.
> *A healthy baby:*
> - Born blue
> - Good tone
> - Cries seconds after delivery
>
> - Good heart rate (120–150 bpm)
> - Rapidly becomes pink during the first 90sec
>
> *A less healthy baby:*
> - Blue at birth
> - Less good tone
>
> - ± slow heart rate (<100 bpm)
> - ± inadequate breathing by 90–120 sec.
>
> *An ill baby:*
> - Born pale
> - Floppy
>
> - Slow/very slow heart rate (<100 bpm)
> - Not breathing

Heart rate: Best judged by listening with a stethoscope. In many cases it can also be felt by palpating the umbilical cord. Feeling for peripheral pulses is not helpful.

Airway
- Open the airway by placing the head in a neutral position – where the neck is neither extended nor flexed.
- If the occiput is prominent and the neck tends to flex, place a support under the shoulders – but don't overextend the neck.
- If the baby is very floppy, apply jaw thrust or chin lift as needed.

Breathing: Inflation breaths are breaths with pressures of ~30cm of water for 2–3sec.

If heart rate ↑: You have successfully inflated the chest. If the baby doesn't then start breathing alone, continue to provide regular breaths at a rate of ~30–40 breaths/min. until the baby starts to breathe on its own.

If heart rate does not ↑: Either you have not inflated the chest or the baby needs more help. By far the most likely is that you have failed to inflate the chest (the chest does not move). *Consider:*
- Is the baby's head in the neutral position?
- Do you need jaw thrust?
- Do you need a longer inflation time?
- Do you need a second person's help with the airway?
- Is there an obstruction in the oropharynx e.g. meconium (laryngoscope and suction)?
- What about an oropharyngeal (Guedel) airway?

Chest compressions: Only commence after inflation of the lungs.
- Grip the chest in both hands in such a way that the thumbs of both hands can press on the sternum at a point just below an imaginary line joining the nipples and with the fingers over the spine at the back.
- Compress the chest quickly – ↓ the AP diameter of the chest by ~$\frac{1}{3}$ with each compression. The ratio of compressions to inflations is 3:1.

Drug support: For a few babies inflation of the lungs and effective chest compression are not sufficient to produce effective circulation. IV or interosseous drugs may be helpful. Doses:

- Adrenaline (epinephrine):10mcgm/kg (0.1ml/kg of 1:10,000 solution), increasing to 30mcgm/kg (0.3ml/kg of 1:10,000 solution) if ineffective
- Sodium bicarbonate: 1–2mmol/kg (2–4ml 4.2% bicarbonate solution)
- Dextrose: 250mg/kg (2.5ml/kg of 10% dextrose).

For emergency volume replacement (e.g. history of a bleed): use 10ml/kg 0.9% saline given over 10–20sec. Repeat if needed.

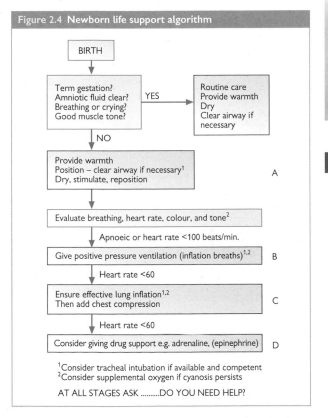

Figure 2.4 Newborn life support algorithm

BIRTH

Term gestation?
Amniotic fluid clear?
Breathing or crying?
Good muscle tone?

YES →

Routine care
Provide warmth
Dry
Clear airway if necessary

NO

Provide warmth
Position – clear airway if necessary[1]
Dry, stimulate, reposition   A

Evaluate breathing, heart rate, colour, and tone[2]

Apnoeic or heart rate <100 beats/min.

Give positive pressure ventilation (inflation breaths)[1,2]   B

Heart rate <60

Ensure effective lung inflation[1,2]
Then add chest compression   C

Heart rate <60

Consider giving drug support e.g. adrenaline, (epinephrine)   D

[1]Consider tracheal intubation if available and competent
[2]Consider supplemental oxygen if cyanosis persists

AT ALL STAGES ASK ....DO YOU NEED HELP?

Further information
Resuscitation Council (UK) Resuscitation guidelines (2005) 🖥 www.resus.org.uk

Figure 2.4 is reproduced with permission from the Resuscitation Council UK
🖥 www.resus.org.uk

Coma

Patients in coma/pre-coma nearly always require emergency admission.

When you receive the call for assistance
- Advise the attendant (unless history of possible spinal injury) to turn the patient onto his/her side.
- Call an ambulance to meet you at the scene.

On reaching the patient
- Assess the need for basic life support (📖 p.30):
  - Airway patent?
  - Breathing satisfactory?
  - Circulation adequate?
- Turn into the recovery position (📖 p.33) if no contraindications e.g. spinal injury.
- Call for ambulance support if you have not already done so.
- Ensure the patient is warm.
- Try to establish a diagnosis (see assessment).

As soon as possible
- Insert an airway.
- Give oxygen.
- Establish IV access.
- Transfer to hospital (unless the condition has resolved e.g. hypoglycaemia, fit).

Possible causes
- *Drugs:* Sedatives or hypnotics; opiates; alcohol; solvents; carbon monoxide poisoning
- *CNS:* Fit or post-ictal state; hydrocephalus (e.g. blocked shunt); cerebral oedema (e.g. meningitis, SAH, head injury); concussion; extradural or subdural haematoma
- *Metabolic:* Hypo or hyperglycaemia; hypothermia; hypopituitarism
- *Infection:* Meningitis or septicaemia; pneumonia

Assessment and management: See Figure 2.5

Glasgow coma scale: 📖 p.51

Hypoglycaemia: 📖 p.192

Hyperglycaemia and ketoacidosis: 📖 p.191

Menigitis and encephalitis: 📖 p.48

Overdose and poisoning: 📖 p.52

Figure 2.5 Assessment and management of the unconscious patient

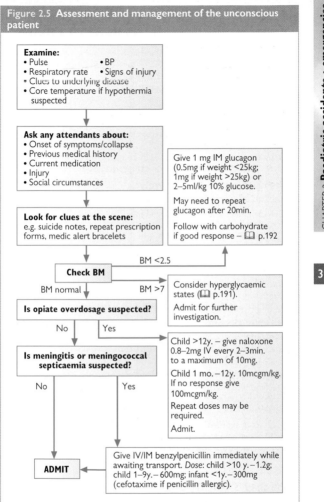

Examine:
- Pulse
- BP
- Respiratory rate
- Signs of injury
- Clues to underlying disease
- Core temperature if hypothermia suspected

Ask any attendants about:
- Onset of symptoms/collapse
- Previous medical history
- Current medication
- Injury
- Social circumstances

Look for clues at the scene:
e.g. suicide notes, repeat prescription forms, medic alert bracelets

Check BM

BM <2.5

Give 1 mg IM glucagon (0.5mg if weight <25kg; 1mg if weight >25kg) or 2–5ml/kg 10% glucose.

May need to repeat glucagon after 20min.

Follow with carbohydrate if good response – 🔲 p.192

BM normal

BM >7

Consider hyperglycaemic states (🔲 p.191).

Admit for further investigation.

Is opiate overdosage suspected?

No   Yes

Child >12y. – give naloxone 0.8–2mg IV every 2–3min. to a maximum of 10mg.

Child 1 mo.–12y. 10mcgm/kg. If no response give 100mcgm/kg.

Repeat doses may be required.

Admit.

Is meningitis or meningococcal septicaemia suspected?

No   Yes

ADMIT

Give IV/IM benzylpenicillin immediately while awaiting transport. *Dose:* child >10 y. – 1.2g; child 1–9y. – 600mg; infant <1y. – 300mg (cefotaxime if penicillin allergic).

Foreign body airways obstruction

⚠ If the child is breathing spontaneously, encourage his own efforts to clear the obstruction. ONLY intervene if these attempts are ineffective.

⚠ Don't perform blind or repeated finger sweeps of the airway as these may further impact a foreign body or cause soft tissue damage.

Is the diagnosis likely? Look for:
- Sudden onset of respiratory distress in a previously well child – often witnessed by the child's carer
- Respiratory distress associated with coughing, gagging or stridor
- Recent history of playing with or eating small objects.

Is the child coughing effectively?
Signs of an effective cough include:
- Fully responsive – crying or verbal response to questions
- Loud cough and able to take a breath before coughing
- ▶▶ *Encourage the child to cough and monitor*

Signs of an ineffective cough include:
- Unable to vocalize
- Quiet or silent cough
- Unable to breathe ± cyanosis
- Decreasing level of consciousness
- ▶▶ *Call for assistance (e.g. dial 999) and assess conscious level*

If the child IS conscious but has absent/ineffective coughing:
- Give up to 5 back blows as needed.
- If back blows don't relieve the obstruction, give up to 5 chest thrusts (infants <1y.) *or* up to 5 abdominal thrusts (children ≥1y.) as needed.

Following back blows, or chest or abdominal thrusts: Reassess:
If the object has not been expelled and the victim is still conscious: Continue the sequence of back blows and chest (for infant) or abdominal (for children) thrusts. ⓘ Don't leave the child.

If the object is expelled successfully: Assess the child's clinical condition (including abdominal examination if abdominal thrusts used). If there is any suspicion part of the object is still in the respiratory tract or there are any intra-abdominal injuries as a result of abdominal thrusts, refer to A&E for assessment.

If the child is UNCONSCIOUS: ⓘ Don't leave the child.
- Place on a firm, flat surface – call out/send for help if not arrived.
- Open the mouth and look for any obvious object. If one is seen, make an attempt to remove it with a single finger sweep.
- *Rescue breaths:* Open the airway and attempt 5 rescue breaths. Assess effectiveness of each breath – if a breath doesn't make the chest rise, reposition the head before making the next attempt.
- If there is no response to the rescue breaths, proceed immediately to chest compression – regardless of whether the breaths were successful. Follow the PBLS sequence (📖 p.31) for 1min. before summoning help if not already there.

If it appears the obstruction has been relieved:
- Open and check the airway.
- Deliver rescue breaths if the child is not breathing.
- If the child regains consciousness and is breathing effectively, place him in a safe side-lying (recovery) position and monitor breathing and conscious level whilst awaiting the arrival of the emergency services.

Figure 2.6 Algorithm for management of paediatric foreign body airway obstruction (PFBAO)

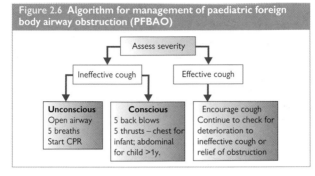

Back blows for small children/infants
- Place the child in a head-downwards, prone position (e.g. across your lap). Support the head if needed by holding the jaw.
- Deliver a smart blow with the heel of one hand to the middle of the back between the shoulder blades. Repeat up to 5 times as needed.

Back blows for older children
- Support the child in a forward-leaning position.
- Deliver a smart blow with the heel of one hand to the middle of the back between the shoulder blades from behind. Repeat up to 5 times as needed.

Chest thrusts for infants <1y.
- Turn the child into a supine position with head down (e.g. by holding the child's occiput and laying the child along your arm, supported on your thigh).
- Deliver 5 sharp chest thrusts (like chest compressions but slower rate ~20/min.) to a point one finger's breadth above the xiphisternum.

Abdominal thrusts for children ≥1y.
- Stand behind the child (kneel if small child). Place your arms under the child's arms and encircle his torso.
- Clench your fist and place it between the umbilicus and xiphisternum.
- Grasp your clenched hand with your other hand and pull sharply inwards and upwards. Repeat up to 5 times as needed.
- ❶ Ensure that pressure is not applied to the xiphoid process or the lower rib cage as this may cause abdominal trauma.

Further information
Resuscitation Council (UK) Resuscitation guidelines 2005
🖥 www.resus.org.uk

Figure 2.6 is reproduced with permission from the Resuscitation Council UK 🖥 www.resus.org.uk

Anaphylaxis

Severe systemic allergic reaction.

Common causes
- *Foods:* nuts, fish and shellfish, sesame seeds and oil, milk, eggs, pulses (beans, peas)
- *Insect stings:* wasp or bee
- *Drugs:* antibiotics, aspirin and other NSAIDs, opiates
- *Latex*

Essential features: 1 or both of:
- Respiratory difficulty e.g. wheeze, stridor – may be due to laryngeal oedema or asthma
- Hypotension – fainting, collapse or loss of consciousness.

Other features: All or some of the following:
- Erythema
- Angio-oedema
- Itching of palate
- Itching of external auditory meatus
- Generalized pruritus
- Rhinitis
- Nausea
- Palpitations
- Urticaria
- Conjunctivitis
- Vomiting
- Sense of impending doom

Examination
- **A**irway: mouth/tongue for oedema
- **B**reathing: chest (wheeze), PEFR
- **C**irculation: pulse, BP
- *Skin:* check for rashes

Algorithm for management of anaphylaxis: Figure 2.7. Admit the patient to hospital until all ill effects have settled.

❶ Give IM injections into the midpoint of the anterolateral thigh. Don't give 1:1000 epinephrine/adrenaline IV.

Follow-up
- Warn patients or parents of the possibility of recurrence.
- Advise sufferers to wear a device (e.g. Medic-Alert bracelet) that will inform bystanders or medical staff should a future attack occur.
- Refer all patients after their first attack to a specialist allergy clinic.
- Consider supplying sufferers (or parents) with an EpiPen or similar which can be used to administer IM epinephrine (adrenaline) immediately should symptoms recur.
- If you supply an EpiPen, teach anyone likely to need to use it how to operate the device. Intramuscular epinephrine (adrenaline) is very safe.

Further information
Resuscitation Council UK Emergency medical treatment of anaphylactic reactions for first medical responders (2005) 🖥 www.resus.org.uk

GMS contract		
Medicines 2	The practice possesses the equipment and in-date emergency drugs to treat anaphylaxis	2 points

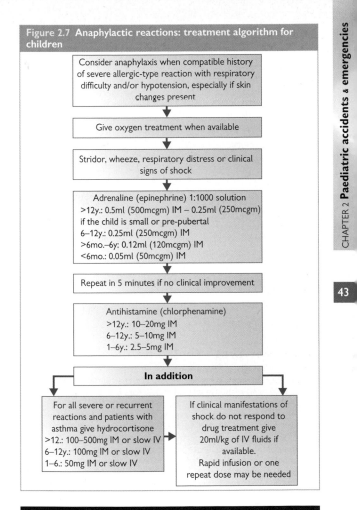

Figure 2.7 Anaphylactic reactions: treatment algorithm for children

Consider anaphylaxis when compatible history of severe allergic-type reaction with respiratory difficulty and/or hypotension, especially if skin changes present

Give oxygen treatment when available

Stridor, wheeze, respiratory distress or clinical signs of shock

Adrenaline (epinephrine) 1:1000 solution
>12y.: 0.5ml (500mcgm) IM – 0.25ml (250mcgm) if the child is small or pre-pubertal
6–12y.: 0.25ml (250mcgm) IM
>6mo.–6y: 0.12ml (120mcgm) IM
<6mo.: 0.05ml (50mcgm) IM

Repeat in 5 minutes if no clinical improvement

Antihistamine (chlorphenamine)
>12y.: 10–20mg IM
6–12y.: 5–10mg IM
1–6y.: 2.5–5mg IM

In addition

For all severe or recurrent reactions and patients with asthma give hydrocortisone
>12.: 100–500mg IM or slow IV
6–12y.: 100mg IM or slow IV
1–6.: 50mg IM or slow IV

If clinical manifestations of shock do not respond to drug treatment give 20ml/kg of IV fluids if available.
Rapid infusion or one repeat dose may be needed

43

Advice for Patients: Information and support for parents

Allergy UK ☎ 01322 619898 🖳 www.allergyuk.org
Anaphylaxis Campaign ☎ 01252 542029 🖳 www.anaphylaxis.org.uk
Medic-Alert Foundation Supply Medic-Alert bracelets ☎ 0800 581 420
🖳 www.medicalert.co.uk

Figure 2.7 is reproduced with permission from the Resuscitation Council UK
🖳 www.resus.org.uk

Acute asthma in children

Assess and record
- Pulse rate – increasing heart rate generally reflects ↑ severity
- Respiratory rate and breathlessness
- Use of accessory muscles – best noted by palpation of neck muscles
- Amount of wheezing
- Degree of agitation and conscious level

Levels of severity
Child >5y.: Figure 2.8
Child 2–5y.: Figure 2.9 📖 p.46
Child <2y.: Assessment of children <2y. can be difficult
- *Moderate wheezing:*
  - O_2 saturation ≥92%
  - Audible wheezing
  - Using accessory muscles
  - Still feeding
- *Severe wheezing:*
  - O_2 saturation <92%
  - Cyanosis
  - Marked respiratory distress
  - Too breathless to feed
- *Life threatening:*
  - Apnoea
  - Bradycardia
  - Poor respiratory effort

⚠ If a patient has signs and symptoms across categories, always treat according to the most severe features.

Management
Child >5y.: Figure 2.8
Child 2–5y.: Figure 2.9 📖 p.46
Child <2y.: Intermittent wheezing attacks are usually in response to viral infection and response to bronchodilators is inconsistent.
- If mild/moderate wheeze:
  - A trial of bronchodilators can be considered if symptoms are of concern – use a metred dose inhaler and spacer with a face mask
  - If no response consider alternative diagnosis (aspiration pneumonitis, pneumonia, bronchiolitis, tracheomalacia, CF, congenital anomaly) and/or admit.
- *If severe wheezing:* Admit to hospital.
- *If any life-threatening features:* Admit immediately as a blue-light emergency.

Follow-up after treatment or discharge from hospital:
- GP review within 1 week.
- Monitor symptoms, PEF and check inhaler technique.
- Written asthma action plan.
- Modify treatment according to guidelines for chronic persistent asthma.
- Address potentially preventable contributors to admission.

Management of chronic asthma: 📖 p.144

Figure 2.8 Management of acute asthma in children >5y

ASSESS ASTHMA SEVERITY		
Moderate exacerbation	Severe exacerbation	Life-threatening asthma
Oxygen saturation ≥92% PEF ≥50% best or predicted Able to talk Heart rate ≤120/min. Respiratory rate ≤30/min.	Oxygen saturation <92% PEF <50% best or predicted Too breathless to talk Heart rate >120/min. Respiratory rate >30/min. Use of accessory neck muscles	Oxygen saturation <92% PEF <33% best or predicted Silent chest Poor respiratory effort Agitation Altered consciousness Cyanosis
β_2 agonist 2–4 puffs via spacer Consider soluble prednisolone 30–40mg	Oxygen via face mask β_2 agonist 10 puffs via spacer ± facemask or nebulized salbutamol 2.5–5mg (or terbutaline 5–10mg) Soluble prednisolone 30–40mg	Oxygen via face mask Nebulize: • salbutamol 5mg or terbutaline 10mg + • ipratropium 0.25mg Soluble prednisolone 30–40mg or IV hydrocortisone 100mg
Increase β_2 agonist dose by 2 puffs every 2min. up to 10 puffs according to response	Assess response to treatment 15min. after β_2 agonist	
IF POOR RESPONSE ARRANGE ADMISSION	IF POOR RESPONSE REPEAT β_2 AGONIST AND ARRANGE ADMISSION	REPEAT β_2 AGONIST VIA OXYGEN-DRIVEN NEBULIZER WHILST ARRANGING IMMEDIATE HOSPITAL ADMISSION

GOOD RESPONSE	POOR RESPONSE
Continue up to 10 puffs or nebulized β_2 agonist as needed (max. every 4h.) If symptoms are not controlled repeat β_2 agonist and refer to hospital Continue prednisolone for up to 3d. Arrange follow-up clinic visit	Stay with the patient until the ambulance arrives Send written assessment and referral details Repeat β_2 agonist via oxygen-driven nebulizer in the ambulance

⚠ *Lower threshold for admission if:*
- Attack in late afternoon or at night
- Recent hospital admission or previous severe attack
- Concern over social circumstances or ability to cope at home

45

Figure 2.8 is reproduced from the British guideline on the management of asthma (2005) with permission from British Thoracic Society and SIGN.

Figure 2.9 Management of acute asthma in children 2–5y. in general practice

ASSESS ASTHMA SEVERITY		
Moderate exacerbation	Severe exacerbation	Life-threatening asthma
Oxygen saturation ≥92% Able to talk Heart rate ≤130/min. Respiratory rate ≤50/min.	Oxygen saturation <92% Too breathless to talk Heart rate >130/min. Respiratory rate >50/min. Use of accessory neck muscles	Oxygen saturation <92% Silent chest Poor respiratory effort Agitation Altered consciousness Cyanosis
β_2 agonist 2–4 puffs via spacer Consider soluble prednisolone 20mg	Oxygen via face mask β_2 agonist 10 puffs via spacer ± facemask or nebulized salbutamol 2.5mg (or terbutaline 5mg) Soluble prednisolone 20mg	Oxygen via face mask Nebulize: • salbutamol 2.5mg or terbutaline 5mg + • ipratropium 0.25mg Soluble prednisolone 20mg or IV hydrocortisone 50mg
Increase β_2 agonist dose by 2 puffs every 2min. up to 10 puffs according to response	Assess response to treatment 15min. after β_2 agonist	
IF POOR RESPONSE ARRANGE ADMISSION	IF POOR RESPONSE REPEAT β_2 AGONIST AND ARRANGE ADMISSION	REPEAT β_2 AGONIST VIA OXYGEN-DRIVEN NEBULIZER WHILST ARRANGING IMMEDIATE HOSPITAL ADMISSION

GOOD RESPONSE
Continue up to 10 puffs or nebulized β_2 agonist as needed (max. every 4h.)
If symptoms are not controlled repeat β_2 agonist and refer to hospital
Continue prednisolone for up to 3d.
Arrange follow-up clinic visit

POOR RESPONSE
Stay with the patient until the ambulance arrives
Send written assessment and refeerral details
Repeat β_2 agonist via oxygen-driven nebulizer in the ambulance

⚠ *Lower threshold for admission if:*
- Attack in late afternoon or at night
- Recent hospital admission or previous severe attack
- Concern over social circumstances or ability to cope at home

Further information

BTS/SIGN British guideline on the management of asthma (2005)
🖳 www.sign.ac.uk

Figure 2.9 is reproduced from the British guideline on the management of asthma (2005) with permission from British Thoracic Society and SIGN.

Meningitis and encephalitis

Meningitis and encephalitis present in similar fashion. Usually rapid onset (<48h.). Typical symptoms may be preceded with a prodrome of fever, vomiting, malaise, poor feeding and lethargy which is often indistinguishable from a viral infection. Particularly significant early signs include:

- Severe leg pain – so bad that the child can't stand/walk
- Cold hands or feet when the child is running a fever
- Pale skin ± blueness around the lips.

Typical symptoms/signs:

Meningism:

- Headache
- Photophobia
- Stiff neck – can't put chin on chest
- Kernig's sign +ve – with hips fully flexed resists passive knee extension

↑ *Intracranial pressure:*

- Irritability
- Vomiting
- Drowsiness/↓ consciousness
- ↓ pulse rate
- Fits
- ↑ BP
- Abnormal tone/posturing
- Bulging fontanelle (baby)

Septicaemia/septic shock:

- Fever
- Tachypnoea
- Arthritis
- Peripheral shut down – cool peripheries, mottled skin, cyanosis
- Hypotension
- Tachycardia
- ± rash – petechiae suggest meningococcus

⚠ Small children or immunocompromised patients may not present with typical signs. Go on gut feeling.

⚠ Action:

- Call an emergency ambulance and get the patient to hospital as soon as possible.
- If shocked, lie the patient flat and raise legs above waist height.
- If symptoms/signs of meningitis or meningococcal septicaemia, give IV/IM benzylpenicillin immediately while awaiting transport. *Dose:*
  - Child ≥10y. – 1.2g
  - Child 1–9y. – 600mg
  - Infant <1y – 300mg.
- Cefotaxime is an alternative for patients allergic to penicillin (child >12y. – 1g; child <12y. – 50mg/kg).
- If possible gain IV access whilst awaiting the ambulance and take blood for cultures. Consider starting IV fluids/plasma expander. Give 10ml/kg rapidly over 10–15min.
- If available give 100% oxygen.

GP Notes: The glass test

If a viral rash is pressed with a glass, it blanches under pressure. A purpuric rash of meningitis won't – Figure 4.5 (📖 p.117).

Contact tracing/prophylaxis for meningococcal meningitis:

- Undertaken by the local public health department.
- For a single case only very close contacts ('kissing contacts'), e.g. immediate family members, require prophylactic antibiotics.
- Prophylaxis – rifampicin 600mg bd for 2d. (child 10mg/kg bd for 2d. unless <1y. when dose is 5mg/kg bd for 2d.) *or* ciprofloxacin 500mg as a single dose (unlicensed and not suitable for children).
- Rifampicin colours urine red.

ⓘ Meningitis and acute encephalitis are notifiable diseases.

Box 2.1 Meningitis vaccination

- Group C strains are responsible for 40% of meningococcal disease.
- Group B strains are responsible for most of the rest.
- Group A strains are common in other parts of the world but rare in the UK.

Meningococcal A&C vaccine: No protection against group B strain. Immunize individuals travelling abroad to high-risk areas with the meningococcal A&C vaccine, even if they have received the meningitis C conjugate vaccine beforehand.

Meningitis C conjugate vaccine:

- For infants doses are given at 2, 3 and 4mo. as part of the routine childhood vaccination programme.
- For infants >4mo. 2 doses are required and >1y. of age only 1 dose is necessary to confer lasting immunity.
- Vaccine may be given to HIV +ve patients.
- A gap of 6mo. is recommended between a dose of the meningococcal A&C vaccine, usually given for travel purposes, and meningitis C conjugate vaccine.
- Do not use meningitis C conjugate vaccine for travel purposes as the greatest risk is from group A infection.

Advice for patients: Telephone helplines for families

Meningitis Research Foundation ☎ 080 8800 3344
🖥 www.meningitis.org.uk
Meningitis Trust ☎ 0800 028 1828 🖥 www.meningitis-trust.org

GMS contract

All routine vaccinations for the under-5s and vaccinations for older children missed by the school vaccination programme, including routine meningitis C vaccination, are provided as an additional service. Opting out of giving vaccinations to the under-5s results in a 1% ↓ in global sum.

Head injury

Severe head injury
- Perform basic life support (📖 p.30).
- Protect the cervical spine (see below and 📖 p.33).
- Transfer to A&E by ambulance.

Less severe head injuries

History: If possible take the history from a witness as well as the patient. Ask about circumstances of injury, loss of consciousness (LOC), seizures, current symptoms and behaviour.

Examination: Check scalp, head for injury, neurological examination (including fundi), other injuries – accompanying neck injuries are common.

⚠ *Refer to A&E if* [N]:
- Glasgow Coma Scale <15 at any time since injury (Table 2.1)
- Loss of consciousness
- Focal neurological deficit since injury – problems speaking, understanding, reading, writing, ↓ sensation, loss of balance, weakness, visual changes, abnormal reflexes, problems walking, irritability or altered behaviour especially in young children
- Any suspicion of skull fracture; penetrating head injury; blood or CSF in the nose, ear or wound; serious scalp laceration or haematoma
- Amnesia for events before or after injury
- Persistent headache
- Vomiting (any vomiting in children >12y.; >1 vomit in children <12y.)
- Seizure
- Any previous cranial neurosurgical interventions
- High-energy head injury (e.g. pedestrian hit by motor vehicle, fall >1m or >5 stairs)
- History of bleeding or clotting disorder or on anticoagulant therapy
- Difficulty in assessing the patient (e.g. very young or epileptic) or concern about diagnosis
- Suspicion of non-accidental injury (📖 p.322)
- Inadequate supervision at home

If there is a history of neck pain/neck injury, immobilize the neck and refer to A&E.

If examination is normal
- Warn the child and parents that the child may suffer mild headaches, tiredness, dizziness, tinnitus, poor concentration and poor memory for the next few days.
- Advise rest and paracetamol (but not codeine-based analgesics) for the headache.
- Young children can be difficult to assess – sleepiness is common and not a worrying sign as long as the child is rousable.
- Give written head injury information regarding warning signs to trigger reconsultation – drowsiness, severe headache, persistent vomiting, visual disturbance and/or unusual behaviour.

Table 2.1 The Glasgow Coma Scale		
Eye opening:	Spontaneous	4
	To voice	3
	To pain	2
	None	1
Best verbal response:	Oriented	5
	Confused	4
	Inappropriate words	3
	Incomprehensive	2
	None	1
Best motor response:	Obeys command	6
	Localizes pain	5
	Withdraws	4
	Flexion	3
	Extension	2
	None	1
Total score = eye opening + best verbal + best motor response scores		

GP Notes

🕐 **Watch out for post-concussion syndrome:** Seen following even quite minor head injury. Due to neuronal damage.

Features include all or some of:

- Headache
- Dizziness
- Poor concentration
- Fatigue
- Depression
- Memory problems

Treatment is supportive and symptoms usually resolve with time (though can take months or even years).

Further information

NICE Triage, assessment investigation and early management of head injury in infants, children and adults (2003) 🖥 www.nice.org.uk

Other paediatric emergencies

The fitting patient

When the call for assistance is received: Instruct attendant to:
- stay with the fitting patient
- move anything from the vicinity of the patient that might cause injury
- turn the patient onto his/her side.

In a child <5y., suspect a febrile cause and advise the attendant to cool the child by stripping off layers of clothing and tepid sponging.

⚠ *Management of a major fit:*
- Ensure that the airway is clear.
- Turn the patient into the recovery position (i.e. as close to the true lateral position as possible – 📖 p.33).
- Prevent onlookers from restraining the fitting patient.
- Do not give drugs for the 1st 10min. – the fit is likely to stop spontaneously. After 10min. treat with diazepam IV or pr (10mg if >12y.; 5–10mg aged 2–12y.; 5mg aged 1mo.–2y.; 1.25–2.5mg if <1mo.).
- If the fit is not controlled treat as status epilepticus.

Admit any child with a fit if:
- There is suspicion that the fit is secondary to other illness e.g. meningitis, subdural haematoma.
- The child doesn't recover fully after the fit (other than feeling sleepy).
- Status epilepticus.

Status epilepticus: If >1 seizure without the patient regaining consciousness or fitting continues >20min.:
- Give diazepam 5–10mg IV or pr (5mg if 2–3y.; 2.5mg if <2y.)
- Repeat every 15min. until fits are controlled
- Check BM to exclude low blood sugar
- Arrange immediate admission even if fits are controlled.

Follow-up: Refer any child who has a first fit not related to fever to paediatrics for urgent assessment[N].

Further information:
- Epilepsy in children: 📖 pp.228–31
- Febrile convulsions: 📖 pp.224–7

Overdose or accidental poisoning: Peak incidence of accidental poisoning is at 2y. – mainly household substances, prescribed or OTC drugs, or plants. Teenagers may take deliberate overdoses, especially of OTC medication e.g. paracetamol (📖 p.315).

⚠ Poisoning can be a form of non-accidental injury (📖 p.322).

On receiving the call for assistance:
- Try to establish what has happened – substances involved, ongoing dangers, state of the patient.
- Advise the caller to stay with the patient until you arrive.
- If the child is unconscious, arrange for an ambulance to meet you at the scene.

Assessment of the unconscious patient: 📖 p.38
Assessment of the conscious patient:

- Note down any information about the exposure: product name (if unidentified tablets see if any are left and send them to hospital with the child in their own container), time of incident, duration of exposure/amount ingested, route of exposure (swallowed, inhaled, injected etc.), whether intentional or accidental.
- Record symptoms and examine pulse, BP, temperature (if necessary), level of consciousness or confusion, any injuries.
- If deliberate exposure, e.g. overdose, assess whether NAI (📖 p.322) or suicidal intent (📖 p.314).
- Take a general history: medical history, current medication, substance abuse, alcohol, social circumstances.

Consider admission if:

- The child's clinical condition warrants it: unconsciousness, respiratory depression etc.
- The exposure warrants admission for treatment or observation:
  - *Symptomatic poisoning:* Admit to hospital
  - *Agents with delayed action:* Aspirin, iron, paracetamol, tricyclic antidepressants, Lomotil (co-phenotrope), paraquat and modified release preparations. Admit to hospital even if the patient seems well.
  - *Other agents:* Consult poisons information.
- You judge there is a possibility of NAI (📖 p.322), serious suicidal intent (📖 p.314) or the patient has another psychiatric condition which warrants acute admission.
- There is a lack of adequate care for the child at home.

Poisons information:
UK National Poisons Information Service ☎ 0870 600 6266
TOXBASE poisons database 🖥 www.toxbase.org

Acute ketoacidosis: 📖 p.191

Hypoglycaemic coma: 📖 p.192

Drowning: 3rd most common cause of accidental death among the under-16s. > ½ those who drown can swim. Children can drown in a few centimetres of water. Hypothermia is commonly associated with drowning and increases risk of asystole and VF during rewarming.

Action:
- Call for help.
- Start basic life support (Airway, Breathing, Circulation) – 📖 p.30.

⚠ Attempted resuscitation of a seemingly dead child is worthwhile as recovery can occur after prolonged immersion.

Prevention: The best way to ↓ drowning is prevention. Supervise children near water. Don't let children go near water alone. Spot the dangers. Take safety advice and learn how to help others.

Common injuries and accidents

Wounds: Most patients with significant lacerations present directly to A&E. If a patient presents to general practice perform immediate care (elevate bleeding limb and apply pressure to arrest bleeding). Advise nil by mouth and transfer to A&E.

Minor lacerations

- Ensure no foreign body is in the wound – if in doubt refer for X-ray/surgical exploration (especially important if injury was with glass).
- Wash wound and clean away debris and any necrotic material.
- Check there is no damage to underlying nerves, tendons, bone or blood supply before dressing or closing a wound.
- Aim to oppose the skin edges without tension to allow healing. For children in primary care, Steri-strips can be used where necessary for small cuts in non-hairy skin which are not under tension. Skin glue e.g. Histoacryl can be used for hairy skin e.g. the scalp.
- Do not attempt to close a wound if you are not confident that you can achieve an adequate result. Refer to A&E if in doubt.
- Check tetanus status.
- Consider non-accidental injury in children – 📖 p.322.

Haematoma of the pinna: Usually after trauma (e.g. rugby). Must be evacuated urgently (aspirated via large-bore needle or surgically) to prevent necrosis of the cartilage and 'cauliflower' ear – refer to A&E.

Nail injuries

- **Avulsed nail:** Protect the nail bed of an avulsed nail with soft paraffin and gauze, check tetanus status and give antibiotic prophylaxis (e.g. flucloxacillin for 5d.). Partially avulsed nails – refer to A&E for removal.
- **Subungual haematoma:** A blow to the finger can cause bleeding under the nail – very painful due to pressure build-up. Relieve by trephining a hole through the nail using a 19-gauge needle (no force required, just twist the needle as it rests vertically on the nail) or a heated point (e.g. of a paper clip or cautery instrument). Of benefit up to 2d. after injury.

Foreign bodies

- **Coin and other foreign body ingestion:** Most coins will pass through the gut without any problems. If asymptomatic, they can be left to take their course (advise checking stools to ensure passed). If symptomatic refer for X-ray and consideration for endoscopic removal. If there is any indication of aspiration refer urgently.
- **In the ear:** Most common in children. Try to remove under direct vision with forceps but avoid pushing objects deeper into the canal and causing damage. Don't poke around with forceps in an uncooperative child. Removal under GA may be needed. Insects can be drowned in oil and syringed out.
- **In the nose:** Common in young children. Refer all children with unilateral offensive discharge for exploration under GA. Do not try to remove a foreign body yourself unless the object is very superficial and the child cooperative. You might push the object further in and cause trauma.

- *Air gun pellets:* Common. Refer for X-ray. Can be difficult to remove – may be left in place if not in a harmful position. If in a joint, refer for removal.

Knocked out teeth: Ask the patient to suck tooth clean, reinsert or store in milk and send to a dentist.

Animal bites: ~200,000 people are bitten by dogs each year in the UK. Animal bites are contaminated and wound infection is common. Clean carefully with soap and water. Check tetanus status. Do not suture unless cosmetically essential and there is minimal tissue damage – refer if in doubt. Give prophylaxis against infection (e.g. with co-amoxiclav or erythromycin).

Human bites: Are especially prone to infection. Also consider risk of hepatitis B and HIV. If HIV prophylaxis is indicated, it needs to be started immediately – refer urgently to A&E for local policy implementation.

Snake bites: The adder is the only poisonous snake in the UK. Bites are only rarely lethal. Attempt to identify the snake species and refer the patient urgently to hospital. Do not apply a tourniquet or try cutting or sucking the wound.

Insect stings and bites: Response depends on the insect involved and the individual's response to the stings. Ranges from blisters through papules to urticarial wheals – 2° infection is common.

Management
Anaphylaxis: Follow algorithm in Figure 2.7, 📖 p.43, and admit to hospital as a blue-light emergency.

Immediately after the sting: Remove any sting present in the wound; often no further treatment is needed.
- *If severe local reaction occurs*: Apply an ice pack; give oral antihistamine (e.g. chlorphenamine); continue antihistamine 4–6 hourly as needed.
- *If 2° bacterial infection occurs*: Treat with oral or topical antibiotics.

Remove sources of insects e.g. remove fleas from carpets with household flea spray (multiple bites on ankles and lower legs).

GP Notes:

Removing a tight ring from a swollen finger:
- Wind cotton tape around the finger advancing towards the ring.
- Then thread tape through the ring and pull on this end to unwind the tape (levers ring over PIP joint).
- If unsuccessful, use a ring cutter.

Removing fish hooks: Infiltrate with lidocaine. Push the hook forwards through the skin until the barb is exposed. Cut the barb off and then ease the hook back through the skin the same way it entered.

Removing ticks: Place a large blob of petroleum jelly (Vaseline™) over the tick. It suffocates over a few hours and can be removed easily with a pair of tweezers.

Weaver fish sting: Common on sandy beaches. The fish lurks under the sand so is usually trodden on – presents with severe pain in the foot. Immerse the affected area in uncomfortably hot (but not scalding) water. Give analgesia. Pain resolves after 2–3d.

Jelly fish sting

- Remove the patient from the sea as soon as possible.
- Scrape or wash adherent tentacles off.
- Alcoholic solutions including suntan lotions should **not** be applied because they may cause further discharge of stinging hairs.
- Ice packs ↓ pain and a slurry of baking soda (sodium bicarbonate), but not vinegar, may be useful for treating stings from UK species.

Fractures

Presentation:
- *Symptoms:* Pain at the affected site made worse by movement; loss of function.
- *Signs:* Swelling; bruising; deformity; local tenderness; impaired function; crepitus; abnormal mobility

Action:
- Immobilize the affected part and give analgesia.
- If available and the patient is shocked, start an IV infusion.
- Refer to A&E for assessment, X-ray and treatment.

Fracture complications
- Often occur after the patient has been discharged from hospital and may present to the GP.
- Patients should not have persistent pain – beware of compartment syndrome.
- Refer back to the fracture clinic or A&E if:
  - Persistent pain
  - Limb swelling that is not settling
  - Offensive odour or discharge
  - If cast edges are abrading the skin or if the cast has deteriorated in structural strength e.g. from getting wet.

Compartment syndrome: Crush injury, fracture, prolonged immobility or tight splints, dressings or casts can result in ↑ pressure within muscle compartments, ultimately resulting in vascular occlusion. Hypoxia and necrosis cause further ↑ pressure.

Signs: Swelling, severe pain – ↑ on passive stretch of muscles, distal numbness, redness, mottling, blisters. ❶ Pulses may be present distally.

Action: Refer as an emergency for orthopaedic assessment – a fasciotomy may be needed to relieve the pressure.

Sports injuries: Exercise is good for children – it stimulates development of the musculoskeletal and cardiovascular systems. It should be fun and not physically or emotionally over-demanding.

Principles of managing sporting injuries
- *First aid (**A**irway, **B**reathing, **C**irculation):* Refer severe injuries to A&E.
- *Confirm the diagnosis:* Clinical examination, X-ray
- *R I C E:*
    - *Rest:* Relative rest of affected part whilst continuing other activities to maintain overall fitness
    - *Ice and analgesia:* Use immediately after injury (wrap ice in a towel and use for maximum 10min. at a time to prevent acute cold injury)
    - *Compression:* Taping or strapping can be used to treat (↓ swelling) and also to prevent acute sprains and strains
    - *Elevation:* ↓ local swelling and dependent oedema enabling quicker recovery.
- *Early treatment:* According to cause. Don't delay. Refer children with suspected overuse or sports injuries, which don't recover rapidly with simple analgesia, for specialist assessment, especially injuries of growth plates, to ensure correct alignment and continued growth.
- *Liaise:* With sports physician, sports physio and coach if élite athlete.
- *Rehabilitation:* Regaining fitness, strength and flexibility. Look for and correct cause of the injury if possible (e.g. poor technique, equipment).
- *Graded return to activity:* Discuss with coach.

Prevention: Suitable preparation and training (e.g. suitable footwear, warm-up and warm-down exercises, safety equipment) can ↓ likelihood of injuries. Equipment must be checked regularly to ensure it fits.

Further information
British Association of Sport and Exercise Medicine
⌂ www.basem.co.uk
ABC of sports medicine (1999) BMJ Publishing ISBN 072 791 3662

Scalds and burns

Assess
- Cause, size and thickness of the burn.
- Estimate extent of the burn by comparison with the area of the child's hand. The area of the fingers and palm ≈1% total body surface area.
- Partial thickness burns are red, painful and blistered; full thickness burns are painless and white or grey.
- Always consider non-accidental injury in children – 📖 p.322.

> ### ⚠ Action
> - Remove clothing from the affected area and place under cold running water for >10min. or until pain is relieved.
> - Do not burst blisters.
> - Prescribe/give analgesia.
> - Refer all but the smallest (<5%) partial thickness burns for assessment in A&E.
> - Refer all electrical burns for assessment in A&E.
> - Refer all chemical burns for assessment in A&E unless burn area is minimal and pain free.
> - Consider referral to A&E for smoke inhalation.
>
> *If managing the burn in the community:*
> - Check tetanus immunity and give immunization ± prophylaxis as necessary.
> - Apply silver sulfadiazine cream (flamazine) or vaseline impregnated gauze and non-adherent dressings and review for healing and infection every 1–2d.
> - Cover burns on hands in flamazine and place in a sterile plastic bag – elevate the hand in a sling and encourage finger movement.
> - Refer if burns are not healed in 10–12d.

Prevention of scalds and burns
- Prevention through public education is important.
- Children often sustain burns by pulling on the flex of boiling kettles or irons, pulling on saucepan handles or climbing onto hot cookers.
- Refer any children who have sustained accidental burns to the health visitor for follow-up.

Smoke inhalation
- Refer all patients who have potentially inhaled smoke for assessment – a seemingly well patient can deteriorate later.
- Smoke can cause thermal injury, carbon monoxide poisoning and cyanide poisoning.
- Airway problems occur due to thermal and chemical damage to the airways causing oedema – suspect if singed nasal hairs, a sore throat or a hoarse voice.
- Carbon monoxide poisoning may result in the classic cherry-red mucosa – but this may be absent.
- Cyanide poisoning is commonly due to smouldering plastics and causes dizziness, headaches and seizures.

Sunburn: Susceptibility depends on skin type.
- Tingling is followed 2–12h. later by erythema.
- Redness is maximal at 24h. and fades over 2–3d.
- Desquamation and pigmentation follow.
- Severe sunburn may cause blistering, pain and systemic upset. Treatment is symptomatic with calamine lotion prn (some advocate application of vinegar) and paracetamol for pain.
- Rarely dressings are required for blisters or, in severe cases, hospital admission for fluid management.
- Predisposes to skin cancer and photoageing.

GP Notes: Burns in special situations

Chemical burns
- Usually caused by strong acids or alkalis.
- Wear gloves to remove contaminated clothing.
- Irrigate with cold running water for ≥20min.
- Do not attempt to neutralize the chemical – this can exacerbate injury by producing heat.
- Refer all burns to A&E unless the burn area is minimal and pain free.

Electric shock
- Causes thermal tissue injury and direct injury due to the electric current passing through the tissue.
- Skin burns may be seen at the entry and exit site of the current.
- Muscle damage can be severe with minimal skin injury.
- Cardiac damage may occur and rhabdomyolysis can lead to renal failure.
- Refer all patients for specialist management.

Advice for patients: The sun safety code

- Take care not to let your child burn in the sun.
- Cover him or her up with loose cool clothing, a hat and sunglasses.
- If you're swimming outdoors or on the beach, dress your child in a UV protective sunsuit for swimming. When your child is out of the water, add a T-shirt, sunglasses and sunhat.
- Seek shade during the hottest part of the day.
- Apply a high-factor sunscreen on any parts of the body exposed to the sun (≥SPF 25).

Chapter 3

Neonates and infants

Problems of prematurity

Any baby born at <37wk. gestation is considered premature, although most born at 36wk. gestation have few problems and babies born as early as 32wk. do very well, many needing only tube feeding and warmth. Although some babies of 23–24wk. gestation now survive, survival is rare and there is a high incidence of disability in these extremely premature babies. Prematurity affects all systems of the body and in general the problems are worse the more premature the baby.

Nutrition: Preterm babies suck and swallow poorly so commonly need nasogastric tube feeding. They are also at particular risk of hypoglycaemia so need frequent feeds. Breast milk (sometimes with calorie supplements) or special low-birth-weight formula is used. Vitamin and iron supplements are routine.

Thermoregulation: Poor in preterm infants, as they have a high surface area:body weight ratio and little subcutaneous fat. A controlled temperature and adequate insulation, with clothes and blankets where appropriate, is important.

Respiration

- *Preterm infants >32wk. gestation:* May have transient tachypnoea at birth due to inability to express fluid from their lungs. Some need oxygen by headbox.
- *Preterm infants <32wk. gestation:* There may be insufficient surfactant produced causing respiratory distress syndrome and requiring mechanical ventilation. Incidence and severity is ↓ by antenatal corticosteroids and by giving exogenous surfactant either as prophylaxis or rescue treatment.
- *Extremely premature babies:* May develop bronchopulmonary dysplasia (chronic lung disease) and be ventilator and oxygen dependent for many months. These babies are often sent home on oxygen via nasal cannulae. They are at higher risk from respiratory infections, particularly RSV, and episodes of bradycardia and apnoea are common. Have a low threshold for readmission. Prolonged intubation can lead to subglottic stenosis (📖 p.276).

Jaundice: The immature liver is less able to process bilirubin so premature babies are at greater risk of developing neonatal jaundice. They are also more likely to develop kernicterus so have a lower threshold to refer for phototherapy.

Infection: The immune system is poorly developed so there is greater risk of infection. Furthermore these babies exhibit few signs, so have a low threshold to refer to paediatrics for a septic screen and antibiotics.

Anaemia: Low iron stores and repeated venepuncture lead to anaemia in premature babies. Some very premature babies may need repeated transfusion, and erythropoietin is often used to ↓ transfusion requirements. Iron supplements are routinely given to most premature babies.

Neurology: Intraventricular haemorrhages are common. Small ones may have few consequences; more extensive haemorrhages may lead to cerbral palsy, hydrocephalus and learning disability. Hypoxia can also lead to cerebral damage.

Vision: Retinopathy of prematurity, the development of abnormal vascularization at the back of the eye, occurs in very premature babies as a result of high partial pressures of oxygen. This may result in visual impairment, even blindness. Babies born at <32wk. gestation should be screened by an ophthalmologist before leaving the neonatal unit but may need follow-up and/or laser treatment once home.

Hearing: Premature babies are at greater risk of hearing problems and should have neonatal screening and appropriate follow-up.

Bonding: Separation of mother and premature baby is often necessary. Poor bonding is common, and the problem is added to by fear of losing the baby. Parents may be (quite understandably) very anxious when their babies first come home after a long period in special care and need more support and reassurance than other parents.

Cot death: Premature babies have ↑ risk of cot death:
- Prevention: 📖 p.11
- Management: 📖 p.80.

> **GP Notes: Avoiding infection**
>
> Advise parents of very premature babies to keep them away from all potential sources of infection when they first come home e.g. doctors' waiting rooms, schools when collecting siblings etc. This might entail making special arrangements for vaccinations and additional requirement for home visits.

> **Advice for patients: Information and support for parents of premature babies**
>
> **Bliss** support line ☎ 0500 618 140 🖥 www.bliss.org.uk
> **Premature Babies** website 🖥 www.premature-babies.co.uk

Minor problems of neonates and small babies

Table 3.1 Minor problems of neonates and small babies

Condition	Features	Management
Milia	Tiny pearly white papules on the nose ± palate – blocked sebaceous ducts.	Disappear spontaneously – reassure.
Erythema toxicum (neonatal urticaria)	Red blotches with a central, white vesicle. Each spot lasts ~24h. Spots are sterile and the baby is well.	If sepsis is suspected, take a swab. Otherwise reassure – resolves spontaneously.
Harlequin colour change	One side of the body flushes red whilst the other stays pale giving a harlequin effect.	A harmless vasomotor effect – reassure.
Single palmar crease	Common abnormality. Associated with several genetic syndromes e.g. Down's.	Usually of no consequence unless associated with other abnormalities.
Milaria (heat rash)	Itchy red rash which fades as soon as the baby is cooled (e.g. by undressing).	Reassure. Keep the baby cool if the rash appears.
Peeling skin	Common among babies born after their due date.	Apply olive or baby oil, or aqueous cream to prevent the skin cracking.
Petechial or subconjunctival haemorrhage and facial cyanosis	May all occur during delivery.	Resolve spontaneously – reassure. Ensure the baby has had vitamin K supplements.
Swollen breasts	Due to maternal hormones. Occur in both sexes and occasionally lactate (witches' milk).	Breast swelling usually subsides spontaneously. May become infected and require antibiotics.
Sticky eye	Common. Usually due to a blocked tear duct. Swab to exclude ophthalmia neonatorum.	Ophthalmia neonatorum – 📖 p.xxx. Blocked tear duct – 📖 p.xxx.
Sneezing	Neonates clear amniotic fluid from their noses by sneezing.	Reassure.
Red-stained nappy	Common in the first few days of life. Usually due to urinary urates but may be due to blood from the cord or vagina (oestrogen withdrawal bleed).	Reassure.

Table 3.1 (Contd.)		
Condition	**Features**	**Management**
The umbilicus	After birth the umbilicus dries, becomes black and separates at about 1wk. of age.	The umbilical stump can become infected – offensive odour, pus, periumbilical flare, malaise – requiring antibiotics.
		If a granuloma forms at the site of separation, exclude a patent urachus (look for discharge of bowel fluid or urine – refer if present) and treat with silver nitrate cautery.
Failure to regain birth weight by 2wk. of age	Usually due to a feeding problem or minor intercurrent illness.	Monitor weight carefully. Examine baby carefully.
		Refer to paediatrics if no cause is apparent or if, despite treatment of the underlying cause, the baby is not gaining weight.
Possetting	Common.	Only of concern if the baby is otherwise unwell or failing to thrive – see gastro-oesophageal reflux.
	The baby effortlessly brings back 5–10ml of each feed during the feed or soon after.	If thriving, advise parents to feed the child propped up and slow down the speed at which feeds are given.
Gastro-oesophageal reflux	Similar to possetting but a greater proportion or all of each feed is brought back.	Advise parents to feed the child propped up.
	Often results in failure to thrive.	Thickening agents (e.g. Carobel, Nestargel) may be helpful as may Gaviscon Infant ± ranitidine.
	More common in babies with cerebral palsy.	Babies usually grow out of the condition after a few months and/or when solids are introduced.
	Rare complications are oesophageal stricture due to acid reflux or aspiration pneumonia.	Refer to paediatrics if failing to thrive despite simple measures, chestiness or anaemia.
Colic	Very common in newborns up to ~3mo.	Cause is unknown and symptoms resolve spontaneously with time.
	Repeated bouts of intense, unsoothable crying commonly attributed to abdominal pain (though there is no objective evidence).	Advise parents to try colic drops or gripe water.
		There is no evidence that changing from cow's milk to soya-based formula is helpful.
	During an attack the baby's body becomes tense and rigid, face goes red and knees draw up.	Refer to paediatrics if diagnosis is in doubt, severe symptoms, other symptoms or signs (e.g. failure to thrive, severe eczema) or fails to resolve by 12wk. of age.
	Usually occurs in early evening.	
	Examination is normal.	
Crying	📖 p.292	📖 p.292

Feeding babies and toddlers

Breast-feeding: Breast-feeding is the preferred way to feed infants from birth until fully weaned or longer. However, ~1:3 mothers who start breast-feeding have stopped by 6wk. Most wish to continue, but problems with painful breasts/nipples, concern regarding amount of milk the baby is getting and lack of support are common reasons for stopping.

Breast-feeding is something some find natural and others find difficult. Teaching a woman and baby to breast-feed takes time and patience. Be supportive and ask a midwife, health visitor or the local breast-feeding advisor to help if needed.

Advantages of breast-feeding
- Encourages a strong bond between mother and baby.
- More convenient than bottle-feeding – the milk is ready-warmed and there is no need for sterilized bottles.
- Cheaper than bottle-feeding.
- Protects the baby from infection.
- ↓ childhood obesity.
- ↓ childhood atopy.
- Possible ↓ risk of DM for the baby.
- ↓ postpartum bleeding.
- Helps the mother ↓ weight after pregnancy.
- Protects the mother against breast and ovarian cancer.

Common problems with breast-feeding: Table 3.2

Bottle-feeding

Cow's milk formula feeds: Prepared from cow's milk altered to simulate the composition of human milk, with added iron and vitamins. Advise parents to choose a formula suitable for their baby and make up the formula exactly as the manufacturer suggests. Feeding bottles and teats should be well washed and, until >6mo. of age, sterilized. Using a cup rather than bottle is advisable from about 6mo. Families on low incomes may be entitled to claim free formula milk for their babies.

Follow-on formula: Not essential unless a child is not taking solids and is >6mo. old. Baby milks suitable from birth can be used until a switch is made to normal cow's milk.

Soya protein-based formula: Available for children with cow's milk allergy, though this group are frequently also intolerant of soya milk. Soya formula is useful for babies who have transient intolerance after gastroenteritis, but be careful – it contains large amounts of glucose syrup and can damage the teeth of babies fed on it long term, and it contains phyto-oestrogens, which may be harmful particularly to male infants. Soya formula is available on NHS prescription.

Special artificial formula: Available for children intolerant to soya and cow's milk formulae – prescribe only on consultant recommendation.

Unmodified cow's milk: Not recommended until the baby is >1y. old as unmodified cow's milk is less digestible, and contains little iron. (semi-skimmed milk <2y.; skimmed milk <5y.)

Table 3.2 Common problems with breast-feeding

Problem	Possible solutions
Painful breasts and/or nipples	Ensure correct positioning. Treat mastitis or thrush if present.
It is difficult to know how much milk the baby is taking at each feed	Encourage demand feeding and tell mothers to exhaust milk supply in one breast before starting the other. Plot weight. If there are concerns about weight gain, consider other causes of failure to thrive – 📖 p.68.
Breast milk does not contain all the nutrients the baby needs	Breast milk has low levels of vitamin K , D and iron. Ensure babies who have had oral vitamin K at birth receive additional vitamin K supplements. Encourage weaning at 6mo. Lactating mothers and babies from 6mo. can be given vitamin D supplements if needed. Iron drops can be given to babies with low iron reserves (e.g. low birth weight, maternal anaemia).
Only the mother can feed the baby	Mothers who anticipate they will be absent from the baby for a period of time can express milk for someone else to feed to the baby in a bottle whilst they are gone. Advise mothers not to attempt this before breast-feeding is well established as the baby might find the 2 techniques confusing. 2 methods are commonly used: • Using a commercially available breast pump or • By hand into a sterile bowl. Breast milk can be frozen (special bags are available) and defrosted when required. Bottles should be sterilized and the milk warmed in the same way as for bottle-feeding.
Disease can be transferred in breast milk	In general breast milk protects the baby from disease. Some diseases can be transferred in breast milk e.g. hepatitis B or HIV. Bottle-feeding is recommended where uncontaminated water is available.
Drugs taken by the mother may have adverse effects on the baby	Mothers should take medical advice before taking any drugs (including herbal remedies). For most conditions drugs safe for use whilst breast-feeding are available. Rarely breast-feeding is contraindicated e.g. for women taking lithium or on chemotherapy.

Advice for patients: Sources of support for breast-feeding mothers

National Childbirth Trust ☎ 0870 444 8708 🖥 www.nctpregnancyandbabycare.com
La Leche League ☎ 0845 120 2918 🖥 www.laleche.org.uk
Baby Café 🖥 www.thebabycafe.co.uk
Association of Breast-feeding Mothers ☎ 0870 4017711 🖥 www.abm.me.uk
Breast-feeding Network 🖥 www.breastfeedingnetwork.org.uk ☎ 0870 9000 8787

Weaning: Current guidelines recommend solids should be introduced at 6mo. of age, although they stress individual needs of infants and choices of parents should be considered and supported. Earlier introduction of solids is linked with ↑ rates of infection and ↑ incidence of allergy/intolerance to certain foods e.g. gluten or eggs.

Feeding problems: Parents commonly complain their child is not eating enough or eating the wrong foods. Usually the child continues to grow and develop normally. If so, reassure the parents. Consider referral to the health visitor for advice/support. Advise parents to:
- Restrict snacks between meals
- Show little emotion when putting food in front of the child at meal times and remove the food after 15–20min. without comment about what is or isn't eaten.

If the child is not growing or developing normally, look for reasons for failure to thrive (below).

Failure to thrive: Common problem. The result of insufficient nutrition to allow weight ↑. Defined as:
- Weight consistently <3rd centile for age
- Progressive ↓ in weight to <3rd centile or
- ↓ in expected rate of growth based on the child's growth curve.

Usually head circumference is preserved relative to length and length relative to weight.

Causes: Many and varied.

Non-organic causes
- Lack of food due to neglect, lack of education, poverty or famine
- Emotional problems e.g. emotional neglect, unhappy family or other difficulties at home.

Organic causes
- Chronic infection
- Gastrointestinal disease e.g. coeliac disease, chronic diarrhoea
- Metabolic disease e.g. DM
- Respiratory disease e.g. severe asthma, cystic fibrosis
- Heart disease
- Physical feeding problems e.g. cleft palate.

Presentation: Usually detected by the health visitor when performing routine weighing or developmental checks.

Assessment
- Ask how the child is fed – quantities and times of the day. Check the parent is making up formula feeds correctly.
- Ask about problems feeding the child – specifically about regurgitation of food and vomiting.
- Ask about other physical problems e.g. breathlessness, diarrhoea.
- Examine the child carefully from top to toe looking for any physical abnormalities or signs of developmental delay.

- Watch the way the child interacts with you and the parent. Look for evidence of neglect or maltreatment.
- Look to see how large the parents are – 2 small parents will probably have a small child.

Management: Treat any reversible causes. Continue to measure weight, length and head circumference regularly. Try to use the same scales on each occasion.

Refer urgently to paediatrics

- If no cause for failure to thrive is found
- If an abnormality requiring specialist paediatric care is found
- If, despite treatment of a reversible cause, the child continues to lose or fails to gain weight

Advice for parents on weaning

- Introduce solids to your baby's diet at about 6 months of age.
- Your baby is ready when he or she:
  - Can sit up
  - Is always hungry even soon after a feed
  - Mouths objects
  - Is interested in food and chewing.
- Sterilize feeding bowls and cutlery before use until your baby is more than 6 months old.
- It is not essential to use ready-made baby meals – often babies like home prepared purées better and they are cheaper. If making purées don't add salt or sugar.
- Start with one flavour of finely puréed food e.g. baby rice or fruit. Babies take time to learn how to feed from a spoon and it is usual for most of the food to ooze out of his or her mouth at first and for your baby to play with the spoon, spilling the contents. Babies often only take 2–3 teaspoonfuls per meal when they start taking solids.
- Gradually offer a wider variety of different foods one by one. Avoid eggs and gluten if your baby is under 6 months old. Don't give your baby raw eggs, shellfish or nuts.
- Introduce lumpy foods gradually if your baby is over 6 months old and once your child has got used to the finely pureed food. Introduce 'finger foods' your baby can feed him or herself – such as pieces of toast, rusks or biscuits – at the age of 7–9 months.
- Continue giving your baby breast or formula milk. This is your baby's main source of food until he or she is a year old.
- It is usual for your baby's stool to change consistency when weaned.

Further information and support for parents

Weaning Information leaflet available from 🖳 www.dh.gov.uk
Lewis S *practical parenting: weaning and first foods – which foods to introduce and when* (2003) Hamlyn ISBN: 0600605647
Parentline ☎ 0808 800 2222 🖳 www.parentlineplus.org.uk

Further information

DoH Infant feeding recommendation 🖳 www.dh.gov.uk
Drugs in Lactation Advisory Service 🖳 www.ukmicentral.nhs.uk
UNICEF Baby Friendly Initiative 🖳 www.babyfriendly.org.uk

Neonatal jaundice and pyloric stenosis

Neonatal jaundice: In the first few days of life, most babies have ↑ serum bilirubin levels as the liver takes over the excretion of bilirubin from the placenta. Mild jaundice from age 2–6d. is physiological. However, very high levels of unconjugated bilirubin are toxic and can cause encephalopathy (*kernicterus*).

Pathological causes of jaundice in neonates

Galactosaemia: Inborn error of metabolism characterized by ↑ plasma galactose. Clinical manifestations depend on the site of enzyme defect:

- *Galactokinase deficiency:* Autosomal recessive inheritance. *Incidence:* 1:40,000. Presents in childhood with cataracts. Treatment involves a galactose-free diet.
- *Classic galactosaemia:* Autosomal recessive inheritance. *Incidence:* 1:44,000. The child appears normal at birth but becomes anorexic and jaundiced within a few days or weeks of consuming breast milk or lactose-containing formula. Vomiting, poor growth, hepatomegaly and septicaemia are common and can be rapidly fatal. Treatment involves eliminating all sources of galactose in the diet. Long-term complications – poor growth, learning difficulty, infertility, speech and neurological abnormalities – are common.

Neonatal hepatitis: Presents with persistent neonatal jaundice. Always requires specialist investigation and management. Possible causes:
- Congenital infection e.g. hepatitis B
- Galactosaemia
- Cystic fibrosis
- Glycogen storage diseases.

Biliary atresia: The end stage of a sclerosing process in an initially patent biliary tree. Cause is unclear. Presents with jaundice in the neonate. Prognosis has improved with laparotomy and porto-enterostomy which can relieve the problem in ~50–70% of babies. The operation must be carried out within 2mo. of birth to stand any chance of success.

Gilbert syndrome: Inherited metabolic disorder causing unconjugated hyperbilirubinaemia. *Prevalence:* ~1–2%. Onset is shortly after birth, but the condition may go unnoticed for years. Jaundice occurs during intercurrent illness. ↑ bilirubin on fasting can confirm the diagnosis. Liver biopsy is normal. No treatment is required and prognosis is excellent.

Other causes
- Infection – particularly UTI – 📖 p.186
- Hypothyroidism – 📖 p.18
- Haemolysis – 📖 p.112

Pyloric stenosis: Infantile hypertrophic pyloric stenosis usually develops in the first 3–6wk. of life (rare >12wk.). Failure of the pyloric sphincter to relax results in hypertrophy of the adjacent pyloric muscle. Typically affects first-born, male infants. Pyloric stenosis runs in families and is associated with Turner's syndrome, PKU and oesophageal atresia.

Presentation
- *Projectile vomiting:* Milk – no bile. The child is still hungry after vomiting and immediately feeds again. Rarely there is haematemesis.
- *Failure to thrive*
- *Dehydration and constipation* ('rabbit pellet' stools)
- A *pyloric mass* (feels like an olive) is palpable in the right upper abdomen (95%), especially if the child has just vomited.
- After a test feed, there is *visible peristalsis* of the dilated stomach in the epigastrium.

Differential diagnosis
- Posseting/reflux
- Overfeeding
- Gastroenteritis
- Milk allergy
- Other causes of intestinal obstruction
- Infection – especially UTI
- ↑ intracranial pressure
- Uraemia
- Adrenal insufficiency

Management: Admit or refer urgently to paediatric surgery. After rehydration and investigation to confirm diagnosis, treatment is surgical with a Ramstedt's pyloroplasty. There are usually no long-term consequences.

GP Notes: Which babies with jaundice need referral?

Refer to paediatrics if:

Jaundice <24h. after birth: Any jaundice in the first 24h. is assumed to be pathological and needs immediate referral back to hospital to determine cause (usually haemolysis or infection) and for treatment with phototherapy or, in rare, severe cases, exchange transfusion.

Significant jaundice within 1wk. of birth: This may be difficult to assess, particularly in a dark-skinned baby. The opinion of midwives who are dealing with neonates daily can be very valuable. If necessary, arrange bilirubin estimation either by asking the community midwife to take a heel prick sample or by contacting the neonatal on-call doctor. High levels require further investigation and phototherapy. The level at which phototherapy is necessary varies with maturity, age and may differ slightly between paediatric units. Discuss ↑ levels with the neonatal registrar if worried.

Jaundice persisting >10d.: Although physiological jaundice may persist for some time, particularly in breast-fed babies, it is important to rule out pathological causes:
- Hypothyroidism
- Mild haemolysis
- Infection
- Liver disease – results in high levels of conjugated bilirubin
- Galactosaemia.

Early diagnosis is particularly important in congenital biliary atresia so that surgery can be carried out before the liver is irreversibly damaged.

Congenital infections and infections transmitted during birth

Congenital infections are acquired by the fetus from the mother *in utero*. They often have profound consequences on intrauterine and subsequent development. Serious infections may also be passed from mother to baby during passage through the birth canal. TORCH (Figure 3.1) is an acronym used to describe the more common infections.

Toxoplasmosis

- Caused by a parasite found in raw meat and cat faeces.
- 70% of women have not had toxoplasmosis before pregnancy and ~ 2/1000 will catch it during pregnancy. 30–40% of infected women pass it to their fetus. Prevention – see advice for pregnant women (opposite).
- Risk of transmission to the fetus is related to gestation at the time of infection – 3rd trimester ≈ 70%, 1st trimester ≈ 15%.
- Infection may result in miscarriage, stillbirth, growth problems, blindness, hydrocephalus, brain damage, epilepsy and/or deafness.
- If infection is suspected refer for specialist advice.

Listeriosis: Rare.

- Infection of the mother is usually via infected food e.g. pâté, soft cheese, milk.
- Maternal symptoms: fever, shivering, myalgia, headache, sore throat, cough, vomiting, diarrhoea, vaginitis.
- Consequences: abortion (may be recurrent), stillbirth, premature labour, transmission to the fetus (in 2nd/3rd trimester).
- Infection in the newborn infant manifests in pneumonia ± meningitis.
- Detection is with blood cultures. Suspect if unexplained fever >48h. and refer for expert advice.
- Prevention – see advice for pregnant women opposite.

Parvovirus

- Risk of infection in pregnancy ≈ 1/400; risk for a non-immune mother with a child who has Fifth disease (slapped cheek) ≈ 50–90%.
- Maternal infection <20wk. gestation results in a 4% ↑ in miscarriage. Infection between 9–20wk. may also cause anaemia of the fetus (3% of those infected). Hydrops fetalis develops 2–17wk. afterwards.
- If known contact check immune status.
- If parvovirus infection is suspected (especially if known contact) refer for fetal monitoring. Early transfusion improves survival of the baby.
- There are no long-term effects from an infection which doesn't cause miscarriage or hydrops.

Syphilis: ~70–100% of pregnant mothers with primary syphilis transmit the disease to the fetus (1:3 die *in utero*). In the early latent phase, risk of transmission is ~40% and ~10-15% in the late latent phase. Neurological abnormalities as a result of congenital syphilis include encephalopathy and sensorineural deafness. Expert advice is needed. Treatment is with benzylpenicillin given to the mother and neonate.

Figure 3.1 'TORCH' congenital infections

T	Toxoplasmosis
O	Other • Listeria • Chickenpox • Parvovirus • HIV • Syphilis
R	Rubella
C	CMV
H	Hepatitis Herpes

Advice for patients: Preventing infections

Advice for pregnant women on prevention of toxoplasmosis and listeriosis

- Only eat well-cooked meat.
- Wash hands, cooking utensils and food surfaces after preparing raw meat.
- Keep raw meat and cooked foods on separate plates.
- Wash all soil from fruit and vegetables before eating.
- If possible, get someone else to clean cat litter or use gloves and wash hands afterwards.
- Use gloves when gardening and wash hands afterwards.

Information for parents on preventing hepatitis B

Department of Health Hepatitis B: how to protect your baby. Available from 🖥 www.dh.gov.uk

Further information

RCOG 🖥 www.rcog.org.uk
- Chicken pox in pregnancy (2001)
- Management of genital herpes in pregnancy (2002)
- Prevention of early-onset neonatal group B streptococcal disease (2001)

Chickenpox[G]: Contact with chickenpox in pregnancy is common. If the mother has definitely had chickenpox there is no risk to herself or the baby. If she doesn't recall having chickenpox:

- Check her immunity with a blood test – 80% have antibodies from silent infection. In cases of 'at risk' exposure arrange for varicella-zoster immunoglobulin (VZ-Ig) to be given to mother and/or baby. It must be given ≤10d. after exposure.
- If mother develops chickenpox, treat with aciclovir if she presents <24h. after the rash appears and the mother is >20wk. gestation.

Risks to the baby

- *<20wk. Gestation:* Risk of chickenpox syndrome (eye defects, hypoplasia, microcephaly) is 1–2%. If a woman has VZ-Ig treatment after being exposed, risk is even lower.
- *Mother's rash develops <1wk. prior to delivery – 1mo. after delivery:* Risk of overwhelming infection. Baby may need VZ-Ig treatment.

HIV: Up to 50% of infants of HIV seropositive mothers are pre- or peri-natally infected with HIV, accounting for 90% of HIV infections in childhood. Risk can be ↓ to <5% by giving zidovudine to the mother antenatally, during delivery and to the neonate for the 1ˢᵗ 6wk., together with elective LSCS and advice against breast-feeding.

Fetal abnormalities include: wide-set eyes, short nose, patulous lips, 'box' forehead and growth failure. However, diagnosis is usually made between 6mo. and 2y. of age. when the child presents with lymphade-nopathy, recurrent or opportunistic infections, failure to thrive or progressive encephalopathy. Expert advice is needed throughout pregnancy and for neonatal follow-up.

Rubella

- Asymptomatic reinfection of women who have received vaccination can occur so serology is essential in all pregnant rubella contacts.
- 50% of mothers who are infected with rubella are asymptomatic.
- Transmission rates depend on gestation of the fetus at the time of infection: 50–60% are affected if infection occurs in the 1ˢᵗ month; <5% at 16wk. Risk of transmission is much lower with reinfection (<5%).
- Abnormalities that can occur include: cataract, deafness, cerebral palsy, mental retardation, microcephaly, microphthalmia.
- If infection is suspected get expert advice.

Cytomegalovirus (CMV): More frequent cause of birth defect than rubella in the UK – 5/1000 live births – 10% develop handicap. The fetus is most vulnerable when infection occurs in early pregnancy. Maternal disease may be asymptomatic or a mild flu-like illness. No effective prevention strategy and usually not detected until a child with multiple abnormalities is born.

Hepatitis C: Prevalence 0.1–6%. Except when initial infection of the mother occurs during pregnancy (when transfer rate is much higher), transmission rate to the fetus is 5%. To date there is no evidence HCV can be transferred to the child by breast-feeding. Infants at risk can be screened for HCV infection at 12mo. (RNA screen) or 18–24mo. (HCV antibody test). The majority of infants who acquire HCV infection via their mothers develop chronic hepatitis. Treatment is with interferon and achieves viral clearance rates of ~40%.

Hepatitis B: Women are routinely offered screening for hepatitis B infection in pregnancy. Transmission to the baby occurs during labour (10–20 % of infants of women seropositive for HBsAg and 90% of infants of women seropositive for both HBsAg and HBeAg). Infants infected are at high risk (~90%) of becoming chronic carriers and of developing chronic liver disease ± premature death.

Postnatally: Refer infected women for hepatology assessment. Infected mothers should not donate their milk.

Immunization: Give hepatitis B vaccine as soon as possible after birth to babies born to carrier mothers with the addition of immunoglobulin (HBIG) if the mother carries the hepatitis B e-antigen or had acute HBV infection during pregnancy. 85–95% effective in preventing neonatal hepatitis B infection. Further doses of vaccine are required at 1 and 2mo. of age, and a booster dose at 1y. at the same time as follow-up testing.

Herpes simplex infection: Neonatal herpes is usually the result of infection acquired from the birth canal when the mother has active genital herpes. Neonatal infection is uncommon. It may be localized to the skin, mouth or eyes. Disseminated disease may occur with CNS involvement. Mortality is then ~60–70%, with high degrees of morbidity amongst survivors. Consider in any ill baby <1mo. old, regardless of maternal history – genital herpes may be silent in the mother.

Group B streptococcus^G (GBS): Bacterium carried by 15–20% of pregnant women in the vagina, usually causing no problems. Rarely transmission to the baby during delivery results in septicaemia. Prophylactic treatment is advised in 'high risk' scenarios: early labour (<37wk.); prolonged or early rupture of the membranes; if the woman has a temperature during labour or if a previous baby has been affected with the condition. Treatment involves IV antibiotics during labour.

Sexually transmitted infection: Both chlamydia (5% pregnancies) and gonorrhoea (<1/1000 pregnancies) can pass to the baby during delivery, causing eye infections (📖 p.270). Chlamydia can also cause neonatal chest infections. Both are treatable with antibiotics – follow-up with swabs to confirm eradication.

Others

- *Malaria:* Serious complications of malaria are more common if a woman is infected whilst pregnant. Malaria can also result in IUGR.
- *Urinary tract infections:* 1:25 women develop UTI in pregnancy. Both untreated bacteriuria and frank UTI are associated with preterm delivery and IUGR.
- *Bacterial vaginosis:* Associated with ↑ risk of preterm delivery. Risk returns to normal if the mother is treated.

Genetic problems

There are 46 chromosomes – 22 matching pairs with matching genes (autosomes) and one pair of sex chromosomes which may match (XX–♀) or differ (XY–♂). Genetic abnormalities are the most common cause of developmental delay. There are a huge number of genetic syndromes, many of them extremely rare. Categorize by the nature of the defect.

Chromosome number

- *Alteration in number of chromosomes:* Example: Down's syndrome (extra chromosome number 21).
- *Sex chromosome abnormalities:* A sex chromosome is duplicated or deleted. Examples : Turner's syndrome (XO).

Gross structural changes in chromosomes:

- *Translocation:* A portion of one chromosome is transposed or translocated onto another. If no genetic information is lost there is no clinical effect (balanced translocation), though offspring of affected individuals often have problems. 6% Down's syndrome is due to translocation.
- *Deletion*: Loss of a portion of chromosome. *Example:* Cri du chat syndrome (deletion of the short arm of chromosome 5).

Single gene abnormalities

- *Autosomal dominant:* >1000 diseases are known to be inherited in this way. Individually they are rare and together account for <1% of all disease. Heterozygotes demonstrate the disease. 1:2 pregnancies of an affected individual will be affected – usually ♂=♀. Expression of the gene in a given individual may vary. *Examples:* neurofibromatosis, myotonic dystrophy.
- *Autosomal recessive:* >700 known diseases. Only manifest in the homozygote. Heterozygotes may be asymptomatic or show milder abnormalities. To develop severe disease, the affected gene must be inherited from both parents who must both be heterozygotes. The risk of an affected pregnancy is 1:4 – usually ♂=♀. Affected individuals have unaffected children unless their partner is a heterozygote. *Example:* phenylketonuria, CF.
- *Sex-linked disorders:* ~100 are recognized. Most are recessively inherited from the mother and affect only ♂ offspring. A ♂ child of a heterozygote mother has a 1:2 chance of developing the disease. A ♀ child of a heterozygote mother has a 1:2 chance of carrying the disease. A ♀ child can only be affected by the disease if the father has the disease and mother is a carrier, when she has a 1:2 chance of being affected and, if not affected, will be a carrier. *Examples:* fragile X syndrome, Duchenne's muscular dystrophy.

Polygenic inheritance: Familial trends of disease are often seen but there is no simple inheritance pattern. Usually due to the combination of genes inherited (polygenic inheritance). *Example:* neural tube defect.

Management: Depends on specific problems of each child. A multi-disciplinary approach is essential. Support the child and family. Ensure receipt of all available benefits. Tell carers about local facilities, voluntary and self-help organizations. Review regularly.

Table 3.3 Structural chromosome problems seen in general practice

Genetic problem	Features
Down's syndrome Trisomy 21 (92%) Translocation (6%) Mosaicism (2%) *Affects 1:600 births*	Facial abnormalities: flat occiput, oval face (mongoloid facies); low-set eyes with prominent epicanthic folds Other abnormalities: single palmar crease; hypotonia; congenital heart disease Developmental delay Life expectancy is ↓ but ~½ live to 60y
Edward's syndrome Trisomy 18 *Affects 1:6000 births* ♀:♂≈2:1	Facial abnormalities: low-set malformed ears, receding chin, protruding eyes, cleft lip or palate Other abnormalities: short sternum makes the nipples appear too widely separated; fingers cannot be extended and the index finger overlaps the 3rd digit; umbilical/inguinal hernias; rocker-bottom feet; rigid baby with flexion of limbs Developmental delay Life expectancy is ~1mo
Patau's syndrome Trisomy 13 *Affects 1:7500 births*	Facial abnormalities: small head and eyes; cleft lip and palate Other abnormalities: skeletal abnormalities e.g. flexion contractures of hands ± polydactyly with narrow fingernails; brain malformation; heart malformation; polycystic kidneys. 50% die in <1mo. Usually fatal in the first year
Cri du chat syndrome Deletion of short arm of chromosome 5 *Affects 1:50, 000 births*	Facial abnormalities: microcephaly; marked epicanthic folds; moon-shaped face; alert expression Other abnormalities: abnormal cry (cat-like) Developmental delay Usually fatal in the first year
Turner's syndrome XO – deletion of 1 X chromosome. Mosaicism may occur (XO, XX) *Affects 1:2500 births*	Female appearance Facial abnormalities: ptosis; nystagmus; webbed neck Other abnormalities: short stature (<130cm); hyperconvex nails; wide carrying angle (cubitus valgus); inverted nipples; broad chest; coarctation of the aorta, left heart defects; lymphoedema of the legs; ovaries rudimentary or absent Lifespan is normal
Klinefelter's syndrome XXY or XXYY polysomy *Affects 1:1000 live births*	Male appearance Often undetected until presentation with infertility in adult life Clinical features: may present in adolescence with psychopathy; ↓ libido, sparse facial hair, gynaecomastia, small firm testes Associations: hypothyroidism; DM; asthma Specialist management: androgens and plastic surgery may be useful for gynaecomastia

Glycogen storage diseases: Incidence ~1:25,000. A group of hereditary disorders caused by lack of ≥1 enzyme involved in glycogen synthesis or breakdown and characterized by deposition of abnormal amounts or types of glycogen in tissues. Inheritance is autosomal recessive for all forms except type VI, which follows an X-linked inheritance. Symptoms and age of onset vary considerably:

- Predominantly liver involvement (types I, III, IV, VI) → hepatomegaly, hypoglycaemia, metabolic acidosis
- Predominantly muscle involvement (types V, VII) → weakness, lethargy, poor feeding, heart failure.

Treatment: Involves frequent small carbohydrate meals; allopurinol (to prevent renal urate stone formation and/or gout) ± limiting anaerobic exercise. A high-protein diet is also helpful for some patients.

Tuberous sclerosis: Autosomal dominant inheritance but $^2/_3$ arise from new mutations. The abnormalitiy is localized on chromosome 9. Incidence 5–7/100, 000. Characterized by hamartomatous lesions in the skin, nervous system and internal organs. Usual presentation is with:

- Adenoma sebaceum (angiofibromas of the skin – seen as red – brown papules on the face – appear aged 5–10y.)
- Epilepsy and developmental delay.

Other features: Coarsened skin over the sacrum (shagreen patch); nail fold fibromas; hypopigmented oval patches (ash leaf spots); cardiac, renal, lung and eye abnormalities.

Friedreich's ataxia: The most common inherited ataxia (autosomal recessive). Prevalence 1:50,000. Presents in adolescence with progressive gait and limb ataxia, loss of proprioception, pyramidal weakness and dysarthria. Extra-neurological involvement includes hypertrophic cardiomyopathy (most patients) and DM (10%). Treatment is supportive. Most patients become chairbound within 15y. and die in the 4th or 5th decade from cardiac or pulmonary complications.

Sturge-Weber syndrome: Congenital syndrome inherited as an autosomal dominant trait, though most new cases are sporadic mutations. Characterized by:

- Unilateral capillary naevus (port wine stain) – usually over the forehead and eyelid
- Epilepsy (90%)
- Developmental delay (50%)
- Hemiparesis and/or homonymous hemianopia (30%)
- Glaucoma in the affected eye.

Fragile X syndrome: Affects 1:1250 ♂ births and 1:2500 ♀ births. Genetic abnormality carried on the X-chromosome comprising:

- Low IQ (20–70)
- Large testes
- High forehead
- Large jaw
- Facial asymmetry
- Long ears
- Short temper

½ of carrier females have a normal IQ, ½ are affected. Consider fragile X syndrome in any child with developmental delay of unknown cause.

Management: There is some evidence that folic acid supplements ↓ hyperactive and disruptive behaviour tendencies in children with fragile X. Antenatal testing is possible for future pregnancies.

Other genetic conditions covered elsewhere:

- Phenylketonuria (PKU): 📖 p.16
- Duchenne's muscular dystrophy: 📖 p.236
- Neurofibromatosis: 📖 p.236
- Ataxia telangectasia: 📖 p.107
- Sickle cell disease and thalassaemia: 📖 p.114
- Haemophilia: 📖 p.118
- Cystic fibrosis: 📖 p.162
- Marfan syndrome: 📖 p.126

GP Notes: General principles of primary care management

- Support the child and family. Ensure receipt of all available benefits.
- Find out about the condition the child is suffering from.
- Liaise with the primary health care team and community and specialist services to ensure prompt provision of equipment and services.
- Tell carers about local facilities, voluntary and self-help organizations.
- Make referrals for new problems promptly.
- Liaise with specialist services to provide ongoing care.
- Refer parents of any child affected by a genetic problem for genetic counselling and offer prenatal diagnosis, if available, for any subsequent pregnancies.

ℹ There are associations between:
- Down's syndrome and leukaemia
- Neurofibromatosis and CNS tumours
- Other rare syndromes and some cancers.

⚠ Be alert to the potential significance of unexplained symptoms in children with such syndromes[N].

Advice for patients: Information and support

Parent experiences of caring for a disabled child: 📖 p.327

Advice and support for parents

Contact a Family ☎ 0808 808 3555/6 🖥 www.cafamily.org.uk
Genetics Interests Group ☎ 020 7704 3141 🖥 www.gig.org.uk
Unique Rare Chromosome Disorder Support Group
☎ 01883 330766 🖥 www.rarechromo.org
Down's Syndrome Association ☎ 0845 230 0372
🖥 www.downs-syndrome.org.uk
Turner's Syndrome Support Society ☎ 0845 230 7520
🖥 www.tss.org.uk
Association for Glycogen Storage Disease (UK) 🖥 www.agsd.org.uk
The Tuberous Sclerosis Association ☎ 0121 4456970
🖥 www.tuberous-sclerosis.org
Sturge-Weber Foundation UK ☎ 01392 464675
🖥 www.sturgeweber.org.uk
Fragile X Society ☎ 01371 875100 🖥 www.fragilex.org.uk
Ataxia UK ☎ 0845 644 0606 🖥 www.ataxia.org.uk

Sudden infant death syndrome

~1:1500 babies/y. are found unexpectedly dead in the 1st year of life in the UK. These deaths are most common in winter months and at night (midnight–9a.m.). An identifiable cause for the death can be found for 1:10 deaths – the rest remain unexplained ('*cot death*'). Theories include cardiac arrhythmia and apnoeic attacks. *Peak age:* 1–4mo., ♂>♀.

Risk factors for cot death

- Baby sleeping face down
- Smoking (mother and other family members)
- Overheating
- Minor intercurrent illness
- Twin or multiple pregnancy
- Low birth weight
- Social disadvantage
- Young mother
- Large numbers of siblings

Reducing the risk of cot death: 📖 p.11

Management

If you are the first person contacted

- Check an ambulance is on its way and go immediately to the scene. If in doubt, start resuscitation. Continue until the baby gets to hospital.
- If it is clear the baby is dead and can't be resuscitated, inform the parents sympathetically. Contact the police/coroner. Arrange for the baby to be taken to A&E, not to a mortuary. Contact the paediatrician designated for cot deaths who may wish to see the baby and parents as soon as they get to A&E.
- Take a brief history and record the circumstances of death immediately (e.g. position when found, bedding, vomit etc.). Your notes might be helpful later. Spend time listening to the parents. Mention the baby by name and don't be afraid to express your sorrow.
- If the baby is a twin, the surviving twin is at ↑ risk of cot death and should be admitted to hospital for observation.

If you learn later that a baby has died: Consider:

- A prompt visit to express sympathy and stress that no one is to blame. There may be some anger directed towards you as often babies have been seen in general practice within a few days or weeks of the death. Do not be defensive or become angry.
- Explain about formalities – necessary post-mortems and coroner's inquests, arranging a funeral, registering the death etc.
- Discuss suppression of lactation if breast-feeding offer carbegoline 250mcgm bd for 2d.
- Encourage taking photographs of the baby and other mementoes i.e. lock of hair, hand and foot prints.

🕛 Babies who die at <28d. of age require a special death certificate.

Follow-up

- Cancel outstanding appointments for the baby (e.g. developmental screening, immunizations) and inform other involved health/social care professionals.
- Review within a few days. Advise parents about likely grief reactions – guilt, anger, ↓ appetite, sleeplessness, hearing the baby cry. Don't forget siblings – they can be deeply affected too. Continue

regular review as long as it is needed and wanted. Be sensitive to anniversaries. Watch for serious psychiatric illness.

- Ensure parents have received written information about cot death including details of self-help organizations and helplines. Consider referral for counseling – ideal timing for referral varies.
- Ensure you get a copy of the post-mortem findings and try to attend the case discussion which should be held ~1mo. after death.
- Parents should have an opportunity to speak to a consultant paediatrician about the death.
- Refer for specialist obstetric assessment early in the next pregnancy and make sure parents are put in touch with the Care of Next Infant (CONI) scheme. Discuss the use of apnoea alarms.

Apnoea alarms: Commonly issued to or purchased by parents if they are worried about the risk of cot death. An apnoea alarm cannot be useful unless parents are taught basic life support to a proficient standard. An alarm should not be supplied without this training. There is no evidence that apnoea alarms prevent cot deaths.

Near-miss cot deaths: Parents may rush a child to A&E or the GP after an episode of pallor ± floppiness. Parents may have attempted mouth-to-mouth resuscitation before the baby starts to respond to them or may have simply touched the baby or lifted him up and received a response. Usually there are no residual symptoms or signs.

Management: Difficult. Parents may have misinterpreted normal irregularities in sleep or the child might be unwell and have a physical cause for symptoms e.g. early stages of a viral infection. Usually parents are very anxious by the time you see the child. Take a careful history and examine the child from top to toe. Treat any cause of symptoms found. Be as reassuring as possible and play down anxieties.

> △ If the child has any risk factors for cot death, comes from a diffi-cult social background or parents are unable to cope following the episode, admit the child for observation and further assessment.

Further information and parent support

Foundation for the Study of Infant Deaths (FSID) Guidelines for general practitioners when a baby dies suddenly and unexpectedly (2003); Information, support and administration of the CONI scheme ⊟ www.sids.org.uk

Child Bereavement Trust ☎ 0845 357 1000
⊟ www.childbereavement.org.uk

Child Death Helpline ☎ 0800 282 986
⊟ www.childdeathhelpline.org.uk

Chapter 4

Childhood infection, haematology and immunology

Immunization

Immunity can be induced in 2 ways

- *Active immunity:* Induced using inactivated or attenuated live organisms or their products. Acts by inducing cell-mediated immunity and serum antibodies. Generally long-lasting.
- *Passive immunity:* Results from injection of human immunoglobulin. The protection afforded is immediate but lasts only a few weeks.

Childhood immunization: Table 4.1

Contraindications: Box 4.1. For specific contraindications to individual vaccinations see manufacturer's leaflet or the Green book.

Table 4.1 UK schedule of childhood immunization

Disease (vaccine)	Age	Comment
Tuberculosis (BCG)	High risk neonates	1 injection
Diphtheria/Tetanus/Pertussis/ Haemophilus influenzae type b/ Inactivated Polio (DTaP/IPV/Hib)	2, 3 and 4mo.	Primary course (3 doses, a month between each dose)
Pneumococcal vaccine	2, 4 and 13mo.	Primary course
Meningococcus type C (men C)	3, 4 and 12mo.	Primary course
Haemophilus influenzae type b (Hib)	12mo.	Booster dose
Measles/Mumps/Rubella (MMR)	13mo.	1st dose, 1 injection
Diphtheria/Tetanus/Acellular pertussis/inactivated Polio (DTP/IPV)	3y. 4mo.–5y. (3y. after completion of the 1st course)	Booster dose 1 injection
Measles/Mumps/Rubella (MMR)	3y. 4mo.–5y.	2nd dose, 1 injection
Tetanus/low dose diphtheria (Td/IPV)/inactivated Polio	13–18y.	Booster dose 1 injection

Advice for patients: Information for parents

Immunization NHS website for patients 🖥 www.immunisation.org.uk

Box 4.1 Which children should not be immunized?

Acute illness: Delay until fully recovered. Minor ailments without fever or systemic upset are not reasons to postpone immunization.

Severe local reaction to a previous dose: Extensive area of redness and swelling which becomes indurated and involves much of the antero-lateral surface of the thigh or a major part of the circumference of the upper arm.

Severe generalized reaction to a previous dose
● Fever ≥39.5°C <48h. after vaccination
● Anaphylaxis, bronchospasm, laryngeal oedema and/or generalized collapse
● Prolonged unresponsiveness
● Prolonged high-pitched or inconsolable screaming for >4h.
● Convulsions or encephalopathy <72h. after vaccination

Live vaccines: Don't give live vaccines to:
● *Immunocompromised patients:* Patients on high-dose steroids for >1wk. (e.g. >1mg/kg/d. prednisolone), with haematological malignancy, who have had radiotherapy or chemotherapy in the last 6mo. or who have another immunodeficiency syndrome
● *<3wk. after another live vaccine,* but 2 live vaccines may be given together at different sites
● *With immunoglobulin:* From 3wk. before – 3mo. after.

❶ Patients with HIV infection may receive live vaccines except BCG and yellow fever. Do not give MMR whilst severely immunosuppressed.

GP Notes: Giving immunizations

Only GPs and nursing staff suitably trained should give immunizations.
● Check immunization is necessary and the child is fit and well.
● Check consent has been given (written consent is usually obtained for childhood vaccinations but this only consents for the child to be included in the vaccination programme – check verbally that parents are aware of the nature of the vaccination and agree to its administration).
● Check immunizations are the correct ones and in date.
● Ensure resuscitation facilities are available.
● Reconstitute the vaccine (if necessary) and give according to manufacturer's instructions.
● Record vaccine expiry date and batch number, date of vaccination and site in the child's medical notes.

Further information
DoH The Green Book: immunization against infectious disease 🖳 www.dh.gov.uk
Health Protection Agency (HPA) Information on vaccines and vaccination schedules 🖳 www.hpa.org.uk

Vaccinating children as additional and directed enhanced services

Childhood vaccination as an additional service: 2 additional service payments are available for vaccinating patients registered as either permanent residents or temporary residents within the practice area:

- *Childhood vaccinations and immunizations:* Includes all necessary childhood vaccinations and immunizations – Table 4.1 📖 p.84
- *Vaccinations and immunizations:* Includes all necessary vaccinations and immunizations (except the influenza and pneumococcal immunization directed enhanced services, childhood vaccinations and immunizations and certain travel vaccines that can be charged for privately) provided by the NHS.

In all cases the practice must

- Provide enough information to enable informed choice about whether to have a vaccination.
- Record in the patient's notes any refusal to routine vaccination.
- Record in the patient's notes any contraindications to administration.
- Where the offer of vaccination is accepted, record the patient's consent to the vaccination or the name of the person who gave consent and relationship to the patient.
- Where the offer of vaccination is accepted, administer the vaccination and record the date of administration in the patient's notes together with the title (including manufacturer), batch number and expiry date.
- Where 2 vaccines are administered in close succession, record route of administration and injection site of each vaccine in the patient notes.
- Record in the patient's notes any adverse reactions to the vaccination.
- Ensure all staff involved in administering vaccines are trained in the recognition and initial treatment of anaphylaxis.

Opting out of giving vaccinations

- Routine childhood vaccinations – 1% ↓ in global sum
- Other vaccinations – 2% ↓ in global sum

Childhood vaccination as a directed enhanced service

Requires practices to:

- Develop and maintain a register of registered children aged ≤5y.
- Provide information to parents about the vaccination programme and record that advice has been given in the child's GP notes
- Record any refusal of vaccination in the child's notes
- Perform the immunizations and that they have been given in the child's notes
- Provide all necessary training for staff in order for them to advise on and administer the vaccinations
- Have resuscitation equipment on site in case of anaphylactic shock
- Audit the process, including monitoring of immunization rates in the under-2s, booster rates for the under-5s, and changes in these rates within the year together with possible reasons for those changes.

Payment: Practices must report all immunizations given to their local PCO. Arrangements for doing this vary according to locality.

There are 2 payments available for childhood immunization: one for children aged 2y. and another for children aged 5y. These are paid when children complete their vaccinations.

For children aged 2 this includes:
- Group 1 – Pentavalent vaccine (diphtheria, tetanus, poliomyelitis, pertussis and Hib) (50% of target payment)
- Group 2 – MMR (25% of target payment)
- Group 3 – Meningitis C (25% of target payment)

For children aged 5 this includes: A single booster dose of diphtheria, tetanus, polio and pertussis.

Within each of these 2 payments, there are 2 levels of payment which depend on the % of eligible children who complete their vaccinations. The lower payment is achieved when ≥70% of eligible children have been vaccinated; the higher figure when this proportion is ≥90%.

Payments, adjusted further for the proportion of vaccinations carried out in NHS general practice or elsewhere (such as in private clinics), are made quarterly if, on the first day of the quarter, the proportion of vaccinated eligible patients on the practice list is 70% or more.

ⓘ Exception reporting/informed dissent does not apply.

Influenza and pneumococcal immunizations for at-risk groups as a directed enhanced service: This directed enhanced service aims to provide influenza and pneumococcal vaccination for the elderly and other 'at-risk' groups including children requiring influenza vaccination and 'at-risk' children who have not received pneumococcal vaccine as part of the routine childhood vaccination programme. Practices DO NOT have preferred provider status for this service.

Target group for influenza vaccination: 📖 p.155

Target group for pneumococcal vaccination: 📖 p.97

Qualifications to provide the service
- Practices are expected to use a call–recall system identifying those 'at risk' through existing registers compiled for use within the Quality and Outcomes Framework.
- Practices not participating in the Quality and Outcomes Framework must compile a register to qualify to provide this enhanced service.

Targets
- No target has been set for the proportion of 'at-risk' patients given influenza or pneumococcal vaccination.
- Additional payments are available through the Quality and Outcomes Framework for vaccinating high proportions of 'at-risk' patients against influenza – but most of these targets do not currently apply to children <16y.

Fever and childhood infection

Pyrexia: ↑ temperature – oral >37.5°C; rectal >38°C; axillary >37.3°C; ear >38°C. NICE suggests a traffic light system for assessment – Table 4.2

Table 4.2 Traffic light system for assessment of children with fever		
Red	**Amber**	**Green**
Immediate assessment if life threatening features – in all cases see in <2h.	*See the child the same day. Urgency depends on symptoms/signs reported*	*Give advice on management at home and when to seek further help*
Symptoms/Signs:		
• appears ill • ↓ consciousness/ unresponsiveness • colour – mottled/ ashen/blue • weak, high-pitched or continuous cry • respiratory rate >60 • moderate/severe chest indrawing • ↓ skin turgor • non-blanching rash • bulging fontanelle • neck stiffness • status epilepticus • focal neurological signs/ seizures • bile stained vomiting • high temperature (0–3mo. >38°C; >3mo. >39°C)	• pallor • ↓ response to social cues/excessive drowsiness • ↓ activity/no smile • nasal flaring • ↑ respiratory rate (>50 – aged <6mo.; >40 aged >6mo.) • oxygen saturation ≤95% in air • dry mucous membranes • poor feeding in infants • capillary return ≥3 seconds • ↓ urine output • fever for ≥5d. • swelling of a limb/joint • non-weight bearing/ not using an extremity • new lump >2cm	• normal colour of skin/lips/tongue • responds normally • not excessively drowsy • normal cry/smiles/ content • moist mucus membranes • none of the amber/ red symptoms or signs

Common causes of pyrexia: Childhood infections are the most common cause of fever amongst children in general practice – Table 4.3.

🌓 Don't forget tropical diseases e.g. malaria in children returning from abroad. Think of TB and endocarditis – especially in high risk patients.

Other causes of pyrexia: May present as prolonged fever
• *Cancer:* lymphoma; leukaemia
• *Immunological:* connective tissue and autoimmune disease (e.g. Still's disease); sarcoidosis; Kawasaki disease
• *Drugs* e.g. antibiotics
• *Liver or renal disease*

Febrile convulsions: 📖 p.224

Table 4.3 **A–Z of childhood infection**			
Infection	**Page**	**Infection**	**Page**
Bronchiolitis	📖 p.156	Measles[ND]	📖 p.90
Chicken pox	📖 p.92	Meningitis (all types)[ND]	📖 p.48
Conjunctivitis*	📖 p.270	Meningococcal septicaemia[ND]	📖 p.48
Croup	📖 p.276	Molluscum contagiosum	📖 p.256
Diptheria[ND]	📖 p.99	Mumps	📖 p.90
Encephalitis[ND]	📖 p.48	Otitis media	📖 p.284
Endocarditis	📖 p.134	Pneumonia	📖 p.158
Epiglottitis	📖 p.276	Polio[ND]	📖 p.94
Erythema infectiosum	📖 p.90	Roseola infantum	📖 p.90
Gastroenteritis**	📖 p.176	Rubella[ND]	📖 p.90
Glandular fever	📖 p.277	Scabies	📖 p.260
Hand, foot & mouth	📖 p.90	Scarlet fever[ND]	📖 p.96
Head lice	📖 p.260	Sinusitis	📖 p.278
Hepatitis A[ND]	📖 p.100	Skin infection	📖 p.254
Hepatitis B[ND]	📖 p.75	TB[ND]	📖 p.160
Herpes	📖 p.92	Tonsillitis	📖 p.274
HIV	📖 p.94	URTI	📖 p.154
Impetigo	📖 p.254	UTI in childhood	📖 p.186
Influenza	📖 p.154	Viral warts	📖 p.256
Kawasaki's disease	📖 p.102	Whooping cough[ND]	📖 p.156
Malaria[ND]	📖 p.100		
* Ophthalmia neonatorum is a notifiable disease			
** Suspected food poisoning is a notifiable disease			

Pyrexia of unknown origin: Fever (either intermittent or continuous) which has lasted for >2wk. and for which no cause has been found.
- Re-check history and re-examine carefully.
- Check: FBC, EBV screen, ESR, LFTs, urine (M,C&S), viral titres, blood cultures and CXR. Depending on the age and clinical state of the child, it may be best to refer/admit to hospital for investigations.
- If cause does not become rapidly obvious refer urgently to paediatrics for further investigation.

Notifiable diseases ([ND]): Notification of certain diseases is required under the Public Health (Control of Disease) Act 1984 and Public Health (Infectious disease) Regulations 1988. Notification is made to the local authority's Medical Officer for environmental health (who also provides forms for notification purposes). A fee is payable.

Further information:

NICE Feverish illness in children (2007) 🖥 www.nice.org.uk
Health Protection Agency (HPA) Information on notification of infectious diseases 🖥 www.hpa.org.uk

Viral infections

Table 4.4 Common childhood viral infections		
Condition	**Duration**	**Main symptoms**
Measles[ND]	10d. Figure 4.1(a)	*Incubation:* 10–14d. *Early symptoms:* fever, conjunctivitis, cough, coryza, LNs *Later symptoms:* Koplik's spots (tiny white spots on bright red background found on buccal mucosa of cheeks), rash (florid maculopapular appears after 4d. – becomes confluent) *Complications:* bronchopneumonia, otitis media, stomatitis, corneal ulcers, gastroenteritis, appendicitis, encephalitis (1:1000 affected children), subacute sclerosing panencephalitis (rare)
Rubella[ND] (German measles)	10d. Figure 4.1(b)	*Incubation:* 14–21d. *Symptoms:* mild and may pass unrecognised. Fever, LNs (including suboccipital nodes), pink maculopapular rash which lasts 3d. *Complications:* birth defects if infected in pregnancy; arthritis (adolescents); thrombocytopoenia (rare); encephalitis (rare)
Mumps[ND]	10d. Figure 4.1(c)	*Incubation:* 16–21d. *Symptoms:* subclinical infection is common. Fever, malaise, tender enlargement of 1 or both parotids ± submandibular glands *Complications:* aseptic meningitis; epididymo-orchitis; pancreatitis
Roseola infantum	4–d.	Child <2y. *Symptoms:* high fever, sore throat and lymphadenopathy, macular rash appears after 3–4d. when fever ↓
Erythema infectiosum (5th disease or slapped cheek) *Parvovirus*	4–7d. Figure 4.1(d)	*Symptoms:* erythematous maculopapular rash starting on the face ('slapped cheeks'), reticular, 'lacy' rash on trunk and limbs, mild fever, arthralgia (rare) Contact with parvovirus in pregnancy
Hand, foot and mouth disease *Coxsackie virus*	5-7d. Figure 4.1(e)	*Symptoms:* oral blisters/ulcers, red-edged vesicles on hands and feet, mild fever

Management: For all the infections listed in Table 4.4, management is supportive with paracetamol, fluids ± antibiotics for 2° infection. Teething gels e.g. Calgel may sooth mouth lesions in hand, foot and mouth disease.

Box 4.2 Prevention of measles, mumps and rubella

- Measles, mumps and rubella (MMR) vaccination consists of live attenuated measles, mumps and rubella viruses.
- Vaccine viruses are not transmitted so there is no risk of infection from people who have just been immunized.
- Routinely administered to all children after their 1ˢᵗ birthday and again pre-school. Re-immunization is needed if given to children of <1y.
- Children with chronic illness e.g. CF are at particular risk from measles and should be immunized.
- Malaise, fever and rash are common ~1wk. after immunizations and usually last 2–3d. Advise on fever prevention.

♦ Suggestions that MMR vaccine may be associated with autism and inflammatory bowel disease are controversial. Scientific opinion is strongly in favour of there being no link but ↓ public confidence in MMR has resulted in ↓ vaccination uptake, risk of measles outbreaks and debate over the use of single vaccines.

Figure 4.1 Features of common viral infections

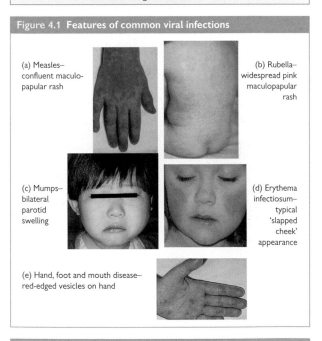

(a) Measles— confluent maculo- papular rash

(b) Rubella— widespread pink maculopapular rash

(c) Mumps— bilateral parotid swelling

(d) Erythema infectiosum— typical 'slapped cheek' appearance

(e) Hand, foot and mouth disease— red-edged vesicles on hand

GMS contract

Childhood vaccination: Can be provided as an additional service and a directed enhanced service (📖 p.86).

Figure 4.1 (a) and (b) are reproduced with permission from the UK Clinical Virology Network.

Chickenpox: Common especially amongst children <10y. and in spring.

- *Presentation:* Incubation period is 10–21d. Presents with rash ± fever. Spots appear in crops for 5–7d. on skin and mucous membranes and progress from macule → papule → vesicle then dry and scab over (usually in <14d.) – Figure 4.2(a). Infectious for 1–2d. before rash develops and for 5d. afterwards.
- *Complications:* Eczema herpeticum (📖 p.243); encephalitis (cerebellar symptoms are most common); pneumonia; birth defects and neonatal infection (📖 p.74).
- *Management:* Supportive. Admit if complications are suspected.

⚠ Non-immune immunosuppressed patients, pregnant women or neonates (📖 p.74) with significant exposure to chickenpox or shingles should receive zoster immunoglobulin (V_Z–IG) as soon as possible (<3d. after contact). Check antibody levels if immune status is unknown.

Shingles: Reinactivation of latent chickenpox virus. Contacts may develop chickenpox but shingles can't be acquired by exposure to chickenpox. Infectious until all lesions have scabbed.

- *Incidence:* 1:25. Any age – more common if immunocompromised.
- *Presentation:* Unilateral pain precedes a vesicular rash by 2–3d. Crops of vesicles appear over 3–5d. and are in the distribution of ≥1 adjacent dermatomes – Figure 4.2(b). The affected area is usually hyperaesthetic – pain may be severe. Lesions scab over and fall off in <14d.
- *Management:* Disease is usually mild in children, so treat as for chickenpox. Oral aciclovir (or similar) is only effective if initiated <48h. after onset of the rash. If immunocompromised admit for IV antivirals.
- *Complications:* Postherpetic neuralgia (rare in children); dissemination to other areas – occurs in immunosuppressed patients – admit for IV aciclovir; eye involvement – refer urgently to ophthalmology; Ramsay Hunt syndrome.

Herpes simplex (HSV) infection: Transmitted by direct contact. Diagnosis is usually clinical but can be confirmed with viral swab:

- HSV-1 causes herpes labialis (cold sore), stomatitis and keratitis
- HSV-2 usually causes genital herpes. If genital herpes presents in a child, suspect abuse.

Primary infection: May be asymptomatic. After <6h. of tingling, discomfort or itching, small tense vesicles appear on an erythematous base. Vesicles then dry, forming a thin yellowish crust and take 8–12d. to heal. Often systemic symptoms too e.g. fever, malaise, tender lymph nodes.

Recurrent infection: After initial infection, HSV remains dormant in the nerve root ganglia. Recurrent eruption may be precipitated by overexposure to sunlight, febrile illnesses, physical/emotional stress or immunosuppression. Trigger stimulus is often unknown. Recurrent disease is generally less severe and more localized.

Complications: Aseptic meningitis or encephalitis (📖 p.48); erythema multiforme (📖 p.264); eczema herpeticum (📖 p.243); generalized infection in immunocompromised patients – oesophagitis, colitis, perianal ulcers, pneumonia and neurological syndromes.

Figure 4.2 Herpes zoster infections

(a) Chickenpox

(b) Shingles on an arm

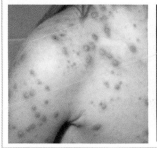
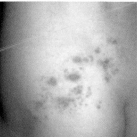

GP Notes: Chicken pox

Chickenpox (varicella) immunization: Single dose. May be given to seronegative healthy children >1y. in close contact with individuals at high risk of severe infection e.g. siblings of a leukaemia sufferer. Vaccination is contraindicated if the child is immunocompromised.

Information for schools about chickenpox: Children can return to school when they are no longer infectious if they are well enough to do so i.e. 5d. after the rash has appeared. National guidance has been produced by the Health Protection Agency and is available at 🖳 www.hpa.org.uk

Advice for patients: Looking after a child with chickenpox

- Chickenpox is an illness which gets better on its own in most children.
- Spots will appear for 5–7 days. When they first appear they are red, then they become blisters which scab over within 2 weeks.
- Spots may cause itching. Itching can be helped by cool baths, and calamine lotion and/or antihistamines (such as Piriton) bought from the chemist. Cotton gloves or socks put on your child's hands can prevent damage from scratching.
- If your child has a fever or complains of pain or discomfort, give paracetamol or ibuprofen syrup. Follow the instructions on the bottle and don't exceed the recommended dose for your child.
- Your child is infectious for 1–2 days before until 5 days after the rash appears. You don't need to wait for all the spots to scab over until your child can go back to school or nursery.
- Whilst your child is infectious, other people might catch chickenpox from him or her. Pregnant women, newborn babies, people on steroid medication and people with serious illnesses e.g. leukaemia can get severe chickenpox, so it is important to avoid contact with them.
- Shingles can't be caught from someone with chickenpox.

Figure 4.2(a) is reproduced with permission from American Academy of Pediatrics 🖳 www.aap.org
Figure 4.2(b) is reproduced with permission from Dr John L. Bezzant.

Management
- *Neonatal infection:* 📖 p.75
- *Severe infection:* e.g. HSV encephalitis, severe eczema herpeticum, immunocompromised patients – admit for treatment with IV aciclovir.
- *Eye involvement:* Refer for urgent ophthalmology assessment. Treatment is with topical ± oral aciclovir.
- *Suppression* of recurrent eruptions: Oral aciclovir (and similar drugs). Take specialist advice.
- *Cold sores:* Topical aciclovir – if started early. Available OTC.
- *Whitlow:* 📖 p.256
- *2° infections:* Topical or systemic antibiotics.

Poliomyelitis^{ND}
- *Spread:* Droplet or faeco – oral. Incubation period is 7d.
- *Presentation:* 2d. flu-like prodrome then fever, tachycardia, headache, vomiting, neck stiffness and unilateral tremor ('pre-paralytic stage'). 65% who experience the pre-paralytic stage go on to develop paralysis (myalgia, LMN signs ± respiratory failure).
- *Management:* Supportive – admit to hospital. <10% of those developing paralysis die but many more are left with permanent disability. Post-polio syndrome (with worsening of neurological deficit) may occur many years later.
- *Prevention:* Box 4.3

Human immunodeficiency virus (HIV): HIV is a retrovirus infecting T-helper cells bearing the CD4 receptor. Up to 50% of infants of HIV seropositive mothers are infected with HIV during pregnancy, childbirth (50%) or breast-feeding, accounting for 90% of HIV infections in childhood. Other infections are usually due to accidental exposure (e.g. contaminated needles or infected blood products).

Presentation:
- Fetal abnormalities: 📖 p.74
- Aged 6mo.–2y. : Failure to thrive, poor feeding, fever, diarrhoea, lymphadenopathy, hepatosplenomegaly, repeated slow-to-clear infections and/or opportunistic infections (e.g. pneumococcus, TB, CMV, *Pneumocystis carinii*, toxoplasmosis and cryptosporidial diarrhoea).

ⓘ HIV testing in children <18mo. is problematic as antibodies are transferred from mother to baby across the placenta – take specialist advice.

Management: Specialist treatment is essential.
- *Antiviral drugs:* A combination of antiviral drugs is usual. Adherence to therapy is essential to avoid resistance. Treatment failure requires switching or increasing therapy.
- *Prophylaxis against opportunistic infection:* Prophylactic antibiotics are used to prevent *Pneumocystis carinii*, toxoplasmosis and *Mycobacterium avium* for children with low CD4 counts.
- *Psychological support:* Due to the stigma attached to HIV infection, patients and parents often lack the support offered by the community for most other serious illness. An important role for the PHCT.

Prevention
- *Prevention of transmission from mother to child:* 📖 p.74
- *Screening blood donors:* Prevents transmission in infected blood products. Seroconversion can take 3mo. so, even with screening, there is still a small risk of transmission
- *HIV vaccination:* Trials of HIV vaccines are in advanced stages.

Influenza: 📖 p.154   **Bronchiolitis:** 📖 p.156

The common cold: 📖 p.154   **Viral skin infections:** 📖 p.256

Further information:
Health Protection Agency (HPA) 🖥 www.hpa.org.uk
- Topics A–Z: Measles, mumps, rubella, polio, herpes simplex and zoster
- MMR information sheet and weblinks
- Guidance on management of communicable diseases in schools and nurseries

Immunisation 🖥 www.immunisation.org.uk
DoH The Green Book 🖥 www.dh.gov.uk
British HIV Association HIV Treatment Guidelines (2006)
🖥 www.bhiva.org

Box 4.3 Prevention of polio

In the UK, inactivated polio vaccine (IPV) has been combined with diphtheria, tetanus, ± whooping cough, ± *Haemophilus influenzae* vaccine to form a single 3, 4 or 5-part vaccine.

Primary immunization in babies and children <10y.: 3 doses of the 5-part vaccine (DTaP/IPV/Hib), each 1mo. apart – usually at 2, 3 and 4mo. of age. If the schedule is disrupted resume the course from where it was stopped.

Booster doses in children: 1 dose of 4-part vaccine (DTaP/IPV) protecting against polio, diphtheria, whooping cough and tetanus >3y. after the 1° course of immunization (usually pre-school) and another dose of 3-part vaccine (Td/IPV) protecting against tetanus, diphtheria and polio between the ages of 13y. and 18y. (usually on leaving school).
Primary immunization in children >10y.: 3 doses of 3-part vaccine (Td/IPV) each 1mo. apart. Booster doses are required 3y. and 10y. after the primary course.

GMS contract

Childhood vaccination: Can be provided as an additional service and a directed enhanced service (📖 p.86).

Advice for patients: Information for parents and children with HIV infection

National AIDS Helpline ☎ 0800 567 123 (24h. helpline)
Terrence Higgins Trust ☎ 0845 1221 200 🖥 www.tht.org.uk
Children with AIDS Charity (CWAC) ☎ 020 7033 8620
🖥 www.cwac.org

Bacterial infections

Streptococcal infection: Several groups are pathogenic to man –
A, B, C, G, D and Viridans streptococci.

Presentation
- Pharyngitis
- Tonsillitis
- Wound/skin infections
- Septicaemia
- Scarlet fever
- Pneumonia
- Rheumatic fever
- Glomerulonephritis
- Neonatal sepsis
- Endocarditis
- Septic arthritis
- Pneumonia
- UTI
- Dental caries

Investigation: Diagnosis is usually clinical. Evidence of infection can be
obtained by measuring changing antibody response to infection (ASO
titres). ASO titres are ↑ in ~80% infections. Wound swabs are +ve if
infection is on the skin and throat swabs may be +ve in pharyngi-
tis/tonsillitis.

Treatment: Most streptococci are sensitive to penicillin though resistance is increasingly common.

Scarlet fever: Gp.A haemolytic *Streptococcus* infection.
- *Incubation:* 2–4d.
- *Presentation:* Fever, malaise, headache, tonsillitis, rash – fine punctate
  erythema sparing face, 'scarlet' facial flushing, strawberry tongue
  (initially white, turning red by $3^{rd}/4^{th}$ d. – Figure 4.3).
- *Treatment:* Penicillin V for 10d.
- *Complications:* Rheumatic fever (📖 p.136), acute glomerulonephritis.

Pneumococcal infection: There are >85 types of *S. pneumoniae*.
Pneumococci are carried in the noses and throats of ½ the population.
In most people they are harmless. Spread is by droplet infection.

Presentations
- Pneumonia
- Acute otitis media
- Sinusitis
- Meningitis
- Endocarditis
- Septic arthritis (rare)
- Peritonitis (rare)

Treatment: Amoxicillin for 7d. (erythromycin in allergic individuals).
Resistance to penicillin in the community is still low.

Prevention: Vaccination.
- Routine vaccination is now offered as part of the childhood
  immunization schedule, in addition offer to high-risk children who
  have not been vaccinated as part of the routine childhood
  vaccination programme (Box 4.4).
- Ineffective in children <2mo.
- Booster doses are not needed except for patients with asplenia or
  nephrotic syndrome, when give a booster after 5–10y.

Box 4.4 Children at high risk of pneumococcal infection

- Asplenia or functional asplenia (📖 p.105) e.g. splenectomy, sickle cell
- Chronic renal disease or nephrotic syndrome
- Immunodeficiency or immunosuppression e.g. lymphoma, Hodgkin's disease, HIV, chemotherapy
- Chronic heart disease
- Chronic lung disease e.g. asthma, CF
- Chronic liver disease
- Coeliac disease
- Cochlear implant
- DM
- CSF shunt
- Children <5y. who have had previous invasive pneumococcal disease

GMS contract

Pneumococcal vaccination may be offered by GMS practices as a directed enhanced service – 📖 p.87.

Figure 4.3 Strawberry tongue of scarlet fever

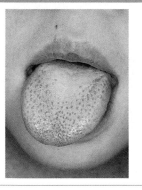

Further information

Health Protection Agency (HPA) Topics A – Z: Streptococcal infections 🖥 www.hpa.org.uk

Staphylococcal infection: Usually *Staph. aureus,* occasionally *Staph. epidermidis.* Antibiotic-resistant strains are common.

Presentation
- Impetigo – 📖 p.254
- Abscesses/furuncles/carbuncles – 📖 p.254
- Wound infection
- Osteomyelitis/septic arthritis – 📖 p.206
- Pneumonia - especially immunosuppressed children
- Neonatal infections – usually appear <6wk. after birth – pustular or bullous skin lesions on neck, axilla or groin
- Septicaemia
- Endocarditis.

Management: Supportive measures, antibiotics (usually flucloxacillin or erythromycin for 7–10d.) ± abscess drainage if appropriate. Where possible obtain specimens for culture before instituting/altering antibiotics.

Methicillin resistant Staph. aureus (MRSA): MRSA acts in exactly the same way as any other *Staph. aureus* – it is carried harmlessly in most but occasionally causes a range of infections. It is only different due to its multiple resistance to antibiotics. Often contracted in hospital.

Toxic shock syndrome: Caused by staphylococcal exotoxin.
- *Risk factors:* Tampon use; staphylococcal wound infection; influenza; osteomyelitis; cellulitis.
- *Presentation:* Sudden onset high fever, vomiting, diarrhoea, confusion and skin rash. May progress to shock ± death.
- *Management:* Admit as an emergency – mortality 8–15%.

Haemophilus influenzae: 99% of infections are due to type b. Rare <3mo. then incidence rises, reaching peak incidence at 10–11mo. Thereafter incidence declines until the age of 4y., after which infection is rare.

Presentation
- Meningitis – 60% – associated with high mortality and incidence of permanent neurological sequelae
- Epiglottitis – 15%
- Septicaemia – 10%
- Osteomyelitis
- Septic arthritis
- Cellulitis
- Pneumonia
- Pericarditis.

Management: Admit patients with severe infections. Organisms are often penicillin resistant and treatment is usually with IV cefotaxime.

Prevention: Box 4.5

Pertussis (whooping cough)^ND: 📖 p.156

Meningococcal meningitis/septicaemia^ND: 📖 p.48

Tuberculosis^ND: 📖 p.160

Gastroenteritis: 📖 p.176

Travel-related illness: 📖 p.100

Diphtheria^{ND}: Caused by *Corynebacterium diphtheriae*. Rare in the UK.
- *Spread:* Droplet infection, contact with articles soiled by an infected person. Incubation 2–5d.
- *Presentation:* In countries where hygiene is poor cutaneous diphtheria is the predominant form. Elsewhere, characterized by an inflammatory exudate which forms a greyish membrane in the respiratory tract (may cause respiratory obstruction). *C. diphtheriae* secretes a toxin which affects myocardium, nervous and adrenal tissues.
- *Management:* Admit for antitoxin and IV erythromycin. Patients may be infectious for up to 4wk. but carriers shed *C. diphtheriae* for longer.
- *Prevention:* Box 4.5

GP notes: Reducing the risk of MRSA transmission^N

- ↓ tendency for multiple resistance by prudent use of antibiotics.
- Wash hands thoroughly with an appropriate antibacterial preparation if they appear soiled.
- If hands appear clean, wash with an alcoholic rub between each and every patient contact.
- Follow local policies for management of patients who are known to be infected with or carry MRSA.

Box 4.5

Prevention of *Haemophilus influenzae* infection: Vaccination is routinely offered to all children (📖 p.84). In addition offer a one-off vaccination to all unimmunized asplenic patients (preferably 2wk. prior to splenectomy) and HIV +ve patients.

Prevention of diphtheria: Vaccination against diphtheria is part of the routine childhood vaccination programme in the UK (📖 p.84). In addition give a booster dose to people in contact with a patient with diphtheria or carrier, or before travel to epidemic or endemic areas.

GMS contract

Childhood vaccination: Can be provided as an additional service and a directed enhanced service (📖 p.86).

Further information

DoH Winning ways: reducing healthcare associated infection in England (2004) 🖥 www.dh.gov.uk
NICE Infection control, prevention of healthcare-associated infection in primary and community care (2003) 🖥 www.nice.org.uk
Health Protection Agency (HPA) Topics A–Z: E. coli enteritis, Hib 🖥 www.hpa.org.uk

Travel-related illness

Children who travel to (or come to the UK from) abroad are exposed to a wide range of illnesses. In all children who have recently returned to the UK from abroad who present unwell, consider imported disease in addition to the usual differential diagnosis. If unsure, seek specialist advice by telephone or admit the child.

Travellers' diarrhoea: 📖 p.176

Malaria[ND]: 2000 cases/y. are notified in the UK.
- *Falciparum malaria:* Caused by *Plasmodium falciparum*. Accounts for ~½ UK cases and may not present for up to 3mo. after return from a malarial area. Can be fatal in <24h. – especially if it occurs in small children (<3y.) – cerebral malaria accounts for 80% deaths.
- *Benign malaria:* Caused by *P. vivax*, *P. ovale* and *P. malariae*. May cause illness up to 18mo. after return. All have very low mortality. Relapse may occur at intervals after initial infection as parasites lie dormant in the liver (*P. vivax* and *P. ovale*) or blood (*P. malariae*).

Presentation: Easy to miss.
- *Symptoms:* Malaria is a great mimic and can present with virtually any symptoms. Usually consists of a prodrome of headache, malaise, myalgia and anorexia followed by recurring high fevers, rigors and drenching sweats – lasting 8–12h. at a time.
- *Examination:* May be normal – look for anaemia, jaundice ± hepatosplenomegaly.

Investigation: In all cases of fever in patients who have returned from a malarial endemic area – even if the plane just landed there and they didn't get off – send a thick and thin film for malaria.

Management: Admit for further investigation and treatment if:
- Very unwell – admit without investigation
- Thick and thin film +ve or unable to check thick and thin film (e.g. presentation out of laboratory hours or at a weekend)
- Persistent fever despite -ve thick and thin film.

Prevention: Avoidance of mosquito bites and chemoprophylaxis.

Hepatitis A (HAV): Common. Spread is via the faeco–oral route with an incubation period of 2–7wk. (average 4wk.). Children are infectious 2 wk. before feeling ill.

Presentation: May be asymptomatic. Symptoms include fatigue, fever, ↓ appetite, nausea ± vomiting, pale stools ± diarrhoea, jaundice, dark urine, abdominal pain ± tender hepatomegaly.

Investigation: LFTs, hepatitis serology – IgM antibodies signify recent infection, IgG remains detectable lifelong.

Management: Supportive. Most recover in <2mo. There is no carrier state and hepatitis A does not cause chronic liver disease. After infection immunity is lifelong.

Prevention: Vaccination (Havrix®) for travellers to high-risk areas.

Typhoid[ND] and paratyphoid[ND]: Spread is by the faeco–oral route. Caused by *Salmonella typhi* and *Salmonella paratyphi*, ~200 cases/y. are notified in the UK. Incubation is 3d.–3wk.

Presentation

- *Symptoms:* Malaise, fever, headache, cough, constipation (or diarrhoea), nose bleeds, bruising and/or abdominal pain
- *Examination:* Pyrexia, relative bradycardia, rose-coloured spots on the trunk (40%), splenomegaly, CNS signs (coma, delirium, meningism)

Management: Admit for further investigation and treatment with antibiotics. 10% die if untreated; <0.1% if treated. 1% become chronic carriers after infection.

GP Notes: Prevention of travel related illness

Consider:

- **Vaccination:** Ensure children are fully vaccinated for the areas they are intending to visit (usually fee payable for vaccination). Charts are available in GP and Pulse magazines and via travel information clinics.
- **Prophylactic medication:** Depending on age of the child and areas to which the child is travelling, consider malaria prophylaxis.
- **Prevention of infection:** Take care to eat and drink uncontaminated food and water – food should be cooked and eaten hot, avoid salads and cold meats/fish and only eat fruit which can be peeled. Stick to drinks made with boiled water/bottled water or drinks with intact seal. Sleep in screened accommodation to prevent insect bites, cover limbs in the evening and spray with a mosquito repellant.
- **Prevention of accidents:** Advise parents not to allow children to perform activities without adequate protective clothing whilst abroad (e.g. riding on motorcycles without helmets). Avoid sunburn.
- **Pre-existing illness:** Don't travel if unwell. Advise patients/parents to take enough supplies of regular medication to last the entire trip.
- **Insurance:** Advise parents to ensure all children travelling abroad are covered by comprehensive medical insurance including repatriation expenses.

Further information

Health Protection Agency (HPA) Guidelines for malaria prevention in travellers from the UK (2003) ⊞ www.hpa.org.uk

DoH Health advice for travellers ⊞ www.dh.gov.uk

National Travel Health Network and Centre (funded by DoH) Information for travellers and health professionals including yellow fever vaccination centres. Advice line for health professionals ☎ 0845 602 6712 ⊞ www.nathnac.org

Fit for Travel NHS (Scotland) travel site ⊞ www.fitfortravel.scot.nhs.uk

Medical Advisory Service for Travellers Abroad (MASTA) ⊞ www.masta.org

Kawasaki disease

Kawasaki disease was first reported by Tomisaku Kawasaki, a Japanese paediatrician, in 1967. He observed and described a systemic vasculitic illness predominantly affecting children <5y.

Kawasaki disease is the commonest cause of acquired heart disease in children in developed countries. Epidemiology suggests an infectious aetiology but cause is, as yet, unknown. *Incidence in the UK:* 3.4/100,000 children aged <5y.

Diagnosis

- There is no diagnostic test and many cases are missed.
- Diagnosis is based on clinical criteria – Table 4.5.
- Difficulty arises due to the similarity of features of Kawasaki disease with those of many other childhood infections and the possibility of atypical presentation of Kawasaki disease.
- Remain alert to the possibility of the diagnosis in any child, particularly if very miserable or with fever for >5d. Poor response to antipyretics heightens suspicion.

Less characteristic features

- Rhinorrhoea
- Cough
- Abdominal pain
- Vomiting
- Diarrhoea
- Pain/swelling of joints
- CNS involvement
- Jaundice
- Sterile pyuria

Complications

- Coronary arteritis with formation of aneurysms (20–30% untreated patients).
- In the acute phase these may cause thrombosis within an aneurysm, MI or dysrhythmias and even death.
- Long-term morbidity results from scarring of coronary arteries, intimal thickening and accelerated atherosclerosis.

Management: If suspected refer for urgent paediatric assessment. Early treatment (<10d. after onset) with IV immunoglogulin and aspirin ↓ incidence and severity of aneurysm formation as well as giving symptom relief. The role of treatment after this time is unclear though IV immunoglobulin is often given >10d. after onset of symptoms if there is evidence of ongoing inflammation.

Table 4.5 Diagnostic criteria for Kawasaki disease

Presence of ≥5 of the following:

- Fever for ≥5d.
- Bilateral (non-purulent) conjunctivitis
- Polymorphous rash
- Changes in lips and mouth:
  - Reddened, dry, or cracked lips
  - Strawberry tongue
  - Diffuse redness of oral or pharyngeal mucosa
- Changes in extremities:
  - Reddening of palms or soles
  - Indurative oedema of hands or feet
  - Desquamation of skin of hands, feet and groin (in convalescence)
- Cervical lymphadenopathy: >15mm diameter. Usually unilateral, single, non-purulent and painful

Exclusion of diseases with similar presentation:

- Staphylococcal infection (such as scalded skin syndrome, toxic shock syndrome)
- Streptococcal infection (e.g. scarlet fever, toxic shock-like syndrome)
- Rickettsial disease
- Leptospirosis
- Stevens-Johnson syndrome
- Drug reaction
- Measles and other viral exanthems
- Juvenile rheumatoid arthritis

🚫 Throat carriage of group A streptococcus does not exclude Kawasaki disease.

Infections in immunocompromised patients

Infections in patients whose host defence mechanisms are compromised range from minor to fatal. They are often caused by organisms that normally reside on body surfaces.

Opportunistic infections: Infections from endogenous microflora that are non-pathogenic or from ordinarily harmless organisms. Occur if host defence mechanisms have been altered by:

- Infection
- Burns
- Neoplasms
- Irradiation
- Metabolic disorders e.g. DM
- Foreign bodies
- Corticosteroids
- Immunosuppressive or cytotoxic drugs
- Diagnostic/therapeutic instrumentation

The precise character of the host's altered defences determines which organisms are likely to be involved. These organisms are often resistant to multiple antibiotics.

Organisms commonly involved:

- Non-pathogenic streptococci
- *E. coli*
- Herpes viruses
- Cytomegalovirus
- Cryptococcal infection
- Toxoplasma
- Mycobacteria
- Pneumocystis
- Candida

Management: Expert care is always required – refer promptly to the consultant responsible for the patient.

Prophylaxis

Antibiotics: Used for prevention of:
- Rheumatic fever and bacterial endocarditis
- TB and meningitis in exposed patients
- Recurrent UTIs and otitis media
- Bacterial infections in granulocytopenic patients
- Pneumocystis (if CD4 count <200 cells/mm^3), toxoplasma (if CD4 count <100 cells/mm^3) and mycobacterium avium (if CD4 count <50 cells/mm^3) in AIDS patients.

⚠ Watch for signs of superinfection with resistant organisms.

Active immunization
- *Influenza vaccine:* Give annually – see 📖 p.155 for list of indications.
- *Haemophilus influenzae type b vaccine:* For asplenic/hyposplenic patients – children should complete routine Hib vaccinations. Individuals immunized in infancy who then become asplenic should receive 1 booster dose aged >1y. Unimmunized children >10y. should receive a single dose of Hib.
- *Meningococcal vaccine:* Give to close contacts of patients with type A or C meningococcal meningitis. In some cases also given to patients with immunosuppression – take specialist advice.

- *Pneumococcal vaccine:* Single dose – give to chronically ill, or asplenic and elderly patients and those with sickle cell and HIV disease. Booster doses are not required except for patients with asplenia or nephrotic syndrome when a booster should be given after 5–10y.
- *Hepatitis B vaccine:* Give to patients who repeatedly receive blood products.
- *Chickenpox vaccination:* Give to non-immune close contacts of immunosuppressed patients e.g. siblings of children with leukaemia.

Passive immunization: Can prevent or ameliorate herpes zoster (VZ-Ig), hepatitis A and B, measles and cytomegalovirus infection in selected immunosuppressed patients. If a patient is in contact with any of these diseases ask advice from the consultant looking after the patient or a consultant in communicable disease control.

Immunoglobulin administration: Effective for patients with hypogamma-globulinaemia. Given on a regular basis by IV infusion.

⚠ Any febrile episode in a neutropenic child requires immediate referral to a specialist unit.

Asplenic patients: All asplenic patients (or functionally asplenic patients e.g. patients with sickle cell disease) are at ↑ risk of bacterial infection. Ensure patients have:
- *Vaccinations:* Haemophilus influenzae b, pneumococcal, influenza and, in some cases, meningococcal vaccine. If possible vaccinations should be given >2wk. prior to splenectomy
- *Prophylactic antibiotics:* Oral penicillin continuously until age 16y. or for 2y. post-splenectomy – whichever is longer
- *Stand-by amoxicillin:* To start if symptoms of infection begin
- *Patient-held card:* Alerting health professionals to infection risk.

⚠
- Warn patients about risk of malaria and other tropical infections.
- Admit if infection develops despite prophylactic measures.

GP Notes: Asplenism/hyposplenism:

Patient cards and information sheets about asplenism/hyposplenism are available from: Department of Health, PO Box 410, Wetherby LS23 7LL. Encourage patients to wear a Medic-Alert bracelet or necklace.

GMS contract

Vaccinations can be provided as
Childhood vaccinations can be provided as an *additional service* or as a *directed enhanced service* (📖 p.87)

Immune deficiency syndromes

A group of diverse conditions caused by immune system defects and characterized clinically by ↑ susceptibility to infections.

> ⚠ Consider an immunodeficiency disorder in anyone with infections that are unusually frequent, severe, resistant or due to unusual organisms.

History: Ask about:
- Family history: immune deficiency, early death, similar disease, autoimmune illness, early malignancy
- Adverse reaction to immunization or viral infection
- Splenectomy, tonsillectomy or adenoidectomy
- Prior prophylactic antibiotic or immunoglobulin therapy.

Primary immunodeficiency: Since many 1° immunodeficiencies are hereditary or congenital, they appear initially in infants and children – ~80% of those affected are <20y. old and, owing to X-linked inheritance, ♂>>♀. Genetic screening is available for some conditions. Refer all suspected cases to paediatrics/immunology.

Classification: >70 primary immunodeficiencies have been described. They are classified into 4 groups depending on which component of the immune system is deficient:
- B cells
- T cells
- Phagocytic cells
- Complement

Prevalence: Selective IgA deficiency (usually asymptomatic) occurs in 1:400 people. All other primary immune deficiencies are rare. Excluding IgA deficiency, ½ of affected patients have B-cell deficiency; 30% – T-cell deficiency; 18% – phagocytic deficiencies; 2% – complement deficiency.

Presentation: Table 4.6 lists some of the more common immune deficiencies. All immune deficiencies present with increased tendency to infections. Type of infection varies according the the component of the immune system involved.

Secondary immunodeficiency: Impairment of the immune system resulting from illness (including drug therapy e.g. with cytotoxics or steroids) or removal of the spleen in a previously normal person. Often reversible if the underlying condition or illness resolves. 2° immunodeficiencies are common – most prolonged serious illness interferes with the immune system to some degree. Treat the cause.

Asplenia and splenectomy: 📖 p.105

Infection in the immunocompromised: 📖 p.104

Advice for patients: Information and support

Immune Deficiency Foundation 🖥 www.primaryimmune.org

Table 4.6 Immune deficiency syndromes

Type	Syndrome	Clinical details
B-cell deficiency Prone to infection with Gram +ve organisms (e.g. streptococci)	Selective IgA deficiency & IgG subclass deficiencies	Variable symptoms with most only mildly affected. When more severely affected, early treatment of infection may be required
	Congenital X-linked hypogamma-globulinaemia & Common variable immunodeficiency	Not inherited – cause unknown ↓ immunoglobulins Treatment is with IV immunoglobulin ↑ risk of leukaemia/lymphoma
T-cell deficiency Prone to viral, fungal and opportunistic infections	DiGeorge's syndrome	Defect on chromosome 22 → absent/hypoplastic thymus (and ↓ T cells), absent parathyroid glands ± cardiac and/or facial abnormalities Mild (80%) – treated supportively Severe – requires thymus/bone marrow transplant
	HIV	📖 p.94
Combined B & T cell deficiency	Severe combined immunodeficiency	Autosomal or X-linked recessive Absence of both T-cell and B-cell immunity Presents <6mo. old with frequent infections Treatment is with bone marrow transplant. Untreated most die at <1y.
	Ataxia telangectasia	Autosomal recessive Selective IgA deficiency or hypogammaglobulinae-mia and T-cell dysfunction Characterized by telangectasia, cerebellar ataxia and recurrent chest infections Treatment is supportive ↑ risk of leukaemia/lymphoma
	Wiskott-Aldrich syndrome (partial combined immunodeficiency syndrome)	X-linked recessive ↑ IgA and IgE; normal or ↓ IgG; ↓ IgM Presents with eczema, thrombocytopenia and recurrent infections Treatment is with bone marrow transplant – rarely survive beyond teens without ↑ risk of leukaemia/lymphoma
Phagocytic deficiency Prone to Staphylococcal and Gram –ve infections	Chronic granulomatous disease	X-linked ($^2/_3$) or autosomal recessive Phagocyte dysfunction Usually presents <6mo. of age with fungal pneumonia, lymphadenopathy, hepatosplenomegaly and/or osteomyelitis Treatment is supportive with prophylactic antibiotics and early treatment of infections
	Agranulocytosis	Usually caused by drugs e.g. carbimazole Absence of neutrophils Sudden onset of fever ± rigors, sore throat, mouth ulcers, headache and malaise → septicaemia If suspected check urgent FBC and/or admit

Allergies

Allergic diseases result from an exaggerated response of the immune system to external substances. Affects 1:6 of the British population – and is increasing. Allergic problems include:

- Asthma – 📖 p.138
- Eczema – 📖 p.242
- Anaphylaxis – 📖 p.42
- Urticaria – 📖 p.248
- Rhinitis – both seasonal and perennial – 📖 p.280
- Conjunctivitis – 📖 p.271

Assessment

- Age
- Symptoms – past and present, main problem, frequency and severity, seasonal/perennial, provoking factors
- Impact on lifestyle – time off school, sleep
- Activities/hobbies
- Treatment – past and present
- Home environment – pets, damp, dust, smoking
- Allergies in the past
- Family history of allergic illness
- Examination will depend on main symptoms (e.g. asthma – 📖 p.140)

Investigation

Skin prick testing: Identifies IgE sensitivity to common allergens, allowing diagnosis or exclusion of atopy. An alternative is measurement of serum IgE levels. In most places this is a 2°care procedure though a pilot study has shown it is feasible in general practice. Patients should avoid using antihistamines before skin prick testing.

Patch testing: Identifies substances causing contact allergy. A battery of allergens on discs are applied to the skin – usually on the back – and stuck in place with tape. The skin response is then monitored. Only done in specialist allergy or dermatology clinics.

Management

- Allergen avoidance
- Medication – see individual conditions
- Consider referral to a specialist allergy clinic:
  - For investigation and management of anaphylaxis
  - If the diagnosis of allergy is in doubt
  - Food allergy
  - Urticaria in which allergic aetiology is suspected
  - For consideration of immunotherapy

Bee/wasp sting allergy: Accounts for ~4 deaths/y. in the UK. May result in a local or generalized reaction of varying severity. Intensity of reaction is also variable – because someone has had 1 bad reaction they will not necessarily get another. Treat local or mild generalized reactions with antihistamine. Supply patients with more severe reactions with an EpiPen and teach them, and close contacts, to use it. Refer to an allergy clinic for consideration of desensitization.

Food allergy: Affects 5–7% of children. Types of adverse reaction to foods include:
- Type 1 food allergy – acute allergy e.g. acute peanut allergy
- Type IV food allergy – delayed e.g. milk causing eczema
- Non-allergic food intolerance:
  - pharmocological e.g. tyramine in cheese may provoke migraine
  - Metabolic e.g. lactase deficiency
  - Toxic e.g. reaction to preservative rather than food
  - Food aversion – symptoms non-specific and unconfirmed by blinded food challenge.

A limited number of foods are responsible for the vast majority of cases of true food allergy: nuts (especially peanuts), wheat, eggs, fish, shellfish and cow's milk (📖 p.178).

Management:
- Avoid the offending food.
- If the reaction is severe, refer to an allergy clinic for confirmation of diagnosis and dietary advice.
- If anaphylactic reaction, supply an EpiPen and teach the child (where possible) and close contacts to use it.

Advice for patients: Allergies

Avoiding allergens: If your child has an allergy, avoiding the substance or situation which causes it will prevent your child having symptoms and, in the case of severe allergic reaction, may be life-saving.

Common allergies include:
Pets: Exclude the offending animal.

Pollens: If the pollen count is high:
- Keep windows shut (including car windows)
- Wear glasses or sunglasses to prevent pollen getting in eyes
- Avoid grassy spaces
- Fit a pollen filter on the car.

Foods or drugs:
- Avoid the food or drug which causes the reaction.
- Avoid hidden exposure (check labels carefully).
- Inform your child's school, nursery or any clubs your child attends.
- Take food with you wherever possible.
- Ensure any drug allergies are recorded in your child's GP notes.

🛈 If your child has a severe allergy (for example, has had an anaphylactic reaction) he or she should wear a bracelet or necklace alerting anyone who might be called in an emergency.

Further information and support
Allergy UK ☎01322 619898 🖥 www.allergyuk.org
Anaphylaxis Campaign ☎01252 542029 🖥 www.anaphylaxis.org.uk
Medic-Alert Foundation Supply Medic-Alert bracelets
☎ 0800 581 420 🖥 www.medicalert.co.uk

Anaemia

Anaemia is lack of sufficient red blood cells and thus haemoglobin. In children normal values of haemoglobin vary considerably with age – neonates are relatively polycythaemic with high MCV. Hb and MCV then fall – reaching their lowest levels from 3mo.–1y. – and rise again reaching typical adult levels at puberty.

Causes of anaemia: Anaemia results if there is:
- ↓ *red cell production:* Defective precursor proliferation and/or maturation – usually caused by nutritional deficiencies (particularly iron), marrow failure (aplastic anaemia) or infiltration (leukaemia)
- ↑ *loss or rate of destruction:* Bleeding (e.g. Meckel's diverticulum, clotting disorders) or haemolysis (haemoglobinopathy, spherocytosis)
- ↓ *tissue requirement for oxygen:* In practice – hypothyroidism.

Presentation:
- If slow onset, may be asymptomatic until very anaemic.
- Symptoms and signs include tiredness, lethargy and pallor (may be noticed by parents).
- Examination is often normal but may give clues to underlying cause.

Finding a cause for anaemia: Figure 4.4

Iron deficiency anaemia: Most common form of anaemia in children. As well as the usual presentations of anaemia, may present as a miserable baby, with poor growth and/or delayed psychomotor development.

❗ Consider checking serum ferritin. Some children are low in iron without being anaemic but still have symptoms (e.g psychomotor delay). These symptoms improve with iron supplementation.

Specific signs of iron deficiency:
- Koilonychia (spoon-shaped nails)
- Glossitis
- Angular stomatitis

Causes:
- *Dietary:* Accounts for the vast majority of cases and a particular problem amongst inner-city Asian populations. Occurs >6mo. of age – usually when unmodified cow's milk is given as the main milk source to a child <1y. and if intake of solids is delayed or poor.
- *Blood loss:* Unusual cause of anaemia in children. May occur with Meckel's diverticulum, reflux or recurrent epistaxis.
- ↑ *demand:* Adolescence and infants (especially premature infants).
- *Malabsorption:* Can be the first sign of coeliac disease (📖 p.180).

Management:
- Treat the underlying cause where possible.
- Consider referral to a dietician.
- Give oral iron supplements e.g. Sytron®
- Monitor response – Hb should increase by 1g/dL/wk.
- Continue treatment until iron stores are replenished (usually about 3mo.).

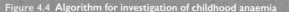

Figure 4.4 Algorithm for investigation of childhood anaemia

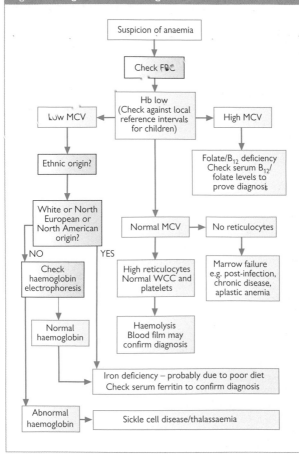

Suspicion of anaemia
→
Check FBC
→
Hb low
(Check against local reference intervals for children)

Low MCV

High MCV → Folate/B₁₂ deficiency
Check serum B₁₂/folate levels to prove diagnosis

Low MCV → Ethnic origin?

White or North European or North American origin?
NO — Check haemoglobin electrophoresis
YES

Normal MCV → No reticulocytes → Marrow failure e.g. post-infection, chronic disease, aplastic anemia

High reticulocytes Normal WCC and platelets → Haemolysis Blood film may confirm diagnosis

Check haemoglobin electrophoresis → Normal haemoglobin → Iron deficiency – probably due to poor diet Check serum ferritin to confirm diagnosis

Abnormal haemoglobin → Sickle cell disease/thalassaemia

GP Notes: Dietary sources of iron

- Iron is found in red meat, leafy green vegetables, chick peas, baked beans, dried fruit, breakfast cereals and formula infant milks.
- Iron absorption, particularly from vegetable sources, is improved by taking vitamin C (e.g. orange juice) at the same time.
- Although iron levels are low in breast milk it is well absorbed.

Folate and vitamin B₁₂ deficiency: B$_{12}$ and folate deficiencies commonly coexist. Both vitamins are absorbed in the gut. B$_{12}$ absorption takes place by active and passive mechanisms – the latter being dependent on intrinsic factor, a protein produced by gastric parietal cells.

Presentation:
- Anaemia
- Sore mouth (glossitis, angular cheilosis and/or mouth ulcers)

Causes of deficiency:
- *Inadequate dietary intake:* e.g. vegans – give dietary advice and/or dietary supplements
- *Malabsorption:* Crohn's disease, coeliac disease

Isolated B$_{12}$ deficiency:
- *Pernicious anaemia:* Due to congenital absence of or antibodies to intrinsic factor.

Isolated folate deficiency:
- *Excess use:* Prematurity, ↑ cell turnover (e.g. haemolysis)
- *Drugs:* Anticonvulsants, trimethoprim

Management: Refer for identification and treatment of cause. Treatment is with folic acid supplements and B$_{12}$ injections.

Haemolysis: Normal red cells survive 120d. before being removed from the circulation – mainly by the spleen. In haemolytic anaemia red cells are destroyed faster than they are produced and anaemia develops.

Presentation:
- May be a family history
- Neonatal jaundice
- Anaemia ± splenomegaly (older children)

Causes: Table 4.7

Management: Refer to paediatrics for advice on management. Rarely splenectomy is required.

Aplastic anaemia^G: Bone marrow failure and pancytopoenia.

Presentation:
- Anaemia
- Thrombocytopoenia – bruising, petechial rash
- Neutropoenia – recurrent infection
- FBC reveals pancytopoenia and lack of reticulocytes.

Causes: Unknown (idiopathic) in 50%
- Congenital
- Drug induced

Management: Refer urgently to paediatrics. Treatment is:
- *Supportive:* transfusions and antibiotics; or
- *Definitive:* Aims to restore a healthy, working bone marrow. Bone marrow transplant is curative. Immunosuppressive therapy is an alternative when transplant is not an option.

Haemoglobinopathy: 📖 p.114

Table 4.7 Causes of haemolytic anaemia

Cause	Examples
Congenital:	
Membrane abnormalities	Hereditary spherocytosis or elliptocytosis
Haemoglobin abnormalities	Abnormal Hb e.g. sickle cell anaemia – 📖 p.114 Defective synthesis e.g. thalassaemia – 📖 p.114
Metabolic abnormalities	Glucose-6-phosphate dehydrogenase (G6PD) or pyruvate kinase deficiency
Acquired:	
Immune	Associated with viral infection Haemolytic disease of the newborn due to Rhesus incompatability of the neonate and mother Drug induced
Hypersplenism	Malaria Glycogen storage disorders – 📖 p.78
Red cell fragmentation	Haemolytic uraemic syndrome – 📖 p.184
Secondary	Renal or liver disease
Miscellaneous	Burns, chemicals, toxins, drugs

GP Notes: Dietary sources of B₁₂ and folate

- **Vitamin B$_{12}$** is found in meats, particularly liver, kidney chicken, fish, eggs and dairy products. Vegans are particularly prone to deficiency.
- **Folate** is found in highest concentrations in liver and yeast but is also found in spinach, other green vegetables and nuts.
- ❗ Most breakfast cereals have folate and vitamin B$_{12}$ added.

Advice for patients: Information and support for patients with aplastic anaemia

Aplastic Anaemia Trust ☎ 0870 487 0099 🖳 www.theaat.org.uk

Further information

British Committee for Standards in Haematology
🖳 www.bcshguidelines.com
- Diagnosis and management of acquired aplastic anaemia (2003)
- Diagnosis and management of hereditary spherocytosis (2004)

Haemoglobinopathy

Thalassaemia: Common in populations from Africa, the Middle East, Mediterranean, Indian subcontinent and SE Asia. Results from ↓ production of either the α (α thalassaemia) or β (β thalassaemia) globin chains of haemoglobin. 2 main types of each are recognized:

- α° and β° thalassaemia: no α or β chains are produced
- α^{+} and β^{+} thalassaemia: α and β chains but produced at ↓ rate.

β thalassaemia

- Defective β chain production → excess α chain synthesis.
- Excess α chains precipitate in red cell precursors causing their destruction in bone marrow and spleen → proliferation of marrow, bony deformity (mongoloid facies, bossing of skull, thinning of long bones) and progressive splenomegaly.
- Homozygotes develop profound anaemia from 3mo. of age and without repeated transfusions would die in <1y.
- Children who receive repeated transfusions grow and develop normally but iron accumulates. Treatment is with desferrioxamine infusions to ↑ iron excretion but iron still accumulates and death is usual in the $2^{nd}/3^{rd}$ decade due to iron overload.

Management: If suspected in an infant refer urgently to paediatrics. Specialist ongoing care is essential. Consider referring family members for genetic counselling. Prenatal and antenatal diagnosis is possible.

α thalassaemia

- The homozygous state for α° thalassaemia is associated with fetal death at ~38wk. (Barts hydrops).
- Haemoglobin H results from inheritance of α° from 1 parent and α^{+} from the other. Patients are moderately anaemic with splenomegaly and have haemoglobin H (4 β chains combined with a haem molecule) in their red cells. Specialist management is needed.

❗ Antenatal screening for α thalassaemia is routinely offered in high-prevalence areas and will be extended to the whole UK in 2006. Meanwhile, refer for antenatal testing if family history.

Asymptomatic patients: Heterozygotes for α and β thalassaemia and homozygotes for α^{+} thalassaemia are usually asymptomatic. These patients may have mild anaemia with hypochromic and microcytic red cells.

❗This anaemia can be confused with iron deficiency but ferritin is normal and it does not respond to iron supplements.

The sickling disorders: Most common amongst people originating from areas in which malaria is endemic – Africans (1–2% newborns) and certain Mediterranean, Middle Eastern and Indian populations.
Varieties:

- Heterozygous state for haemoglobin S (sickle cell trait – AS)
- Homozygous state (sickle cell anaemia/disease – SS)
- Heterozygous states for haemoglobin S and haemoglobins C, D, E or other structural variants
- Combination of haemoglobin S with any form of thalassaemia

Mechanism: Haemoglobin S undergoes liquid crystal formation as it becomes deoxygenated, causing sickling of affected blood cells. The effect of sickling is:
- to shorten survival of red cells → haemolytic anaemia
- to cause aggregation of the sickled cells.

Aggregation of the sickled cells leads to:
- Tissue infarction – resulting in pain and/or tissue damage e.g. stroke (10% children with sickle cell anaemia have a stroke – ½ of those have recurrent strokes) *and/or*
- Sequestration in the liver, spleen or lungs – producing sudden and profound anaemia.

Diagnosis: FBC and film – chronic anaemia with sickling on film. Confirm diagnosis with haemoglobin electrophoresis.

Sickle cell trait: Patients with <40% haemoglobin S have no symptoms unless they are subjected to anoxia e.g. anaesthesia.

Sickle cell anaemia
- Low Hb level (typically 8–9g/dL) with high reticulocyte count – though generally patients compensate well.
- Illness is due to complications arising as a result of acute exacerbations or 'crises' and by the effects of recurrent tissue damage due to microinfarction over a long period of time.
- Prognosis is variable. In Africa children usually die within 1y. In the UK patients frequently survive into adulthood (average survival 42–48y.). Commonest cause of death is infection.

Management
- There is no medication to prevent sickling.
- Treat as if hyposplenic – give Hib and pneumococcal vaccination, annual influenza vaccination ± prophylactic antibiotics (📖 p.135).
- Advise patients to avoid cold and maintain adequate hydration.
- Warn about the dangers of anaesthetics (a Medic-Alert bracelet is helpful).
- Treat infection early.
- Give analgesia for painful crises – admit if severe.
- Admit if significant crisis of any sort (e.g. stroke, dyspnoea, acute abdomen, aplastic anaemia).
- Refer for early management of long-term complications (e.g. renal failure, epilepsy).

Advice for patients: Information and support for patients and their families

UK Thalassaemia Society 🖳 www.ukts.org
Sickle Cell Society ☎ 0800 001 5660 🖳 www.sicklecellsociety.org

The purpuras

Purpura is blue–brown discolouration of the skin due to bleeding within it. Petechiae are small dot-like purpura whilst ecchymoses are more extensive.

> ⚠ Refer any child with purpura for a same-day paediatric opinion. Although ITP and Henoch Schlönlein purpura are usually benign, more serious causes (e.g. leukaemia) need to be excluded.

Vascular purpura: Results from damage to the vessel wall. *Due to:*
- Infection (e.g. meningococcal septicaemia, EBV)
- Immune dysfunction (e.g. Henoch-Schönlein purpura)
- Vitamin C deficiency
- Drug reaction (e.g. steroid-induced purpura).

Thrombocytopoenic purpura: Pupura is related to the level of the platelet count. Bleeding is inevitable if platelet count ↓ to $<5–10×10^9/l$.
- *Non-immune thrombocytopoenic purpura:* Results from conditions which damage the bone marrow e.g. aplastic anaemia (📖 p.112), leukaemia (📖 p.120).
- *Immune thrombocytopoenic purpura:* Usually idiopathic (ITP). May rarely be associated with SLE, transfusions or drug reactions.

Idiopathic thrombocytopoenic purpura (ITP): Often occurs after viral illness or immunization. The child is purpuric with a platelet count of $<10–20×10^9/l$. Despite this severe bleeding is rare.

Management: Refer to paediatrics as an emergency. Often no specific treatment is needed once leukaemia has been excluded. Severe cases are treated with steroids and immunoglobulin. Usually remits spontaneously in <6–8wk. but becomes chronic in 15–20% (particularly ♀ >10y.).

Impaired platelet function: May occur with any haematological malignancy resulting in bleeding – even if the platelet count is normal.

Henoch-Schönlein purpura (HSP): Presents with a purpuric rash over buttocks and extensor surfaces. Often follows a respiratory infection. ♂>♀. *Other features:*
- Urticaria
- Nephritis
- Joint pains
- Abdominal pain (± intussusception) – may mimic an acute abdomen
- Platelet count is normal

Management and prognosis: Refer to paediatrics for confirmation of diagnosis. Most children recover fully over a few months – a few develop long-term renal problems.

Further information

British Committee for Standards in Haematology Guidelines for the investigation and management of idiopathic thrombocytopoenic purpura in adults, children and pregnancy (2003) 🖥 www.bcshguidelines.com

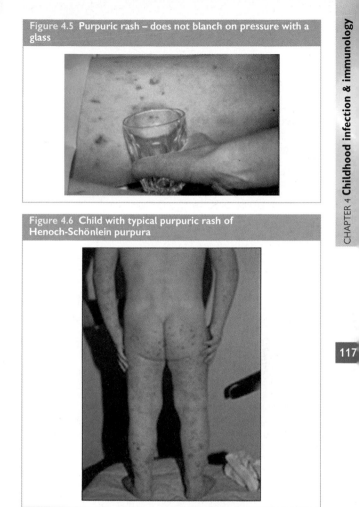

Figure 4.5 Purpuric rash – does not blanch on pressure with a glass

Figure 4.6 Child with typical purpuric rash of Henoch-Schönlein purpura

Advice for patients: Information and support for patients with ITP

ITP Support Association 🖳 www.itpsupport.org.uk

Figure 4.5 is reproduced with permission from the Meningitis Research Foundation UK
🖳 www.meningitis.org
Figure 4.6 permission sought from Healthopaedia.com (🖳 www.healthopaedia.com).

Clotting factor deficiencies

Clotting factor deficiencies may be congenital or acquired.
- **Congenital:** Genetic deficiencies of every clotting factor have been described but the majority of them are rare. The most common disorders of clotting factors are factor VIII deficiency (haemophilia A) and factor IX deficiency (haemophilia B).
- **Acquired clotting factor deficiencies:** Include vitamin K deficiency in newborns (📖 p.14) and liver disease.

Haemophilia: 2 common forms. Both are sex-linked recessive disorders. ♂>>♀.
- **Haemophilia A** (factor VIII deficiency): Prevalence 90/million population
- **Haemophilia B** (factor IX deficiency – Christmas disease): Prevalence 16/million population

Classification
- **Carrier** (♀ heterozygotes – >25% clotting factor activity)
- **Mild** (5–25% clotting factor activity)
- **Moderate** (2–5% clotting factor activity)
- **Severe** (50% haemophiliacs – ≤1% clotting factor activity)

Clinical features
- Bleeding into joints or muscles is often delayed following trauma. If untreated it can result in permanent damage.
- Pressure effects occur if bleeding takes place in a confined space e.g. intracranial bleed.
- Severity of bleeding is related to levels of clotting factors.

Management
- All haemophiliacs need long-term follow-up via a specialist haemophilia centre.
- Prenatal and antenatal screening is available – refer to genetics.
- Treatment can be 'on demand' or 'prophylactic'.

On-demand treatment:
- Transfusion of factor VIII or IX preparation as soon as possible after bleeding has started
- Symptomatic treatment of bleeds e.g. rest, analgesia ± physiotherapy for bleeds in muscles/joints

Prophylactic: Prevents bleeds and their consequences.
- Tranexamic acid: Prevents bleeding after minor surgical procedures for patients with mild haemophilia/carriers with symptoms.
- Desmopressin: Stimulates production of factor VIII (not factor IX). Prevents bleeding in patients with mild/moderate haemophilia A.
- Factor VIII or IX: Factor VIII 3x/wk. or factor IX 2x/wk.

Problems with treatment:

Inhibitors: 25% of patients have antibodies to factor VIII or IX products. These patients are treated with intravenous factor VIIa or with an 'immune tolerization programme' involving daily administration of factor VIII/IX.

Infection from blood products: ~1500 UK haemophiliacs have been infected with HIV through contaminated blood products; more with hepatitis B and C. Whenever possible genetically engineered 'recombinant' products are used rather than blood products.

von Willebrand's disease:

- Autosomal dominant deficiency of a clotting factor (vW factor).
- ♂=♀. *Prevalence:* 1% population.
- Most are mildly affected with easy bruising, nose bleeds and/or menorrhagia. Severe cases may bleed into joints.
- FBC – normal platelets; clotting screen – ↑ bleeding time.
- In all cases, refer to haematology for specialist management.
- Mild cases are managed with tranexamic acid, desmopressin and/or COC pill (for menorrhagia).
- Severe cases may need treatment with vW factor. No recombinant form available as yet.

Advice for patients: Information and support for patients and their families

Haemophilia Society ☎ 0800 018 6068 🖳 www.haemophilia.org.uk

Haematological malignancy

Acute leukaemia: The acute leukaemias are clonal malignant disorders (derived from a single cell) affecting all age groups. In children the peak age of onset is 2–4y. Rarely leukaemia in children is associated with other syndromes e.g. Down's syndrome, Wiskott-Aldrich syndrome and ataxia telangectasia. 2 major types of leukaemia affect children:

- *Acute lymphoblastic leukaemia (ALL):* 310 cases/y. in England and Wales (~85% of childhood leukaemia). Abnormal proliferation of the lymphoid progenitor cells. Usual age range: 2–10y. with a peak at 3–4y.
- *Acute myeloid leukaemia (AML):* 60 cases/y. Derived from abnormal proliferation of a myeloid progenitor cell. There are at least 7 different subtypes. Risk factors include previous chemotherapy or radiotherapy and exposure to radiation.

Presentation: Short history (weeks). Syptoms/signs arise from:

Bone marrow failure:
- Anaemia – pallor, lethargy, dyspnoea
- Neutropoenia – infections of the mouth, throat, skin, fever
- Thrombocytopoenia – spontaneous bruising, menorrhagia, bleeding from wounds, bleeding of gums or nose bleeds

Organ infiltration:
- Superficial lymphadenopathy (>50%)
- Hepatosplenomegaly (70%)
- Bone pain (ALL only)
- Skin infiltration (AML only)
- Testicular enlargement
- Respiratory symptoms due to mediastinal LNs
- Gum hypertrophy
- Unexplained irritability

Differential diagnosis:
- Infections e.g. EBV
- Other blood conditions e.g. aplastic anaemia, ITP
- Other malignancies e.g. lymphoma, neuroblastoma
- Juvenile rheumatoid arthritis

Investigations: Indications for FBC and blood film – Box 4.5.
- *FBC* normal or ↓ Hb and platelets; WCC <1x10^9/l to >200x10^9/l.
- *Blood film* is abnormal with presence of blast cells.

Management: In all cases refer for urgent specialist management – for referral guidelines see Box 4.5.

Lymphoma: Malignant transformation of lymphocytes. In children the peak age of onset is 10–14y. Rarely it is associated with rare syndromes e.g. Wiskott-Aldrich syndrome and ataxia telangectasia.

Hodgkin's lymphoma: 50 cases/y. in England and Wales.
- Characterized by the presence of Reed-Sternberg cells.
- Presents with non-tender cervical/supraclavicular lymphadenopathy. A minority have systemic symptoms.
- History tends to be long.

Non-Hodgkin's lymphoma: 70 cases/y. in England and Wales.
- Presents with cervical and/or supraclavicular lymphadenopathy and/or disease in the abdomen (hepatosplenomegaly) or mediastinum, pleural effusion, SVC obstruction or dyspnoea.
- There tends to be a rapid progression of symptoms.

Differential diagnosis: Infection causing lymphadenopathy (e.g. EBV), acute leukaemia.

Management: In all cases refer urgently for specialist management. Referral guidelines — Box 4.5.

Box 4.5 Referral guidelines[N]

Acute leukaemia
Refer immediately
- Hepatosplenomegaly or
- Unexplained petechiae

Check FBC and blood film if:
- Pallor and/or fatigue
- Unexplained irritability
- Unexplained fever
- Persistent or recurrent URTIs
- Generalized lymphadenopathy
- Persistent or unexplained bone pain
- Unexplained bruising

🛈 If the blood film or FBC indicates leukaemia, make an *urgent referral.*

Lymphoma
Refer immediately
- Hepatosplenomegaly or
- Mediastinal or hilar mass on CXR

Refer urgently (particularly if there is no evidence of local infection):
- non-tender, firm or hard lymph nodes
- lymph nodes >2cm in size
- lymph nodes progressively enlarging
- other features of general ill-health, fever or weight loss
- any axillary nodes (in the absence of local infection or dermatitis)
- any supraclavicular nodes
- shortness of breath (particularly if not responding to bronchodilators)

GMS Contract: Cancer targets — 📖 p.189

Advice for patients: Information and support for patients and families

Children with Leukaemia ☎ 020 7404 0808
🖥 www.leukaemia.org.uk
Lymphoma Association ☎ 0808 808 5555 🖥 www.lymphoma.org.uk

Further information
NICE Referral guidelines for suspected cancer (2005)
🖥 www.nice.org.uk

Chapter 5

Cardiac and respiratory problems in children

123

Congenital heart disease

Common affecting ~6:1000 live births. Congenital heart disease is the major cause of heart disease in children – Table 5.1

Detection:

Antenatal screening: Congenital heart disease may be detected *in utero* by USS. If detected during the routine 10–13wk. or 18wk. anomaly scan, amniocentesis is routinely offered to screen for Down's syndrome (~1:20 have heart disease—especially PDA, ASD and/or VSD) and other chromosomal abnormalities.

❶ The exact nature of heart defects detected on antenatal USS is often not clear until birth—this can present parents with difficult decisions if there is any question of termination.

Examination: Neonatal examination detects ~44% of cardiac malformations detected <1y. of age. The rest are detected during routine developmental checks, if a murmur is detected incidentally when examining the child for another reason, or when the child becomes symptomatic.

Common presentations

Murmur on routine examination: Table 5.2, 🕮 p.129

Ventriculoseptal defect (VSD): Harsh pansystolic murmur with splitting of the 2nd heart sound. Isolated VSD is the commonest congenital lesion in children (about 2:1000 births). Also occurs as a result of other complex lesions (e.g. Fallot's tetralogy).

Atrioseptal defect (ASD): Systolic murmur in the pulmonary area with fixed splitting of the 2nd heart sound. May also present with heart failure or arrhythmia in a young adult,

Patent ductus arteriosus (PDA): Loud, continuous 'machinery' murmur.

Aortic stenosis: Ejection systolic murmur at the apex & left sternal edge with a soft and delayed 2nd heart sound. Slow rising pulse, ↓BP. Rarely dizziness, faintness or loss of consciousness on exertion.

Pulmonary stenosis: Ejection systolic murmur with ejection click.

Coarctation of the aorta: Ejection systolic murmur over the left side and back; absent/delayed femoral pulses and upper limb hypertension.

Innocent murmurs: Murmurs are a common finding in childhood, particularly when examining a febrile child. The majority are not associated with heart disease—so-called 'innocent murmurs'. *Features:*
• Asymptomatic
• Soft, systolic murmur—may vary with position and does not radiate
• Normal 2nd heart sound
• No other associated signs of heart disease (normal pulses, no thrill)

⚠ Unless a child is febrile when a murmur is heard—and the murmur disappears once afebrile—refer all children with murmurs for Echo or paediatric evaluation.

Table 5.1 Congenital cardiac abnormalities

Condition	Features
Coarctation of the aorta	📖 p.130
Tetralogy of Fallot	Large VSD and pulmonary stenosis. In the newborn period may present with a murmur. Progressive cyanosis then develops over the next weeks/years ± ↓ exercise tolerance ± squatting after exercise. Treatment is surgical.
Hypoplastic left heart	Left ventricle ± mitral valve, aortic valve and aortic arch are underdeveloped. Presents within the 1st few days of life with heart failure. Treatment is surgical. Prognosis is poor without heart transplant.
Patent ductus arteriosus (PDA)	The ductus arteriosus fails to close after birth. ♀>♂. Associated with prematurity. Symptoms depend on the size of the shunt. Presents with murmur ± failure to thrive ± heart failure. Treatment is usually surgical closure.
Transposition of the great arteries	The aorta arises from the right ventricle and the pulmonary artery from the left. Progressive cyanosis develops within a few hours of birth. Treatment is surgical.
Valve disease	📖 p.128
ASD	📖 p.130
VSD	📖 p.130

GP Notes: Innocent murmur

❶ Once a murmur has been assessed as being innocent, explain what that means to the parents—otherwise there may be unnecessary ongoing anxiety.

Advice for patients: A parent's experience of antenatal diagnosis

'Every time we went to the hospital we were told, "Well this is what we think is wrong." Which I know must be very, very difficult because at the end of the day they're scanning your baby through your tummy and it's very hard...Unfortunately for our daughter she couldn't have corrective surgery...But they still said to us, "Well we think this is the problem, but you know we may be slightly not quite right, and when she's born we may be able to correct her heart depending on how certain things are." So when we were given the option of termination that was always in the back of our minds. Well how could we consider terminating a baby when the baby could have corrective heart surgery and everything could be fine? So we found that really, really hard.'

Patient experience information is reproduced with permission from Oxford University and DIPEx™ (UK Charity 1087019) 🖰 www.dipex.org.uk

Heart failure:
- Breathlessness, particularly when crying for feeding
- Failure to thrive
- Sweating
- Fast respiratory and pulse rates
- Heart enlargement
- Liver enlargement
- Weight increased due to fluid retention

Causes of heart failure in the 1st week of life include: Left outflow obstruction; severe aortic stenosis; coarctation of the aorta; hypoplastic left heart

Later causes: Large VSD; PDA; ostium primum VSD

Cyanosis:
- **<48h. old:** Likely to be due to transposition of the great arteries or severe pulmonary stenosis.
- **Later presentation:** Mostly due to *Tetralogy of Fallot* (Table 5.1, 📖 p.125).

Management: In all cases, if new congenital heart disease is detected, refer for specialist paediatric and/or cardiology opinion. Specialist treatment of valve lesions depends on the gradient measured across the valve. Most other congenital cardiac lesions (except VSD and ASD) require surgery–staged for complex lesions.

Prevention of endocarditis: An episode of endocarditis may be the presenting feature of congenital heart disease. There is ↑ risk of developing endocarditis in patients with valve lesions, septal defects (which persists after repair), PDA and particularly in those with prosthetic valves. All these patients require antibiotic prophylaxis for dental and surgical procedures–📖 p.135.

Marfan's syndrome: Autosomal dominant connective tissue disease causing abnormalities of fibrillin (a glycoprotein in elastic fibres). If suspected refer to cardiology ± genetics. *Features include:* Arachnodactyly (long spidery fingers); high-arched palate; arm span > height; lens dislocation ± unstable iris; aortic dilatation (β-blockers appear to slow this); aortic incompetence can develop; aortic dissection may cause sudden death–Echo screening may be helpful for affected individuals.

Further information
Journal of the Royal College of Physicians of London Hunter S Congenital heart disease in adolescence (2000) **34**(2) pp.150–2

Advice for patients: Parents' experiences of diagnosis of congenital heart disease

Problems feeding

'Alex was born due to a normal delivery...She fed well and put on weight for the first two or three weeks of life and then she started to have problems feeding. I was breast-feeding at the time and I knew that there was something wrong...Health visitors and midwives didn't really pick up on it and felt that I was just having trouble breast-feeding...I tried bottle-feeding her and she continued not to put on weight...My health visitor said that it was because it was hot weather and things like that and not to worry...Towards the fifth week I was worried because she still hadn't put any more weight on from two weeks old. In fact she'd lost and I was very worried about this. So I took her to see the GP at 5 weeks old and my GP looked at her briefly, made a phone call to the hospital, sent me immediately up to the hospital and said that she could have a heart problem.'

Cyanosis

'And it all came to a head when she was four and a half months...and the little one, the baby, started with a cold so she was all runny-nosed and very snuffly and not right at all...I managed to get an appointment, didn't see our usual GP and saw a female doctor who I hadn't seen before...and she said, "How long has she been like this?". "What do you mean? She's got a cold. You know, the cold sort of started a couple of days ago but she's getting really snuffly." "No, how long has she been cyanosed?", which is blueness, and I said, "Oh she's been like this ever since she was born." She said, "Well she's definitely cyanosed" and she sounded her chest and I could see the alarm bells ringing for her...And she said, you know, "I want her to go hospital now."...And then he [the hospital doctor] said, "I think, I think that her heart is, she's in heart failure."'

Breathlessness

'We were on holiday...we noticed that she was quite breathless...we returned back and I took my daughter to the doctor's, to my local GP...She checked her over and gave her some antibiotics for her chest infection and she asked me, she didn't alarm me at all, but she asked me to come back the following week...We returned the following week and the doctor mentioned that she could hear a heart murmur and she said, "Don't be alarmed. You know, it's found in many children. Don't worry about it but just to, you know, to have it double-checked she needs to be referred to the hospital."...The doctor sounded her and he said yes that there was definitely a murmur there...and they took the ultrasound...and they said that yeah, [our daughter] had a hole in her heart.'

Patient experience information is reproduced with permission from Oxford University and DIPEx™ (UK Charity 1087019) 🖳 www.dipex.org.uk

Valve lesions

The heart valves can become narrowed (stenosis) or leak (regurgitation). In both circumstances, the blood flow through the heart is disrupted and a murmur results. Other effects depend on which valve is affected and the degree to which the valve lesion affects the function of the heart as a pump.

Presentation: Valve disease usually presents with a murmur ± symptoms of dyspnoea, fatigue and/or palpitations.

Valve lesions

Mitral regurgitation (incompetence): In children almost always primary and due to valve disease. Causes include:
- Congenital including mitral valve prolapse ('floppy mitral valve')— commonest cause
- Rheumatic fever–often other valve lesions too
- Cardiomyopathy
- Endocarditis.

Mitral valve prolapse: Prevalence ~1:20. Usually no symptoms. A rare complication is ventricular arrhythmia.

Mitral stenosis: Usually due to rheumatic fever. May cause pulmonary hypertension which presents with right heart failure, haemoptysis and/or recurrent bronchitis.

Aortic stenosis: May be congenital e.g. bicuspid aortic valve (~1:1000) or due to rheumatic fever or hypertrophic cardiomyopathy.

Aortic regurgitation: May be congenital e.g. due to VSD or bicuspid aortic valve or due to rheumatic fever, endocarditis, cardiomyopathy or connective tissue abnormalities e.g. Marfan's or Ehlers-Danlos syndrome.

Right heart valve disease:
- *Tricuspid stenosis:* Mitral valve disease always coexists. Usually caused by rheumatic fever.
- *Tricuspid regurgitation:* Causes include right ventricular enlargement, rheumatic fever and congenital valve abnormalities.
- *Pulmonary stenosis:* Causes include Fallot's tetralogy and rheumatic fever.
- *Pulmonary regurgitation:* Caused by pulmonary hypertension.

Management: Unless a child is febrile when a murmur is heard, and the murmur disappears when the child becomes afebrile, in all cases refer for confirmation of diagnosis by Echo and/or paediatric evaluation. Specialist treatment of valve lesions depends on the gradient measured across the valve.

⚠ Give antibiotic prophylaxis (📖 p.135) for dental or surgical procedures for all children with valve lesions with the exception of mitral valve prolapse where antibiotic prophylaxis should be given if there is regurgitation or thickened (myxomatous) mitral valve leaflets.

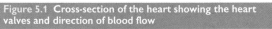

Table 5.2 Differential diagnosis of heart murmurs

Type of murmur	Description	Causes
Ejection systolic murmur	↑ to reach a peak midway between the heart sounds.	• Flow murmurs e.g children, pregnancy, with fever, during/after exercise • Aortic stenosis • Pulmonary stenosis • HOCM (🕮 p.136)
Pan-systolic murmur	Uniform intensity between the 2 heart sounds. Merges with 2nd heart sound.	• Mitral valve regurgitation or prolapse • Tricuspid regurgitation • VSD (🕮 p.130) • ASD (🕮 p.130)
Early diastolic murmur	Occurs just after the 2nd heart sound. High pitched and easily missed.	• Aortic regurgitation • Pulmonary regurgitation • Tricuspid stenosis (mitral stenosis co-exists)
Mid-diastolic murmur	Midway between 2nd heart sound of 1 beat and 1st of the next. Rumbling and low pitched.	• Mitral stenosis • Aortic regurgitation

Figure 5.1 Cross-section of the heart showing the heart valves and direction of blood flow

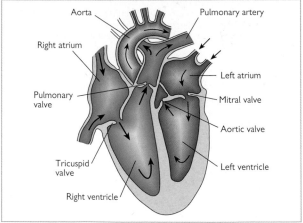

Aorta

Pulmonary artery

Right atrium

Left atrium

Pulmonary valve

Mitral valve

Aortic valve

Tricuspid valve

Left ventricle

Right ventricle

Figure 5.1 is reproduced with permission from the Patient UK website 🖳 www.patient.co.uk

Other structural heart abnormalities

Coarctation of the aorta: Figure 5.2. Localized narrowing of the descending aorta usually distal to the origin of the left subclavian artery.

Presentation: Heart failure; ↑ BP; murmur heard incidentally (ejection systolic murmur over the left side of the chest radiating to the back); lack of femoral pulses or radio-femoral delay; rarely presents with complications e.g. subarachnoid haemorrhage, endocarditis.

Management: Refer to cardiology—surgery to remove the narrowed portion of the aorta is usually indicated.

Atrial septal defect (ASD): A hole connects the 2 atria. Common—occurs in 2:1000 live births. Holes high in the septum (*ostium secundum*) are most common (Figure 5.3); holes lower in the septum (*ostium primum*) are associated with atrio-ventricular valve abnormalities. Blood flows from left → right through the shunt and the right heart takes the burden.

Presentation:
Ostium secundum defects:
- Symptoms are rare in infancy and uncommon in childhood. If detected in these groups presents as a murmur (systolic—loudest in the 2nd left interspace) found incidentally, or with breathlessness/tiredness on exertion, or recurrent chest infections.
- Presentation is usually in the 3rd or 4th decade with heart failure, pulmonary hypertension or atrial arrhythmias.

Ostium primum defects: Heart failure commonly develops in infancy/childhood ± severe pulmonary hypertension. In addition to the ASD murmur, there may be a pansystolic murmur signifying mitral or tricuspid valve regurgitation.

Management: Echo is diagnostic. Refer to cardiology. Cardiac surgery to close the defect is usually indicated. Mortality from percutaneous repair is low. Give all patients with ostium primum defects prophylactic antibiotics—📖 p.135.

Ventricular septal defect (VSD): A hole connects the 2 ventricles (Figure 5.4). Blood flows initially from left → right through the hole. Usually presents with a murmur (thrill may be palpable at the left sternal edge and pansystolic murmur). Other symptoms depend on the size of the defect—patients with small defects ('maladie de Roger') often have no symptoms. Patients with larger defects may present with breathlessness on feeding/crying, failure to thrive, cyanosis, heart failure and/or recurrent chest infections.

🚫 As the child gets older symptoms improve (as the relative size of the defect ↓).

Management: Diagnosis is confirmed on echo. Refer to cardiology (or admit to paediatrics if very unwell)—surgery is usually indicated.

⚠ All patients with VSD require prophylactic antibiotics (📖 p.135).

Figure 5.2 Coarctation of the aorta

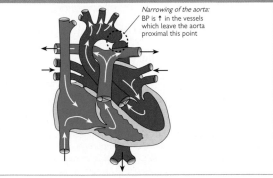

Narrowing of the aorta:
BP is ↑ in the vessels
which leave the aorta
proximal this point

Figure 5.3 Ostium secundum atrial septal defect

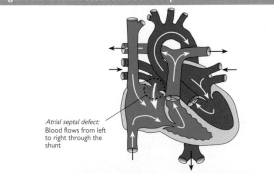

Atrial septal defect:
Blood flows from left
to right through the
shunt

Figure 5.4 Ventricular septal defect

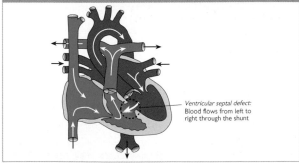

Ventricular septal defect:
Blood flows from left to
right through the shunt

Figures 5.2, 5.3 and 5.4 are reproduced from the Report of the Manitoba Pediatric Cardiac Surgery Inquest with permission.

Palpitations and arrhythmias

Children's hearts beat faster than adults. What would be a tachycardia in an adult can be normal in a child.

Normal pulse rate in children:

- **≤1y.:** 110–160 beats/min.
- **2–5y.:** 95–140 beats/min.
- **5–12y.:** 80–120 beats/min.
- **>12y.:** 60–100 beats/min.

Palpitations: Take a history of the symptoms and examine the child carefully to try to exclude arrhythmia. Symptoms suggestive of arrhythmia are palpitations associated with breathlessness or collapse. A history of cardiac abnormality e.g. congenital heart disease or cardiomyopathy also makes arrhythmia more likely.

Arrhythmia: Abnormal heart rhythm. Whilst arrhythmias are uncommon in children, they are a cause of sudden death in this age group. They are more common in children with pre-existing heart disease or where there is a family history of early death from arrhythmia.

History: Ask about:

- *Palpitations*—the sensation of rapid, irregular or forceful heartbeats. Ask about duration, frequency and pattern, and rhythm (ask the child to tap it out if not present when seen)
- *Precipitating/relieving factors*
- *Associated symptoms*—chest pain, collapse or funny turns, sweating, breathlessness or hyperventilation
- *Past history* e.g. previous episodes, heart disease, thyroid disease
- *Lifestyle (teenagers)*—drug history, caffeine/alcohol intake, smoking.

> ⚠ **Red flag symptoms:**
> - Pre-existing cardiovascular disease
> - Family history of syncope, arrhythmia or sudden death
> - Arrhythmia associated with falls and/or syncope

Examination

- *General examination:* For anaemia, thyrotoxicosis, anxiety, other systemic disease
- *Cardiovascular examination*: Heart size, pulse rate and rhythm, JVP, BP, heart sounds and murmurs, evidence of left ventricular failure

Investigations

- *First-line:* Resting ECG is all that is needed for many patients. If abnormal refer.
- *Further investigations:* Consider ambulatory ECG or cardiac memo; *Blood:* TFTs, FBC, ESR, U&E, fasting blood glucose, Ca^{2+}, albumin.

Common childhood arrhythmias: Table 5.3.

Further information

British Heart Foundation Factfile Palpitations: their significance and investigation (04/2004) 🖳 www.bhf.org.uk
National Service Framework (NSF) for Coronary Heart Disease (2005) 🖳 www.dh.gov.uk

Table 5.3 Common arrhythmias in childhood

Arrhythmia and characteristics	Management
Ventricular ectopic beats Additional broad QRS complexes, without P waves, superimposed on regular sinus rhythm. Common in children and usually of no clinical significance. Rarely may be the presenting feature of viral myocarditis.	*Frequent ectopics (>100/h.) on ECG: Refer urgently to paediatrics.* No *sinister features on ECG*: Explain the benign nature of the condition. Advise avoidance of caffeine and fatigue.
Sinus tachycardia Fast heart rate with normal ECG	Consider infection, pain, shock, exercise, emotion (including anxiety), heart failure, thyrotoxicosis, drugs.
Paroxysmal supraventricular tachycardia Narrow QRS complex tachycardia with a regular rate >180bpm on ECG.	*If seen during an attack*: Get an ECG if possible. Try carotid sinus massage, the Valsalva manoeuvre and/or ice on the face or immersing the face in iced water (especially effective for children—explain to parents what you are doing and why). *Admit as an emergency* if the attack continues. *If the attack stops or diagnosed from history or ambulatory ECG*: Refer for confirmation of diagnosis and initiation of treatment—urgent referral if chest pain, dizziness or breathlessness during attacks. Enclose the ECG trace during an attack if available. *Treatment options*: Treatment is not always required. When needed options are medical treatment with anti-arrhythmics or, in severe cases, surgical ablation of the bypass tract.
Wolff-Parkinson-White syndrome Due to an accessory conduction pathway. Predisposes to SVT and AF. *ECG*: short P-R interval followed by slurred upstroke ('delta wave') into the QRS complex.	Refer. Treatment is with anti-arrhythmics ± ablation of the accessory pathway.
No tachycardia and no ECG abnormalities	Reassure. Explore the possibility of anxiety disorder.

The NSF for Coronary Heart Disease recommends:
- **Referral to a heart rhythm expert:** All 1st degree relatives of sudden cardiac death patients who died <40y.
- **Referral to a paediatric cardiologist:** Any child with:
  - recurrent loss of conciousness or collapse on exertion
  - atypical seizure and normal EEG
  - documented arrhythmia

Infective endocarditis

Infective endocarditis occurs when there is infection of a heart valve. Although uncommon, consequences may be disastrous and endocarditis is often detected late. The valve is usually congenitally abnormal or rheumatic but may be normal. Endocarditis can be the presenting feature of congenital heart disease. In children, common causative organisms include *Strep. viridans* and *Staph. aureus*.

Presentation: May be acute with heart failure and/or septicaemia, or subacute with fever, anaemia and leucocytosis. Usually a new or changed murmur is audible. Classic signs such as splinter haemorrhages and Osler's nodes are uncommon in children, but microscopic haematuria may occur.

Management: Have a high index of suspicion in children with known heart disease and fever. Admit as an emergency if suspected. Avoid starting antibiotics prior to admission as this might cause delay in diagnosis by rendering the blood cultures sterile. Hospital treatment is with prolonged IV broad-spectrum antibiotics (≥2wk.).

Prevention: Those at high/moderate risk of infective endocarditis (Table 5.4) should take prophylactic antibiotics prior to any procedure that might cause a transient bacteraemia (Tables 5.5 & 5.6). Good dental hygiene is also important including regular dentist check-ups.

Further information

British Heart Foundation Factfiles Infective endocarditis (12/2003 & 1/2004) 🖳 www.bhf.org.uk

Table 5.4 **Risk of developing infective endocarditis**		
Risk	**Condition**	**Antibiotic prophylaxis**
High	Prosthetic heart valve Past history of infective endocarditis Complex cyanotic congenital heart disease	Required
Moderate	Significant mitral valve prolapse (take consultant advice) Valvular dysfunction (e.g. following rheumatic heart disease, congenital valve disease especially bicuspid aorta) Ventricular septal defects Primum atrial septal defects HOCM Past history of rheumatic fever	Required
Low	Murmurs not due to valve disease e.g. flow murmurs in febrile children	Not required

Table 5.5 Procedures requiring antibiotic prophylaxis

Procedures requiring prophylaxis		Procedures not requiring prophylaxis
High- & moderate-risk patients	*High-risk patients only*	
Dental procedures which can → gum bleeding (i.e. virtually all dental procedures) Surgery (excluding skin surgery)—warn consultant in referral letter Lower GI or GU endoscopy	All endoscopic procedures including proctoscopy and sigmoidoscopy Insertion of a urethral catheter in a patient with infected urine (ensure infecting organism is sensitive to prophylactic antibiotics)	Routine phlebotomy Insertion of IV cannula (though should be changed frequently)

⚠ If in doubt ask advice from the cardiologist in charge of the child's care or a specialist in infectious diseases.

Table 5.6 Antibiotic regimens for use in primary care BNF 5.1

Patients	Antibiotics
All patients *except:* • those with a past history of endocarditis • those who are penicillin-allergic • those who have had >1 dose of penicillin in the previous month	Child >10y.—amoxicillin 3g po 1h. before the procedure (child <5y.—¼ dose; child 5–10y.—½ dose)
Patients allergic to penicillin *or* Patients who have received >1 dose of penicillin in the previous month	Child >10y.—clindamycin 600mg po 1h. before the procedure (child <5y.—¼ dose; child 5–10y.—½ dose)
Patients with a past history of endocarditis	The procedure should be carried out in hospital with IV gentamicin prior to the procedure then amoxicillin 6h. after the procedure

---

Advice for patients: Information and support for parents and children

Children's Heart Federation ☎ 0808 808 5000
🖳 www.childrens-heart-fed.org.uk

Children's Heart Association ☎ 01706 221 988
🖳 www.heartchild.info

Heartline Association ☎ 01276 707 636 🖳 www.heartline.org.uk

Rheumatic fever, myocarditis and cardiomyopathy

Rheumatic fever: Rare in developed countries but incidence is increasing. Endemic disease in developing countries. *Peak age:* 5–15y. Due to an abnormal immunological response to β-haemolytic strepto-coccal infection (e.g. 2–wk. after sore throat). Diagnosis can be made if Revised Jones criteria are met (Table 5.7).

Management: If suspected refer for specialist care. 60% develop chronic rheumatic heart disease (70% mitral valve; 40% aortic; 10% tricuspid; 2% pulmonary). Likelihood ↑ with severity of initial disease. Recurrence may occur after further streptococcal infection or be precipitated by pregnancy or the COC pill.

2° *prevention:*
- Penicillin bd or sulfadiazine od for ≥5y. to prevent recurrence. Duration of prophylaxis is dependent on whether there was carditis in the initial attack (no carditis—continued for 5y.; if cardiac involvement—continued until ≥25y).
- Once regular prophylaxis has stopped, patients should continue to have prophylactic antibiotics for dental/operative procedures for life (Tables 5.5 & 5.6—📖 p.135).

Cardiomyopathy: Primary disease of the heart muscle.

Dilated (congestive) cardiomyopathy: Dilation of left ± right ventricle and ↓ contractility. Presents with fatigue and ↓ exercise tolerance (mild cases); breathlessness and heart failure (more severe cases) and arrhythmia (rarely). *ECG:* non-specific S-T abnormalities. *CXR:* ↑ heart size and pulmonary venous hypertension. Echo is diagnostic.

Causes:
- Idiopathic or familial (20%)
- Infection (Coxsackie virus)
- Cardiovascular—congenital heart disease, rheumatic heart disease
- Cardiotoxic drugs
- Endocrine disease—myxoedema, thyrotoxicosis
- Metabolic e.g. glycogen storage diseases, haemochromatosis
- Muscular dystrophy

Management: Refer for specialist management. Treatment is symptomatic. The most severe cases may eventually require heart transplant.

Hypertrophic cardiomyopathy: Familial inheritance (autosomal dominant) but ½ are sporadic—in its commonest form causes asymetrical septal hypertrophy ± aortic outflow obstruction (obstructive hypertrophic cardiomyopathy or HOCM). Many are diagnosed through screening of asymptomatic patients with a FH using echo. *Symptoms/signs:*
- Palpitations—associated with arrhythmia
- Breathlessness on exertion
- Chest pain—may be angina or atypical pain
- Murmur—due to outflow obstruction and/or mitral valve dysfunction
- Faints/collapses

Table 5.7 Revised Jones criteria for diagnosis of rheumatic fever

Evidence of previous streptococcal infection (scarlet fever, +ve throat swab and/or ↑ ASO titre >200u/ml)

and

2 major criteria

or

1 major + 2 minor criteria

Major criteria	Minor criteria
Carditis (45–70%) – arrhythmia, new murmur, pericardial rub, heart failure, conduction defects	Prolonged P-R interval on ECG (but not if carditis is one of the major criteria)
Migratory polyarthritis ('flitting' –75%) – red, tender joints	Arthralgia (but not if arthritis is one of the major criteria)
Sydenham's chorea (St. Vitus' dance – 10%)	Fever
	↑ESR or ↑CRP
Subcutaneous nodules (2–20%)	History of rheumatic heart disease or rheumatic fever
Erythema marginatum (2–10%)	

Investigations: Echo – diagnostic. Refer if suspicious symptoms or family history.

Management and prognosis: Ensure antibiotic prophylaxis (Tables 5.5 & 5.6—📖 p.135). Ongoing specialist care is essential. The major cause of mortality is sudden death which is unrelated to severity of symptoms.

Acute myocarditis: Inflammation of the myocardium. Presents with chest pain, heart failure and/or palpitations. Causes include viral infections (e.g. Coxsackie virus), diphtheria and rheumatic fever.

Management: Admit for specialist care. Treatment is supportive. Some recover spontaneously–others progress to intractable heart failure requiring transplantation.

Heart transplant: Considered in patients with estimated 1y. survival of <50%. Post-operatively patients require lifelong immunosuppression–usually with ciclosporin A. Follow-up is undertaken in specialist clinics.

137

Advice for patients: Patient information and support

Cardiomyopathy Association ☎ 01923 249977
🖳 www.cardiomyopathy.org
Cardiac Risk in the Young (Cry) ☎ 01737 363 222
🖳 www.c-r-y.org.uk

Diagnosis of asthma in children

Symptoms/signs of a severe asthma attack in children >2y.:
- Unable to complete sentences in one breath or too breathless to talk/feed
- Tachycardia:
  - Pulse >120 bpm if >5y.
  - Pulse >130 bpm if 2–5y.
- Tachypnoea:
  - respiratory rate >30 breaths/min. if >5y.
  - respiratory rate >50 breaths/min. if 2–5y.

Life-threatening signs in children age >2y.:
- Central cyanosis
- Silent chest (inaudible wheeze)
- Poor respiratory effort
- Confusion
- Exhaustion
- Hypotension
- Coma

Symptoms/signs of a significant asthma attack if <2y.:
- Audible wheezing
- Using accessory muscles
- Cyanosis
- Marked respiratory distress
- Too breathless to feed

Management of an acute asthma attack: 📖 p.44

Asthma and viral-associated wheeze: Childhood asthma affects ~5% of children in the UK and the prevalence is increasing. Virus-associated wheeze affects up to 20% of children at some point. Peak age of onset is 5y. Most wheezing episodes in infancy are precipitated by respiratory infections and will often resolve spontaneously. It can be difficult to differentiate between asthma and non-asthmatic viral-associated wheeze. Asthma is suggested by persisting symptoms and signs between acute attacks and/or a personal or family history of atopic conditions e.g. eczema, hay fever. Differential diagnosis–Table 5.8.

Risk factors:
- Family history of atopy–particularly mother and/or siblings
- Coexistence of atopic disease–this is also a risk factor for persistence of symptoms
- In prepubertal children ♂:♀=3:2. After puberty ♀>♂. Boys are more likely to 'grow out' of their symptoms
- Bronchiolitis in infancy
- Parental smoking–particularly the mother
- Prematurity
- Age at first presentation–the earlier the onset, the better the prognosis. Most children presenting aged <2y. are free of symptoms by 6–11y.

History: History is the cornerstone of diagnosis. Suspect asthma in any child with a history of ≥1 of:
- Persistent or recurrent dry cough–particularly if worse at night
- Wheeze (or noisy breathing)
- Breathlessness
- Tightness of the chest.

Making a diagnosis of asthma in children: Figure 5.5 📖 p.141

Table 5.8 Differential diagnosis of wheezing in children

Clinical clue	Possible diagnosis
Perinatal and family history	
Symptoms present from birth or with perinatal lung problems	CF, chronic lung disease, ciliary dyskinesia, developmental anomaly e.g. tracheo-oesophageal fistula
Family history of unusual chest disease	CF, developmental anomaly, neuro-muscular disorder
Severe upper respiratory tract disease	Defect of host defence
Symptoms and signs	
Persistent wet cough	CF, recurrent aspiration, host defence disorder
Excessive vomiting or posseting	Reflux ± aspiration
Dysphagia	Swallowing problems ± aspiration
Abnormal voice or cry	Laryngeal problem
Focal signs in the chest	Developmental disease, post-viral syndrome, bronchiectasis, TB
Inspiratory stridor as well as wheeze	Central airways or laryngeal disorder
Failure to thrive	CF, host defence defect, gastro-oesophageal reflux
Investigations	
Focal or persistent radiological changes	Developmental disorder, post-infective disorder, recurrent aspiration, inhaled foreign body, bronchiectasis, TB

GMS contract

Asthma 1	The practice can produce a register of patients with asthma, excluding patients with asthma who have been prescribed no asthma-related drugs in the last 12mo.	4 points	
Asthma 8	% of patients aged ≥8y. diagnosed as having asthma from 1.4.2006 with measures of variability or reversibility	up to 15 points	40–80%

139

Advice for patients: Information and support for parents and children

Asthma UK ☎ 08457 01 02 03 ▥ www.asthma.org.uk

Table 5.8 is reproduced from the British guideline on the management of asthma (2004) with permission from British Thoracic Society/SIGN.

Common precipitating/exacerbating factors:

- Exercise
- Emotion
- Weather–fog, cold air, thunderstorms
- Air pollutants–smoke, dust
- Household allergens–house dust mite, animal fur, feathers
- Infection–commonly viral URTI, chest infection
- Drugs–NSAIDs, β-blockers

Examination: Is often normal.

- When there are signs, the most common is audible wheeze heard within the chest via a stethoscope.
- There may be signs of other associated atopic conditions e.g. eczema or hayfever or triggering conditions e.g. URTI.
- Rarely severe asthma may cause impaired growth/failure to thrive or chest deformity e.g. Harrison's sulcus or pigeon chest.

Investigations:

In schoolchildren: Diagnosis can be confirmed using:
- Bronchodilator responsiveness measured with PEFR or spirometry$^{£}$
- Peak flow variability (and night-time dipping) demonstrated through PEFR diary$^{£}$ or
- Bronchial hyper-reactivity testing$^{£}$.

In younger children: It is often not possible to measure airway function in order to confirm the presence of variable airways obstruction. Trial of medication may be the only way to confirm diagnosis.

Expected PEFR in children: 📖 p.146

Further information:

BMJ Learning Childhood asthma: diagnosis and treatment
🖥 www.bmjlearning.com
Clinical Evidence Keeley & McKean Asthma and other wheezing disorders in children (2004) Accessed via 🖥 www.nelh.nhs.uk
British Thoracic Society/SIGN British Guideline on the management of asthma (revised 2005) 🖥 www.sign.ac.uk

---

GP Notes: Measuring peak expiratory flow rate (PEFR) in children

- Use a low-range meter if predicted or best PEFR is <250l/min.
- Ask the patient to stand up (if possible) and hold the peak flow meter horizontally.
- Check the indicator is at zero and the track clear.
- Ask the patient to take a deep breath and blow out forcefully into the peak flow meter, ensuring lips are sealed firmly around the mouthpiece.
- Read the PEFR off the meter. The best of 3 attempts is recorded.
- If the child is having difficulty practise with a whistle or other suitable musical toy.

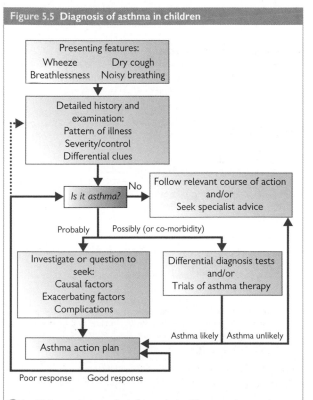

Figure 5.5 Diagnosis of asthma in children

Presenting features:
Wheeze   Dry cough
Breathlessness   Noisy breathing

Detailed history and examination:
Pattern of illness
Severity/control
Differential clues

Is it asthma?   No → Follow relevant course of action and/or Seek specialist advice

Probably   Possibly (or co-morbidity)

Investigate or question to seek:
Causal factors
Exacerbating factors
Complications

Differential diagnosis tests and/or Trials of asthma therapy

Asthma likely   Asthma unlikely

Asthma action plan

Poor response   Good response

141

● In children asthma tends to be extrinsic. Allergy testing may be useful in making a diagnosis of atopy and in seeking causal factors. Absence of allergy should prompt consideration of alternative diagnoses.

Figure 5.5 is reproduced from the British guideline on the management of asthma (2005) with permission from British Thoracic Society/SIGN.

Advice for patients: Frequently asked questions about childhood asthma

What is childhood asthma?

Asthma is a long-term condition which affects the lungs. The lungs allow us to breathe—exchanging old air in the body for fresh air outside. In asthma the lining of the lungs becomes over-sensitive. This prevents them doing their job properly. There are 4 main symptoms: cough, wheeze, breathlessness and chest tightness—you may have one or more of these at different times.

Why have I got asthma?

We don't know exactly why you have asthma. We know you are more likely to get asthma if other members of your family have asthma, especially your mother or her relations. Also we know that people with asthma have lungs which react too much to the environment around them. In children more boys than girls have asthma but boys are more likely to grow out of it as they get older.

Why have I developed asthma now?

Asthma can start at any age, even in adults. In most children asthma starts before the age of 5 but sometimes, if you only have mild asthma, it can take a long time for anyone to make a diagnosis.

What should I do to treat my asthma?

You will normally be started on treatment for your asthma and given instructions on how to use inhalers by your GP. Once your asthma is controlled the asthma nurse from your practice will follow you up at least once a year to check you are not having any problems and do breathing tests, answer your questions about asthma, and check you are using your medicines correctly.

The main inhalers used for treatment of asthma are:

- BLUE INHALER (salbutamol)—this is a reliever inhaler which you need to take when you feel wheezy or short of breath or if your chest is tight. It helps your lungs to expand so that it is easier to breathe
- BROWN INHALER (steroid inhaler)—this is a preventer inhaler which you usually take regularly in the mornings and evenings, and may need to continue taking for months or even years. You will not notice an immediate effect after taking this inhaler. It makes your lungs less sensitive and it less likely that you will get wheezy or short of breath.

There are other inhalers that are sometimes used if your asthma is more difficult to control and your doctor will explain these to you.

ALWAYS take your BLUE INHALER with you wherever you go, and make sure you take any other medicine you have for your asthma with you if you go for a sleepover or overnight school trip.

You may be given a SPACER DEVICE to attach to your inhaler. This makes it easier to take your inhaler, and makes your inhaler work better.

STEROID TABLETS (prednisolone) are sometimes also prescribed. They are usually given for just a short period of time to get your asthma under control. Generally they should be taken every day in the morning.

If your asthma is not as controlled as normal or you have new symptoms then you should make an appointment to see your GP. You should also see your GP before you stop any of your inhalers.

What if I do nothing about my asthma?

It is important to treat asthma and follow your doctor's or nurse's advice about taking the medicines (usually inhalers) you are given. Even people with mild asthma sometimes have severe flare-ups and become ill with their asthma. Every year thousands of people are admitted to hospital as a result of asthma attacks and a few even die.

Even if you never have a flare-up, it is still worth treating your asthma as asthma symptoms can make it difficult to enjoy school and leisure activities. The medicines you are given will prevent this happening.

What can make my asthma worse?

Different things affect different people's asthma in different ways. If you know what makes your asthma worse, it is worth trying to avoid it if possible. Things which can make asthma worse include:

- Having another illness such as a cold
- Air pollution such as cigarette smoke or city fumes
- Things you are allergic to such as pollen or animal fur
- Cold weather
- Stress—for example asthma may be worse during exams
- Some medicines such as ibuprofen.

In some people exercise makes asthma worse. Don't avoid exercise but use your blue inhaler before exercise to prevent symptoms and make sure you warm up before exercise and cool down afterwards. Avoid exercising outside in very cold weather and don't exercise if you have an infection such as a cold.

What will happen in the future?

Roughly:

- ¼ who have asthma as children grow out of it
- ¼ have occasional mild symptoms as adults
- ¼ grow out of their asthma as children but relapse as adults
- ¼ have ongoing symptoms

It is not possible in advance to predict which group you will be in.

Severe asthma attack:

Symptoms: Great difficulty in breathing, feeling panicky, unable to talk in full sentences.

Action:

- Try to keep as calm as possible as getting worried will make it more difficult to breath.
- Take your blue inhaler through a spacer if you have one. Repeat every 2–3 minutes until symptoms improve or help arrives.
- Call for help—if you can breathe with difficulty, but speak in whole sentences, you should call your GP; if you can't speak in sentences, are becoming too tired to continue to breathe properly, are becoming floppy or turning blue then call an ambulance.

Management of chronic childhood asthma

Aims of treatment
- To minimize symptoms and impact on lifestyle (e.g. absence from school; limitations to physical ability)
- To minimize the need for reliever medication
- To prevent severe attacks/exacerbations

Management of acute asthma in children: 📖 p.44

GP services: Ideally routine asthma care should be carried out in a specialized clinic. Doctors and nurses involved in asthma clinics need appropriate training with regular updates. Practices should keep an asthma register of affected patients to ensure adequate follow-up and allow audit[c].

Self-management: All children and parents/carers should receive:
- *Self-management education:* Brief, simple education linked to patient goals is most likely to be successful. Include information about: nature of disease, nature of the treatment and how to use it, self-monitoring/self-assessment, recognition of acute exacerbations, allergen/trigger avoidance, patient's own goals of treatment
- *Written action plan:* Focus on individual needs. Include information about features which indicate when asthma is worsening and what to do under those circumstances. Action plans ↓ morbidity and health costs from asthma[c]
- *PEFR monitoring:* For older children (at least school age), record PEFR at asthma review and if acute exacerbation. Home monitoring in combination with an action plan can be useful, especially for children with severe asthma, brittle asthma (i.e. rapid development of acute asthma attacks) and for those who are poor perceivers of their symptoms.

Reviews and monitoring: Frequency depends on needs. Aim to review all patients with asthma at least annually and more frequently if stepping up or stepping down treatment.
- Check symptoms since last seen. Use objective measures e.g. RCP 3 questions or Revised Jones Morbidity Index–Box 5.1.
- Record smoking status of parents of children with asthma and older children with asthma–advise smokers to stop.
- Record any exacerbations/acute attacks since last seen.
- Check medication–use, concordance (prescription count), inhaler technique, problems, side effects.
- Influenza vaccination is not included in the QoF for under-16s with asthma at present, but may become a requirement in future. Consider for all children >6mo. with asthma.
- Review objective measures of lung function e.g. home PEFR chart, PEFR at review.
- Address any problems or queries and educate about asthma.
- Agree management goals and date for further review.

Advice for patients: Self-help tips

Smoking: Smoking may ↑ symptoms of asthma–children who smoke and have asthma should stop. Cigarette smoke from parents of children with asthma can also make the children's symptoms worse and all parents of children with asthma should try to stop smoking, or at least refrain from smoking in the home and in the child's presence.

Weight: There is some evidence that weight loss in children who are overweight improves asthma control.

Allergen avoidance:

House dust mite: There is little evidence that reducing house dust mite results in improvement of asthma[C]. If you really want to try to exclude house dust mite you need:
- to regularly vacuum the house with a powerful vacuum cleaner with special dust filter
- to fit complete barrier bed coverings remove carpets, and remove soft toys from the bed
- to wash all bed linen at high temperature regularly and apply acaricides to soft furnishings
- to dehumidify the home.

There is no evidence that air ionizers have any beneficial effect.

Pets: There is no evidence that removing pets from a home results in improved symptoms[C] but many experts still advise removal of the pet for patients with asthma who also have an allergy to the pet.

Box 5.1 Objective measures of asthma symptoms: morbidity categories correlate with lung function

The Revised Jones Morbidity Index: *During the last 4 weeks:*
- Have you been in a wheezy or asthmatic condition at least once a week?
- Have you had time off work or school because of your asthma?*
- Have you suffered from attacks of wheezing during the night?

* If the patient does not work/go to school count as a NO answer.

RCP three questions: *In the last month:*
- Have you had any difficulty sleeping because of your asthma symptoms (including cough)?
- Have you had your usual asthma symptoms during the day (cough, wheeze, chest tightness or breathlessness)?
- Has your asthma interfered with your usual activities e.g. housework, work/school etc.?

NO to all questions = low morbidity
1 x YES answer = medium morbidity
2 or 3 x YES answer = high morbidity

🛈 These questionnaires are not designed for use during an acute attack.

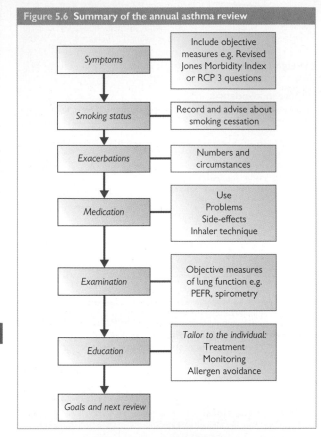

Figure 5.6 Summary of the annual asthma review

Symptoms — Include objective measures e.g. Revised Jones Morbidity Index or RCP 3 questions

Smoking status — Record and advise about smoking cessation

Exacerbations — Numbers and circumstances

Medication — Use / Problems / Side-effects / Inhaler technique

Examination — Objective measures of lung function e.g. PEFR, spirometry

Education — Tailor to the individual: Treatment / Monitoring / Allergen avoidance

Goals and next review

Table 5.9 Predicted PEFR measurements for children in l/min. (EU scale)

Height is the only determinant of PEFR in children. With ↑ age the pattern of adult values takes over.

Height: ft	3'	3'4"	3'8"	4'	4'4"	4'8"	5'	5'4"	5'8"	6'
m	90cm	1	1.1	1.2	1.3	1.4	1.5	1.6	1.7	1.8
PEFR l/min.	88	105	136	172	220	265	313	371	427	487

Drug therapy: Use a stepwise approach (Figures 5.7, 5.8 and 5.9). Start at the step most appropriate to the initial severity of symptoms. The aim is to achieve early control of the condition and then to ↓ treatment by stepping down.

> ⚠ **Exacerbations:** Children still die of asthma–step up rapidly during exacerbations, step down slowly. A rescue course of predni-solone 30–40mg od for 1–2wk. may be needed at any step and at any time.

Stepping down: Review and consider stepping down at intervals ≥3 mo. Maintain on the lowest dose of inhaled steroid controlling symptoms. When reducing steroids, cut dose by 25–50% each time.

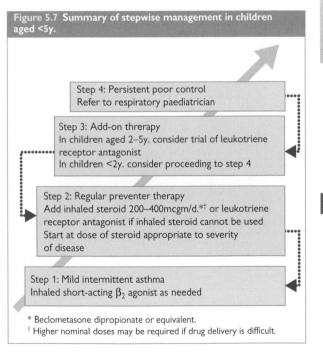

Figure 5.7 **Summary of stepwise management in children aged <5y.**

Step 4: Persistent poor control
Refer to respiratory paediatrician

Step 3: Add-on threrapy
In children aged 2–5y. consider trial of leukotriene receptor antagonist
In children <2y. consider proceeding to step 4

Step 2: Regular preventer therapy
Add inhaled steroid 200–400mcgm/d.*† or leukotriene receptor antagonist if inhaled steroid cannot be used
Start at dose of steroid appropriate to severity of disease

Step 1: Mild intermittent asthma
Inhaled short-acting β₂ agonist as needed

* Beclometasone dipropionate or equivalent.
† Higher nominal doses may be required if drug delivery is difficult.

147

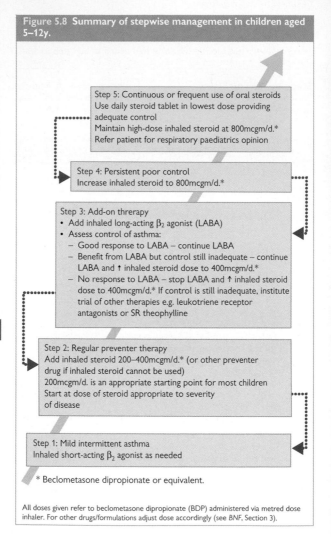

Figure 5.8 Summary of stepwise management in children aged 5–12y.

Step 5: Continuous or frequent use of oral steroids
Use daily steroid tablet in lowest dose providing adequate control
Maintain high-dose inhaled steroid at 800mcgm/d.*
Refer patient for respiratory paediatrics opinion

Step 4: Persistent poor control
Increase inhaled steroid to 800mcgm/d.*

Step 3: Add-on therapy
- Add inhaled long-acting β₂ agonist (LABA)
- Assess control of asthma:
  – Good response to LABA – continue LABA
  – Benefit from LABA but control still inadequate – continue LABA and ↑ inhaled steroid dose to 400mcgm/d.*
  – No response to LABA – stop LABA and ↑ inhaled steroid dose to 400mcgm/d.* If control is still inadequate, institute trial of other therapies e.g. leukotriene receptor antagonists or SR theophylline

Step 2: Regular preventer therapy
Add inhaled steroid 200–400mcgm/d.* (or other preventer drug if inhaled steroid cannot be used)
200mcgm/d. is an appropriate starting point for most children
Start at dose of steroid appropriate to severity of disease

Step 1: Mild intermittent asthma
Inhaled short-acting β₂ agonist as needed

* Beclometasone dipropionate or equivalent.

All doses given refer to beclometasone dipropionate (BDP) administered via metred dose inhaler. For other drugs/formulations adjust dose accordingly (see BNF, Section 3).

Figure 5.9 Summary of stepwise management in children >12y.

Step 5: Continuous or frequent use of oral steroids:
Use daily steroid tablet in lowest dose providing adequate control
Maintain high-dose inhaled steroid at 2000mcgm/d.*
Consider other treatments to minimise the use of steroid tablets
Refer patient for specialist care

Step 4: Persistent poor control
Consider trials of:
- Increase inhaled steroid to 2000mcgm/d.*
- Addition of a 4th drug e.g. leukotriene receptor agonist, SR theophylline, β_2 agonist tablet

Step 3: Add-on threrapy
- Add inhaled long-acting β_2 agonist (LABA)
- Assess control of asthma:

– Good response to LABA – continue LABA
– Benefit from LABA but control still inadequate – continue LABA and ↑ inhaled steroid dose to 800mcgm/d.*
– No response to LABA – stop LABA and ↑ inhaled steroid dose to 800mcgm/d.* If control is still inadequate, institute trial of other therapies e.g. leukotriene receptor antagonists or SR theophylline

Step 2: Regular preventer therapy
Add inhaled steroid 200–800mcgm/d.*
400mcgm/d is an appropriate starting point for many children>12y
Start at dose of steroid appropriate to severity of disease

Step 1: Mild intermittent asthma
Inhaled short-acting β_2 agonist as required

* Beclometasone dipropionate or equivalent.

Figures 5.8 and 5.9 are reproduced from the British guideline on the management of asthma (2005) with permission from British Thoracic Society/SIGN.

Selection of inhaler device:

- If possible use a metred dose inhaler (MDI).
- Spacers or breath-activated devices are useful for children who find activation difficult and essential for children <10y.
- Inadequate technique may be mistaken for drug failure—demonstrate inhaler technique before prescribing and check at follow-ups; emphasize patients must inhale slowly and hold their breath for 10sec. after inhalation.
- Dry powder inhalers are an alternative for older children.

Drugs: *BNF 3.1, 3.2 & 3.3*

Short-acting β_2 agonists: e.g. salbutamol. Use for relieving acute broncho-spasm and before exercise for exercise-induced wheeze. Work more quickly and/or with fewer side effects than alternatives. Use prn unless shown to benefit from regular dosing. Using $\geq$ canister/mo. or >10–12 puffs/d. is a marker of poorly controlled asthma. Side effects include tachycardia, hyperactivity and rarely hypokalaemia with large doses.

Inhaled corticosteroids: Most effective preventer for achieving overall treatment goals. Usual dose is 200–400mcgm of beclometasone/d. –this dose has no effect on the child's growth. May be beneficial even for children with mild asthma. Consider if:
- Exacerbations of asthma in the last 2y.
- Using inhaled β_2 agonists >3x/wk.
- Symptomatic $\geq$3x/wk. or $\geq$1 night /wk.

Oral steroids: Use to treat acute exacerbations. A rescue course of prednisolone 30–40mg od for 1–2wk. may be needed at any step and any time. Don't prescribe long-term oral steroids except under con-sultant supervision.

Add-on therapy: Before initiating a new drug, check compliance, inhaler technique and eliminate trigger factors.
- *Long-acting β_2 agonists:* Inhaled preparations (e.g. salmeterol 50mcgm bd for children >4y.) improve lung function/symptoms. Do not use without inhaled steroids. Only continue if of demonstrable benefit.
- *Theophylline:* ↑ lung function/↓ symptoms. Side effects are common.
- *Leukotriene receptor antagonists:* e.g. montelukast. Provide improvement in symptoms and lung function and ↓ exacerbations.

Inhaled nedocromil: Mast cell stabilizers which ↓ asthma symptoms and severity, bronchodilator use and improve lung function in children aged 6–12y. when compared to placebo. Less effective than inhaled steroids and not included in the British Thoracic Society stepwise approach at present. Doses:
- Nedocromil – 4mg qds, reducing to bd once asthma is well controlled
- Sodium cromoglicate – 20mg qds reducing to 5mg qds for maintenance.

⚠ If poor control, check compliance and inhaler technique before altering medication.

Complementary and alternative therapies: Table 5.10.

Table 5.10 Evidence for use of complementary therapies in asthma

Evidence	Therapy	
Inconclusive but some evidence of benefit	● Acupuncture[C]	– Breathing exercises[C]
	● Physical training[C]	– Herbal medicine[S]
	● Immunotherapy[C] – only in specialized clinics	
Insufficient evidence	● Massage[C]	– Homeopathy[C]
	● Relaxation therapies[S]	
No benefit	● Chiropractic[C]	– Fish oil supplements[C]

GP Notes: Use of spacers with metred dose inhalers

Advantages of using a spacer:
● Allows more time for evaporation of propellant so a larger proportion of active drug is deposited in the lungs.
● There is no need to coordinate actuation with inhalation.
● Less oropharyngeal side effects (e.g. thrush, hoarseness) occur with inhaled steroids if delivered via a spacer.

Choice of spacer: Larger spacers with 1-way valves are most effective (e.g. volumatic) but large spacers are bulky and often not used. Less conspicuous, medium-volume devices (e.g. aerochamber) may be more acceptable/portable, especially for older children, will be used regularly and thus be more effective. Always supply infants with a face mask.

Use of spacer devices: Inhale the drug from the spacer immediately after actuation as effect of the drugs is short-lived. Spacers should be washed and air dried weekly to prevent build-up of electrostatic charge affecting drug delivery, and replaced every 6–12 mo.

Advice for patients: Information and support for parents and children

Asthma UK ☎ 08457 01 02 03 🖥 www.asthma.org.uk

Further information:

Cochrane: Accessed via 🖥 www.nelh.nhs.uk
● Ram et al Physical training for asthma (2005)
● McCarney et al Acupuncture for chronic asthma (2003)
● Dennis & Cates Alexander technique for chronic asthma (2000)
● Abramson et al Allergen immunotherapy for asthma (2003)
● Holloway & Ram Breathing exercises for asthma (2004)
● Thien et al Dietary marine fatty acids (fish oil) for asthma (2002)
● McCarney et al Homeopathy for chronic asthma (2004)
● Hondras et al Manual therapy for asthma (2005)
Thorax:
● Huntley & Ernst Herbal medicines for asthma: a systematic review (2000) 55(11) pp.925–9
● Huntley et al Relaxation therapies for asthma: a systematic review (2002) 57(2) pp.127–31

Psychosocial factors: Asthma severity is associated with life crises and family conflict. When asthma proves difficult to control on usually effective therapy, find out about any family, psychological or social problems which may be interfering with effective management. Family therapy is an effective adjunct to medication in difficult childhood asthma[C].

Referral: Refer to a general or specialist respiratory paediatrician if:
- Severe exacerbation of asthma E
- Failure to thrive U/S
- Unexpected clinical findings e.g. focal signs in the chest, abnormal voice or cry, dysphagia, inspiratory stridor U/S
- Failure to respond to conventional treatment (particularly inhaled steroid >400mcgm/d.) U/S
- Diagnosis unclear or in doubt U/S/R
- Excessive vomiting or posseting S
- Severe upper respiratory tract infections S
- Symptoms present from birth or perinatal lung problem S/R
- Persistent wet cough S/R
- Frequent use of steroid tablets S/R
- Family history of unusual chest disease R
- Parental anxiety or need for reassurance R

E = Emergency admission; U = Urgent; S = Soon; R = Routine

 This is only a rough guide, urgency of referral depends on clinical state.

Prognosis of childhood asthma: Roughly:
- ¼ become asymptomatic
- ¼ have occasional mild symptoms
- ¼ have a remission for ≥3y. but relapse as adults
- ¼ have persistent symptoms.

Factors associated with persistence:
- Family history of atopy
- Coexisting atopic illness
- Female gender
- Presentation age >2y.
- Increased frequency and severity of episodes
- Poor lung function

Further information
British Thoracic Society/SIGN British Guideline on the management of asthma (revised 2005) 🖳 www.sign.ac.uk
Cochrane: Accessed via 🖳 www.www.nelh.nhs.uk
- York & Shuldham Family therapy for chronic asthma in children (2005)
- Bhogal et al Written action plans for asthma in children (2005)
- Gøtzsche et al House dust mite control measures for asthma (2004)
- Kilburn et al Pet allergen control measures for allergic asthma in children and adults (2001)
Clinical Evidence Keeley & McKean Asthma and other wheezing disorders in children (2004) Accessed via 🖳 www.nelh.nhs.uk
BMJ Learning Childhood asthma: diagnosis and treatment 🖳 www.bmjlearning.com

GMS contract			
Asthma 1	The practice can produce a register of patients with asthma, excluding patients with asthma who have been prescribed no asthma-related drugs in the last 12mo.	4 points	
Asthma 3	% of patients with asthma aged 14–19y. in whom there is a record of smoking status in the previous 15mo.	up to 6 points	40–80%
Asthma 6	% of patients with asthma who have had an asthma review in the last 15mo.	up to 20 points	40–70%
Records 22	% of patients aged >15y. whose notes record smoking status in the past 27mo., except those who have never smoked where smoking status need be recorded only once	up to 11 points	40–90%
Information 5	The practice supports smokers in stopping smoking by a strategy which includes providing literature and offering appropriate therapy	2 points	
Medicines 12	A medication review is recorded in the notes in the preceding 15mo. for all patients being prescribed repeat medicines	8 points	Minimum 80%

Upper respiratory tract infection (URTI)

Viral upper respiratory tract infection (URTI): Children have on average 6–8 viral URTIs each year. Peaks in incidence occur when children start nursery, and start or change schools. Caused by:

- *The common cold:* Acute URTI caused by a rhino (30–50%), picorna, echo or coxsackie virus. At any time only a few viruses are prevalent. Spread by contaminated secretions on fingers and droplet infection.
- *Adeno and parainfluenza viruses*

Presentation: Presents with coryza, runny eyes and malaise. The child may also have mild pyrexia and/or a non-specific maculopapular rash.

Management:
- Examine to exclude tonsillitis and otitis media.
- If pyrexia but no other symptoms/signs, check urine to exclude UTI.
- Most viral URTIs settle within a few days with paracetamol and fluids.
- Treat complications e.g. tonsillitis, otitis media, conjunctivitis or exacerbations of asthma as necessary.

Influenza: Sporadic respiratory illness during autumn and winter caused by influenza viruses A, B or C. Spread by droplet infection, person-to-person contact or contact with contaminated items. Incubation is 1–7d.

Presentation:
- In mild cases symptoms are like those of a common cold.
- In more severe cases fever begins suddenly accompanied by prostration and generalized aches and pains.
- Other symptoms follow: headache, sore throat, respiratory tract symptoms (usually cough ± coryza).
- Acute symptoms clear in <5d.—weakness, sweating and fatigue may last longer. 2° chest infection is common.

Management:
- *Patients at high risk of severe disease:* Consider treatment with the antiviral oseltamivir if >1y. old, in a high-risk group for developing severe disease (Box 5.2) and influenza is prevalent in the community[N]. Antivirals are not a 'cure' but may shorten duration of symptoms and ↓ incidence of complications if started <48h. after onset of symptoms.
- *Other patients:* Treat as for viral URTI.

Prevention:
- Influenza vaccine is prepared each year from viruses of the 3 strains thought most likely to cause 'flu' that winter. It is ~70% effective (range 30–90%). Protection lasts 1y.
- Oseltamivir is recommended for prophylaxis in high-risk patients >13y. who are not effectively vaccinated or who live in residential care where a staff member has influenza-like symptoms *only* when influenza is prevalent in the community. Use at a dose of 75mg od for 7–10d. from diagnosis of the latest case in the establishment[N].

❶ Community-based virological surveillance schemes will indicate when influenza is circulating in the community.

GP Notes: Advice for carers of children with viral URTI

- Most coughs and colds are caused by viruses.
- An average 5–10y. old has 6–8 coughs or colds/y. and sometimes several coughs or colds one after another.
- Common symptoms are cough and a runny nose. Cough is often worse at night and sometimes children vomit after a bout of coughing.
- Other symptoms include: ↑ temperature, sore throat, earache (and/or ↓ hearing), headache, tiredness and/or poor appetite.
- Symptoms are worst in the first 2–3d. then ease over a few days. Cough can persist for 2–4wk.
- Antibiotics don't kill viruses, so are of no use.
- Treatment aims to ease symptoms. Give plenty to drink. Give paracetamol to ease aches, pains and fever. Ibuprofen is an alternative.
- Sometimes 2° bacterial infections develop e.g. ear infection, pneumonia. Symptoms/signs to watch for include: wheeze, persistent earache or ↑ temperature, fast/difficult breathing, non-blanching rash, stiff neck, drowsiness and/or chest pain.
- Advise parents to call a doctor/NHS Direct if worried.

Box 5.2

Children at risk of developing severe disease with influenza:

- Chronic respiratory disease including CF and asthma
- Significant cardiovascular disease
- Chronic renal disease
- Immunosuppression (including hyposplenism)
- Diabetes mellitus

Indications for influenza vaccination for children:

- Chronic lung disease e.g. asthma, CF
- Chronic renal or liver disease
- Cardiovascular disease
- Diabetes mellitus
- Immunocompromised or asplenic
- Living in long-term residential care

ⓘ Parents/carers of children with disabilities should also be vaccinated

GMS contract

Influenza vaccination may be offered by GMS practices as a directed enhanced service—📖 p.87.

Further information

NICE Guidance on the use of zanamivir, oseltamivir and amantadine for the treatment of influenza (2003) 🖥 www.nice.org.uk
Health Protection Agency (HPA) Topics A–Z: Influenza
🖥 www.hpa.org.uk

Lower respiratory tract infection (LRTI)

Bronchiolitis: Occurs in epidemics–usually in the winter months. 70% of infections are due to respiratory syncytial virus (RSV) infection. Usually infects infants of <1y. and presents with coryzal symptoms pro–gressing to irritable cough, rapid breathing ± feeding difficulty.

Examination: Tachypnoea, tachycardia, widespread crepitations over the lung fields ± high-pitched wheeze.

Management: Depends on severity of the symptoms.
- *If mild:* Paracetamol as required and fluids. Bronchodilators may give short-term benefit. There is no evidence antibiotics or steroids help.
- *If more severe:* i.e. if the child or parent is distressed, the child is unable to feed, dehydrated and/or there is intercostal recession or cyanosis–admit as a paediatric emergency for oxygen ± tube feeding. Rarely ventilation is required.

Prognosis: A proportion of children who have had broncholitis as babies will wheeze with URTIs as small children.

Pertussis (whooping cough)[ND]: Caused by *Bordetella pertussis* infection. Incubation is 7d.

Presentation:
- *Catarrhal stage:* Symptoms and signs of URTI–lasts 1–2wk.
- *Coughing stage:* Increasingly severe and paroxysmal cough with spasms of coughing followed by a 'whoop'–associated with vomiting, cyanosis during coughing spasms and exhaustion–lasts 4-6wk. then cough improves over 2–3wk. Chest is clear between coughing bouts.

Investigation: Microscopy and culture of pernasal swabs (special swab and culture medium available from the laboratory); FBC–lymphocytosis.

Management: Erythromycin in the catarrhal stage. Once coughing stage has started treatment is symptomatic.

Complications: Pneumonia, bronchiectasis, convulsions, subconjunctival haemorrhages and facial petechiae.

Prevention:
- *Proven contacts:* Treat with erythromycin.
- *Vaccination:* Routinely given in childhood (Table 4.1, 📖 p.84). Children with a personal/family history of febrile convulsion, family history of epilepsy and children with well-controlled epilepsy can be vaccinated–give advice on fever prevention. Defer vaccination for children with any undiagnosed or evolving neurological condition or poorly controlled epilepsy until the condition is stable–if in doubt refer to paediatrics.

Acute bronchitis: Occurs when an URTI spreads down the airways. Presents with coughing ± purulent sputum. Chest examination is nor-mal unless asthma is precipitated by the infection.

Management: Advise parents to treat the child with OTC cough linctus, paracetamol and fluids. Wheeze may respond to bronchodilator therapy. Warn parents that cough may persist for several weeks.

GP Notes: Children at high risk of severe bronchiolitis include

- Premature babies
- Babies <6wk. old
- Children with underlying lung disease e.g cystic fibrosis
- Children with congenital heart disease
- Immunosuppressed children

Have a low threshold for admission.

🛈 Palivizumab is a monoclonal antibody indicated for the prevention of RSV infection in infants at high risk of infection. Prescribe *only* under specialist supervision and on the basis of likelihood of hospitalization. Give the first dose before the start of the RSV season and then give monthly throughout the RSV season.

GMS contract

Pertussis vaccination can be provided as:
- an additional service (📖 p.86)–opting out of giving vaccinations to the under-5s results in a 1% ↓ in global sum and
- a directed enhanced service (📖 p.86)–2 payments are available for reaching vaccination targets, one for children aged 2 and another for children aged 5.

Croup: 📖 p.276
Pneumonia: 📖 p.158
Pneumococcal infection: 📖 p.96
Tuberculosis: 📖 p.160

157

Childhood pneumonia

Presentation: Diagnosis can be difficult in a child as typical signs may not be evident on first presentation. Do listen to the chest again if the child re-presents even shortly after initial assessment. Typical symptoms/signs include all or some of:

- Fever (bacterial cause is likely if <3y. old and fever >38.5°C)
- Malaise
- Anorexia
- Cough ± purulent sputum
- Tachypnoea (respiratory rate: aged 0–5mo.>60 breaths/min.; 6–12mo. >50 breaths/min.; 12mo. >40 breaths/min.) and/or other signs of respiratory difficulty e.g. expiratory grunt, chest recession. For older children difficulty breathing is more helpful than clinical signs.
- Tachycardia
- Pleuritic chest pain
- Abdominal pain due to pleural inflammation and/or mesenteric adenitis
- Focal chest signs – coarse crackles, reduced breath sounds, bronchial breathing. Generalized wheeze is often due to viral infection.

ⓘ Always consider chest infection if the child is ill and there is no other explanation.

Aetiology: Community acquired pneumonia may be caused by:
- Viral infection: 14–35% – more common in younger children
- Bacterial infection: 10–30% – more common in older children. The organism most commonly isolated is Streptococcus pneumoniae followed by mycoplasma then Chlamydia.
- Mixed infection: 8–40%
- No pathogen isolated: 20–60%

Differential diagnosis:
- URTI ± transmitted upper airways noise
- Asthma or other wheezing disorder
- Congenital abnormality e.g. tracheo-oesophageal fistula

Investigations: Often unnecessary in general practice. Consider:
- Pulse oximetry (if available) to assess severity
- CXR – only if diagnostic uncertainty/symptoms are not resolving
- Blood – FBC (↑ WCC); ESR (↑); acute and convalescent titres for atypical pneumonia

Management: Table 5.11
- If symptoms are mild, advise paracetamol and fluids and adopt a watch and see approach, or supply with an interval prescription to use if symptoms are not resolving after 4–5d. or worsening meanwhile.
- Otherwise, treat with a broad spectrum antibiotic. Commonly used antibiotics are amoxicillin or erythromycin (if penicillin allergic or aged >5y. as atypical pneumonia is more common). Advise parents to bring the child back for GP review if not improving in 48h. or worse in the interim.
- If dehydrated, distressed, not responding to simple antibiotics or any complications – admit for paediatric assessment.

Table 5.11 Indicators for hospital admission	
Infants (<1y.)	Older children
Oxygen saturation <92%	Oxygen saturation <92%
Cyanosis	Cyanosis
Respiratory rate >70 breaths/min.	Respiratory rate >50 breaths/min.
Difficulty breathing	Difficulty breathing
Intermittent apnoea	Grunting
Grunting	Signs of dehydration
Not feeding	Family unable to manage
Family unable to manage	Family unable to provide adequate observation/supervision
Family unable to provide adequate observation/supervision	

GP Notes: Recurrent chest infection

Consider further investigation and/or referral to look for an underlying cause if a child has a history of ≥2 probable chest infections. Possible underlying causes include:

- Asthma
- Oropharyngeal aspiration e.g. due to reflux
- Cystic fibrosis
- Post-infective bronchiectasis
- TB
- Congenital heart or lung defects
- Immune disorders e.g. HIV, hypogammaglobulinaemia, leukaemia
- Sickle cell anaemia
- Foreign body in the lung
- Right middle lobe syndrome ● –narrow diameter of right middle bronchus and acute angle → poor drainage and recurrent chest infections. Often associated with asthma/atopy.

GMS contract

Pneumococcal vaccination may be offered by GMS practices to high-risk groups (📖 p.97) as a directed enhanced service–📖 p.87.

Pneumococcal infection: 📖 p.96

Further information
British Thoracic Society Guidelines for the management of community-acquired pneumonia in children (2002) 🖥 www.brit-thoracic.org.uk

Tuberculosis[ND]

Caused by *Mycobacterium tuberculosis*. In the UK 7000 cases of TB are reported each year and 350 patients die. Incidence is increasing and 10% of cases are antibiotic resistant.

Risk factors: In the UK:
- 40% of cases of TB occur in London–TB is an urban disease
- 70% of cases occur in ethnic minority populations–60% in those born abroad ($^1/_2$ are diagnosed <5y. after entering the country)
- Contacts of other patients with TB:
  - If living in the same house risk is 1:3
  - If school/work contact risk is up to 1:50
  - Casual social contact risk is 1:100,000
- Immunosuppressed patients–especially patients with HIV
- Homeless people

Primary TB: Initial infection. Transmitted by droplet infection. A lesion forms (usually pulmonary) which drains to local LNs. Immunity develops and the infection becomes quiescent.

Symptoms/signs: May be none. Fever, night sweats, persistent cough ± sputum/haemoptysis, pneumonia and/or pleural effusion, anorexia and weight loss, erythema nodosum.

Investigations: CXR, sputum samples for culture (state on the form that you are looking for acid-fast bacilli), tuberculin test +ve (may be -ve if immunocompromised).

Management: Refer for treatment and contact tracing.

Post-primary TB: Reactivation of a primary infection. Initial lesions– usually in the upper lobes of the lung–progress and fibrose. Other sites may develop disease. Multiple small lesions throughout the body results in miliary TB and is common in immunocompromised patients. Symptoms and signs relate to the organs infected.

Risk factors:
- Malignancy
- DM
- Steroids
- HIV
- Poor nutrition
- Chronic illness

Management: Refer for specialist treatment.

Treatment[G]:

Asymptomatic people with +ve tuberculin skin test but normal CXR: Treated with isoniazid for 6mo. or isoniazid + rifampicin for 3mo. to prevent development of the clinical disease.

Treatment of symptomatic patients: Combination of 3–4 antibiotics for the 1st 2mo. then 2 antibiotics for a further 4mo. Antibiotics used are rifampicin, isoniazid, pyrazinamide and ethambutol. All have potentially serious side effects and require blood monitoring. Compliance is imperative to prevent antibiotic resistance.

Screening: TB is a notifiable disease. Every time a case of TB is notified, contact tracing is initiated—usually through chest clinics. All contacts are screened for TB with a tuberculin test (Table 5.12). Screen other high-risk groups before vaccination.

Prevention: Vaccination with a live attenuated strain of bacteria derived from *M. bovis* (BCG). BCG is given by intradermal injection into the left upper arm—don't give any other immunizations into the same arm for 3mo. afterwards. Target groups are:

• All infants living in areas where incidence of TB is ≥40/100,000 or whose parents or grandparents were born in a country with TB incidence of ≥40/100,000 and previously unvaccinated new immigrants from countries where there is a high prevalence of TB

• Contacts of known cases.

GP Notes: Tuberculin skin test

Useful in diagnosis of TB and must be carried out before BCG immunization except for infants <3mo. old who have not had any recent contact with TB. The Mantoux test (international standard) replaced the Heaf test as the standard method of tuberculin skin testing in the UK in 2005/2006.

Interpretation: Table 5.12

False results: The tuberculin test can be suppressed by:
• Glandular fever infection
• Viral infections
• Live viral vaccines—don't do a tuberculin test <3wk. after vaccination
• Hodgkin's disease
• Sarcoidosis
• Corticosteroid therapy
• Immunosuppressant treatment or diseases, including HIV.

⚠ If a patient has a +ve tuberculin test—DON'T give BCG vaccination.

Table 5.12 Tuberculin testing and interpretation of results		
Heaf test	**Mantoux test**	**Grade**
No induration at puncture sites	0mm induration	0 – Negative
Discrete induration at ≥4 sites	1–4mm induration	1 – Negative
Ring of induration with clear centre	5–14mm induration	2 – Positive*
Disc of induration 5–10mm wide	≥15mm induration	3 – Refer to chest clinic
Solid induration>10mm wide ± vesiculation or ulceration		4 – Refer to chest clinic

*In schoolchildren, a grade 2 response requires no further action. In other circumstances, refer to a chest clinic.

Further information

NICE Tuberculosis: Clinical diagnosis and management of tuberculosis and measures for its prevention and control (2006) 🖳 www.nice.org.uk

Cystic fibrosis

Cystic fibrosis (CF) is the most common inherited disorder in the UK (prevalence: 1:2500). Median survival has ↑ dramatically and is now >40y. but, of the 7500 CF patients in the UK, 6000 are <25y. old.

Genetics:

- Results from mutation of a single gene on chromosome 7 (cystic fibrosis transmembrane conductance regulator) essential for salt and water movement across cell membranes → thickened secretions. >1200 different mutations have been described.
- Autosomal recessive inheritance—1:4 chance of having a child with CF if both parents are carriers. ~1:25 adults in the UK carries the CF gene (~2.3 million adults).
- Most common in Caucasians—rare in people of Afro-Caribbean origin.

Screening: Several possibilities:

- *Preconceptual screening:* Buccal smears to karyotype prospective parents
- *Antenatal screening:* Chorionic villous sampling at ~10wk.—for parents with an affected child already or where both parents are +ve on karyotyping
- *Neonatal screening:* 📖 p.18.

Presentation: Wide range of clinical presentation and severity:

- Neonatal (meconium ileus)—10%
- Infancy:
  - GI symptoms alone (failure to thrive; steatorrhoea)—30%
  - Recurrent respiratory infections—25%
  - Combination of GI and respiratory symptoms—15%
- <16y.—Variety of presentations (e.g. malabsorption)—10%
- +ve family history or screening—10%.

> ⓘ In future the majority are likely to be detected by screening.

Diagnosis:

- Screening—see above.
- If clinical suspicion of CF, refer to paediatrics. A +ve sweat test (Na^+ >70mmol/l; Cl^- >60mmol/l on 2 occasions) is diagnostic as is ↑ potential difference across the nasal respiratory epithelium.

Common problems associated with CF: Figure 5.10

Further information

UK Newborn Screening Programme CF Screening programme and leaflets about CF screening for parents
🖳 www.newbornscreening-bloodspot.org.uk

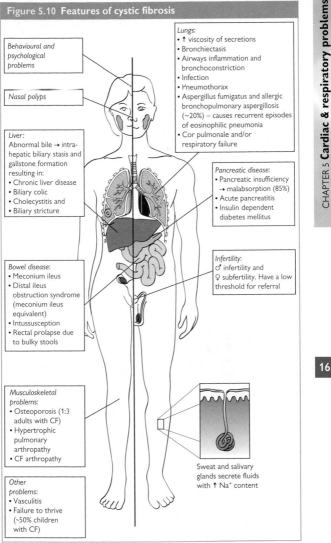

Figure 5.10 Features of cystic fibrosis

Behavioural and psychological problems

Nasal polyps

Liver:
Abnormal bile → intra-hepatic biliary stasis and gallstone formation resulting in:
• Chronic liver disease
• Biliary colic
• Cholecystitis and
• Biliary stricture

Bowel disease:
• Meconium ileus
• Distal ileus obstruction syndrome (meconium ileus equivalent)
• Intussusception
• Rectal prolapse due to bulky stools

Musculoskeletal problems:
• Osteoporosis (1:3 adults with CF)
• Hypertrophic pulmonary arthropathy
• CF arthropathy

Other problems:
• Vasculitis
• Failure to thrive (~50% children with CF)

Lungs:
• ↑ viscosity of secretions
• Bronchiectasis
• Airways inflammation and bronchoconstriction
• Infection
• Pneumothorax
• Aspergillus fumigatus and allergic bronchopulmonary aspergillosis (~20%) – causes recurrent episodes of eosinophilic pneumonia
• Cor pulmonale and/or respiratory failure

Pancreatic disease:
• Pancreatic insufficiency → malabsorption (85%)
• Acute pancreatitis
• Insulin dependent diabetes mellitus

Infertility:
♂ infertility and ♀ subfertility. Have a low threshold for referral

Sweat and salivary glands secrete fluids with ↑ Na^+ content

163

Management: CF is a multisystem disease requiring a holistic approach to care which aims to maintain patients' independence, improve quality of life *and* extend life expectancy. A multidisciplinary team in a specialist CF centre is best placed to achieve this. Patients usually have direct access.

Treatment of lung disease: Aims to prevent chronic infection as long as possible and later stabilize respiratory infection

- **Exercise:** Maintains physical fitness and lung function.
- **↑ viscosity of secretions:** Treated with physiotherapy ± postural drainage ± dornase alpha (nebulized mucolytic enzyme).
- **Bronchiectasis and infection:** Responsible for most morbidity and >90% mortality. In small children, *S. aureus* and *H. influenzae* are common infecting organisms; in older children/adults *Pseudomonas* infection is common. Treat with antibiotics according to sensitivities. Prevention and control of chronic *Pseudomonas* infection minimizes ↓ in lung function and ↑survival.
- **Airways inflammation and bronchoconstriction:** Managed with inhaled bronchodilators and anti-inflammatories.
- **Pneumothorax:** Refer to paediatrics. Treatment depends on size.
- **Cor pulmonale and/or respiratory failure:** Major cause of death. Cadaveric heart–lung transplantation (50% 5y. survival) or partial lung transplant from a related donor is a last resort.

Maintaining good nutritional state: Patients with pancreatic insufficiency require pre-meal oral pancreatic enzymes (e.g. Creon) and a high-calorie diet supplemented with fat-soluble vitamins (A, D and E)—advice from a dietician is essential.

Treatment of complications e.g. DM, osteoporosis

> **GP Notes: Role of the GP**
>
> - Communication and ongoing support
> - Prescribing routine treatment including O_2 as directed by the CF team
> - Providing routine childhood immunizations, pneumococcal vaccination and annual influenza vaccination
> - Managing unrelated illness e.g. URTI
> - Referral for specialist care e.g. for infertility or genetic counselling
> - Certification of illness
> - Support of carers
> - Terminal care

> **GMS contract**
>
> Influenza and pneumococcal vaccination may be offered by GMS practices as a directed enhanced service—📖 p.87.

Further information

CF Trust Standards for the clinical care of children and adults with CF in the UK (2001) 🖳 www.cftrust.org.uk

Advice for patients: Frequently asked questions about cystic fibrosis

What is cystic fibrosis (CF)?
Cystic fibrosis is the UK's most common life-threatening, inherited disease. It affects more than 7500 babies, children and young adults in the UK. It is caused by a faulty gene which causes organs in the body (especially lungs and pancreas) to become clogged with thick, sticky mucus.
- Lung symptoms include troublesome coughs and repeated chest infections.
- Pancreas symptoms include difficulty digesting food, causing abnormal stools and poor weight gain.

Why has my child been affected?
People with one CF gene, or carriers as they are known, are healthy and show no signs of CF. About 2½ million adults in the UK carry the gene which causes CF–that is about 1 in 20 of the population. For a child to be born with CF, both parents must be carriers. A child with CF has inherited 2 altered genes–one from each parent.

What treatment does my child need?
You will be referred to a specialist clinic where experts will supervise your child's treatment, monitor progress and provide you and your child with information and support. Your child will need treatment throughout life–usually with physiotherapy, medicines and special high-energy diets.

What will happen long-term to my child?
At present there is no cure for CF but the faulty gene which causes CF has been identified and doctors and scientists are working to find ways to repair or replace it. As recently as the 1930s, children with CF used to die as babies or small children, but now improved treatment means that children with CF are living much longer. It is now normal for children with CF to live to early or middle adulthood and life expectancy is improving all the time.

If I have one child with CF, what are my chances of having another?
- If the parents of a child with CF have another child together, there is a 1 in 4 chance that child will have CF too.
- If one parent of a child with CF has another child with a different partner, the risk of another child with CF is roughly 1 in 80.

Talk to your GP or health visitor about screening tests available.

Support and further information for patients and parents
Cystic Fibrosis Trust ☎ 0845 859 1000 🖳 www.cftrust.org.uk

Chapter 6

Gastrointestinal, renal and endocrine problems in children

Congenital gastrointestinal and renal abnormalities

Umbilical hernia: Common. Due to a defect in the umbilical ring when the cord separates. ↑ incidence in people of black ethnic origin and associated with certain syndromes (e.g. Trisomy 13 & 18). Usually resolves spontaneously. Advise parents that sticking something over the hernia e.g. a penny does NOT help and may result in abrasion ± infection. Strangulation is rare. Refer for surgery if an umbilical hernia persists >2y. of age.

Inguinal hernia
- **Acute:** Sudden appearance of an irreducible groin or scrotal swelling – necessitates emergency admission for reduction and repair.
- **Non-acute:** History of intermittent groin ± scrotal swelling – the spermatic cord may be thickened on the affected side. Refer to paediatric surgery for repair (herniotomy). ❶ There is a greater risk of incarceration in infants <1y. – request an urgent outpatient appointment.

Diaphragmatic hernia: 1:2500 live births. A defect in one hemidiaphragm allows bowel to herniate into the chest cavity → pulmonary hypoplasia *in utero* or lung compression postnatally. Detected antenatally on USS or postnatally when the child develops respiratory distress soon after birth – CXR confirms diagnosis. Corrective surgery is associated with high mortality but once repaired there are usually no further difficulties.

Exomphalos and gastroschisis: Usually detected antenatally at routine USS. Delivery and surgical repair then takes place at a specialist centre. Once repaired prognosis is good.
- **Exomphalos:** Complete return of the gut into the abdominal cavity fails to occur during intrauterine life. At birth there is a swelling at the umbilicus consisting of gut covered by a membrane.
- *Gastroschisis:* There is a defect in the abdominal wall through which exposed gut prolapses.

Oesophageal atresia and/or tracheo-oesophageal fistula
1:2500 live births. 5% have oesophageal atresia alone; 5% tracheo-oesophageal fistula (TOF) alone; the remainder have both. Risk factor for sudden infant death syndrome.

Presentation:
- *Antenatal:* At routine USS or following investigation of polyhydramnios.
- *Postnatal:* Cough or breathing difficulties in a newborn infant; choking on the first feed; inability to swallow saliva → bubbling of fluid from the mouth developing soon after birth.
- *Later in childhood:* 'H type' fistulas where there is no atresia but just a fistula may present late with recurrent chest infections.

Management: Diagnosis is confirmed with X-ray. Treatment is surgical. Post-operatively children may have a barking cough ('*TOF cough*') and/ or dysphagia – both settle before 2y.

Duodenal atresia: Usually associated with other abnormalities, particularly Down's syndrome. If not detected on antenatal USS, presents postnatally with bile-stained vomiting. Abdominal X-ray reveals a 'double bubble' with air in stomach and first part of duodenum but none beyond. Requires surgical correction.

Anorectal atresia (imperforate anus): 1:4000 live births. Usually the baby fails to pass meconium and no anus is visible. There is often a fistula to the urethra (boys) or vagina (girls). Treatment is surgical. In the period after surgery, anal dilatation is vital to prevent stricture and starts 2wk. post-op. It requires use of graded dilators by the baby's parents for several months. Faecal incontinence may be a problem but can usually be managed using a combination of dietary manipulation, enemas and drug treatment.

Hirschsprung's disease: Absence of the ganglion cells of the myenteric plexus in the distal bowel. Presents with delay in passing meconium, abdominal distension, vomiting and poor feeding in a neonate. If only a short segment is affected, presentation may be much later with chronic constipation. Refer to paediatric surgery. Diagnosis is confirmed with rectal biopsy and the affected area of bowel removed.

Horseshoe kidney, ectopic kidney, double ureter: Common malformations. Usually do not affect kidney function *per se* but predispose to UTI. Recurrent infections may eventually cause renal damage.

Posterior urethral valves: Folds of mucosa inhibit or block passage of urine causing urethral, bladder, ureter and renal pelvis dilatation.

Presentation: Usually detected on antenatal USS. Can present in neonates with urinary retention or dribbling urine + distended bladder, UTI or uraemia or later in childhood with recurrent UTI or incontinence.

Investigation and management: MCUG confirms diagnosis. In all cases refer to urology for surgical disruption of the valves.

Hypospadias: 1:400 male births. The urethral meatus opens on the ventral side of the penis. There is often hooding of the foreskin and ventral flexion of the penis. Refer to urology. Treated with corrective surgery, ideally pre-school.

Undescended testis: Observed in 2–3% of male neonates but most descend during the 1st year. Refer those that don't for surgical descent and fixation to avoid later infertility and ↑ risk of malignancy.

Retractile testis: Usually young boys with active cremasteric reflex. No treatment needed. *Examination:* Scrotum is usually well developed. Try to find the testis and milk it down into scrotum. May be found anywhere from the scrotum to the internal inguinal ring. If not found or unable to bring down into scrotum, assume undescended.

Congenital hydrocoele: Unilateral or bilateral, smooth scrotal swelling which transilluminates. Most congenital hydrocoeles resolve spontaneously in the first year of life. Refer to urology if persists >1y.

Abdominal pain

Abdominal pain is a very frequent symptom in children with many possible causes – Box 6.1.

Recurrent abdominal pain: Occurs in 1:9 children. ♀:♂≈4:3. Rare before 4–5y. Peak age of presentation is 8–10y. with another peak in girls during early adolescence.

Presentation: The child complains of recurrent pain, usually colicky in nature. Site and character is variable though it is most commonly central. There are 2 types of recurrent abdominal pain:
• Those due to organic disease (such as coeliac disease or constipation)
• Those due to functional illness (~90%).

Examination
• If possible, examine the abdomen both whilst the child is in pain and between painful episodes.
• Check for palpable masses and organomegaly – both require urgent investigation.
• Any guarding or rebound tenderness suggests an organic cause.
• If the pain is functional, examination will be normal.

Investigation
• If examination is normal and there are no symptoms suggesting organic disease, check MSU for M,C&S and consider a FBC and ESR. Record the weight of the child at the first assessment and recheck at subsequent visits.
• If there are any accompanying symptoms or signs, consider abdominal ± renal USS and/or referral to paediatrics.

Differential diagnosis: Box 6.1

Management of functional abdominal pain:

• Acknowledge the pain is real and worries of both parents and child. Reassure them there is no serious underlying cause like appendicitis.
• Suggest a balanced diet with plenty of roughage. Encourage adequate fluid intake.
• It might be worthwhile to try excluding milk products for a limited period as lactose intolerance is common – but don't continue if there is no improvement after 2–3wk. Only exclude other foods if a food diary suggests symptoms are linked to ingestion of those foods. There is no scientific basis for food allergy testing using skin resistance devices or postal surveys and a real danger that children with multiple food exclusions can become malnourished.
• Reserve paracetamol for episodes of more severe pain than is usual. Antispasmodics e.g. mebeverine may help children >10y.
• Stress that if the pain changes or is unusually severe or persistent, the child should be reassessed by a doctor.
• Most children recover spontaneously with time, though a proportion develop other recurrent pains, and some continue to have pain as adults when it is termed 'irritable bowel syndrome'.

Box 6.1

Causes of acute abdominal pain

GI causes:

- Gastroenteritis – 📖 p.176
- Constipation – 📖 p.174
- Appendicitis – 📖 p.172
- Meckel's diverticulum – 📖 p.173
- Intussusception - 📖 p.178

- Strangulated hernia
- Inflammatory bowel disease e.g. Crohn's, UC – 📖 p.173
- Functional pain – See opposite page

Gynaecological causes (teenage girls)

- Ectopic pregnancy
- Dysmenorrhoea

- Pelvic inflammatory disease

Other causes

- Mesenteric adenitis – 📖 p.172
- UTI – 📖 p.186
- Otitis media – 📖 p.284
- Abdominal migraine – 📖 p.173
- Pneumonia – 📖 p.158

- Sickle cell crisis – 📖 p.114
- Diabetic ketoacidosis – 📖 p.191
- Henoch – Schönlein purpura – 📖 p.116
- Torsion of the testis – 📖 p.187

Causes of chronic and/or recurrent abdominal pain

- Constipation – 📖 p.174
- Functional abdominal pain – see opposite page
- Abdominal migraine – see opposite page
- Dysmenorrhoea (teenage girls)
- Coeliac disease – 📖 p.180
- Inflammatory bowel disease – 📖 p.173

GP Notes: How can I differentiate functional and organic pain?

- The further away the pain is from the umbilicus, the more likely it is to be organic.
- Investigate all children with loin pain to exclude renal causes.
- Accompanying symptoms (e.g. weight ↓, dysuria or ↑ frequency, regular periodicity) also make an organic cause more likely.
- Other behavioural or psychological problems (e.g. school refusal, irrational fears) make a functional diagnosis more likely.

NICE recommends

- Any child who presents several times (≥3x) with the same problem but with no clear diagnosis should be referred urgently for specialist assessment.
- Persistent parental anxiety is sufficient reason for referral, even where a benign cause is considered most likely.

Further information

NICE Referral guidelines for suspected cancer – quick reference guide (2005) 🖥 www.nice.org.uk

Acute appendicitis: Commonest surgical emergency in the UK – lifetime incidence ≈6%. *Peak age:* 10–30y.

Presentation
- Central abdominal colic progresses and localizes in the right iliac fossa, becoming worse on movement (especially coughing, laughing)
- Anorexia, nausea ± vomiting
- Dysuria
- Constipation or rarely diarrhoea.

Examination
- Discomfort on walking (tend to walk stooped)
- Discomfort on coughing
- Flushed and unwell
- Pyrexia (~37.5°C)
- Furred tongue and/or foetor oris
- Tenderness and guarding in the right iliac fossa (especially over McBurney's point – $^2/_3$ of the distance between the umbilicus and anterior superior iliac spine)
- Pain in the right iliac fossa on palpation of the left iliac fossa (Rovsing's sign)
- Rectal examination – tender high on the right.

Investigation: Urinalysis – normal or +ve for protein and/or white cells but -ve for nitrites.

Differential diagnosis:
- Mesenteric adenitis
- UTI
- Gastroenteritis
- Meckel's diverticulum
- Intussusception
- Crohn's disease
- Gynaecological cause (particularly pelvic inflammatory disease in teenage girls)
- Non-abdominal cause e.g. otitis media, diabetic ketoacidosis, pneumonia

Management: Admit as a surgical emergency – expect to be wrong ~½ the time.

Complications:
- Generalized peritonitis 2° to perforation; appendix abscess; appendix mass; female infertility.

Mesenteric adentitis: Inflammation of the mesentric lymph nodes causing abdominal pain. May follow URTI and can mimic appendicitis. Check MSU to exclude UTI. If guarding/rebound tenderness, refer for acute surgical assessment to exclude appendicitis. Settles spontaneously with simple analgesia and fluids. If not settling in 1–2wk. refer for paediatric assessment – urgency depends on severity of symptoms.

GP Notes: Diagnosing children with appendicitis

⚠ Symptoms and signs of appendicitis may be atypical – especially in very young children – as children localize pain poorly and signs of peritonitis can be difficult to ellicit.
- If unsure of diagnosis and the child is unwell, admit.
- If unsure of diagnosis and the child is well, either arrange to review a few hours later or ask the carer to contact you if there is any deterioration or change in symptoms.

Meckel's diverticulum: Remnant of the attachment of the small bowel to the embryological yolk sac. It is 2 inches (~5cm) long, ~2 foot (100cm) proximal to the appendix and present in 2% of the population. A Meckel's diverticulum may not cause any problems or cause an appendicitis-like picture, acute intestinal obstruction or GI bleeding. Symptoms can occur at any age but are most common in children.

Abdominal migraine or periodic syndrome: Stereotyped attacks in which nausea, vomiting and headache accompany abdominal pain. Treat as for migraine (📖 p.216). A proportion of affected children develop classical migraine later.

Inflammatory bowel disease: Ulcerative colitis (UC) and Crohn's disease are collectively termed inflammatory bowel disease. They are chronic, relapsing – remitting conditions of unknown cause characterized by acute, non-infectious inflammation of the gut. Both are rare in childhood.

Features:
- Ulcerative colitis: inflammation is limited to the colorectal mucosa. Extent varies from disease limited to the rectum (proctitis) to disease affecting the whole colon (pancolitis).
- Crohn's disease: any part of the gut from mouth to anus can be affected with normal bowel between affected areas (skip lesions).

Presentation and management: Presentation is variable. Children can present with non-specific features (e.g. failure to thrive), GI symptoms (e.g. malabsorbtion, bloody diarrhoea, acute abdomen) or complications (e.g. arthropathy or iritis). If suspected refer for confirmation of diagnosis and specialist management.

Abdominal distension[N]: If persistent or progressive, examine the abdomen:
- If a mass is found, refer immediately
- If the child is uncooperative and abdominal examination is not possible, or if examination is difficult, consider referral for urgent abdominal ultrasound.

Advice for patients: Information and support for children with inflammatory bowel disease

National Association for Colitis and Crohn's Disease (NACC)
☎ 0845 130 2233 (info); 0845 130 3344 (support)
🖥 www.nacc.org.uk

Further information
NICE Referral guidelines for suspected cancer – quick reference guide (2005) 🖥 www.nice.org.uk

Vomiting and change in bowel habit

Vomiting and diarrhoea: Most episodes are due to viral infection, short-lived and self-limiting. Differential diagnosis – Table 6.1.

History: Determine nature and duration of symptoms; whether there is blood/mucus in the stool, contact with anyone else with similar symptoms or history of recent foreign travel; other accompanying symptoms.

Examination
- **Assess level of hydration:** Sunken eyes, dry tongue, sunken fontanelle and ↓ skin turgor are all late signs
- **Examine the abdomen:** Masses, distention, tenderness, bowel sounds
- **Look for sources of infection:** e.g. ENT and chest infection; UTI

Management: ⚠ Never give children antidiarrhoeal agents.
- **Treat any identified cause.**
- **If diarrhoea, send a stool sample for M,C&S if:** fever, blood in stool, recent return from a tropical climate, immunocompromised, resident in an institution and/or persists >7d.
- **Rehydration:** Encourage clear fluid intake (small amounts frequently) ± rehydration salts (use commercial preparations e.g. Dioralyte®).
- **Food:** Stick to a bland diet avoiding dairy products until diarrhoea has settled. Babies who are breast-fed or have not been weaned should continue their normal milk.
- **If dehydrated and unable to replace fluids:** e.g. concomitant vomiting, child refusing to drink – admit.
- **If no cause found and lasts >3wk. or any atypical features:** Refer for urgent investigation or admit.

Constipation: Differentiate normal stools a few days apart (normal, needs no treatment) and infrequent hard stools (suggests constipation).

Infants: Bowel habit varies according to diet (and mother's diet if breast-fed). Babies often change colour and look like they are straining when passing stool, even if it is liquid, and it is usual for stool to change colour/consistency (becoming harder/more formed) when switching from breast milk to artificial feeds and/or solids. Constipation can result from hunger, poor hydration or overstrength feeds. If it causes pain on defaecation, this can result in withholding of stool – a vicious cycle hard to break. *Rare causes include:* Congenital abnormalities e.g. spinal cord lesions, imperforate anus (after surgical repair); Hirschsprung's disease; hypothyroidism; cerebral palsy.

Older children: Constipation often accompanies acute febrile illness. Once hard stool causes an anal tear, pain on defaecation results in withholding of stool to avoid pain. Symptoms include abdominal pain, anorexia, vomiting, failure to thrive and predisposition to UTIs. Eventually soft stool leaks out around the hard faecal mass causing faecal soiling.

Management: Advise adequate fluid intake and a high roughage diet. Treatment involves regular senna liquid ± a softener e.g. lactulose. If not controlled with simple laxatives and diet, refer for paediatric assessment.
❶ Faecal soiling may initially get worse before getting better.

Rectal bleeding: Common. Usual causes are constipation, anal fissure or threadworms. Only refer if profuse or if simple treatment for constipation fails. *Rarer causes include:*

- **Neonates:** Necrotizing enterocolitis, volvulus
- **Infants:** Intussusception (📖 p.178), cow's milk intolerance (📖 p.179), rectal prolapse
- **Older children:** Campylobacter/Shigella infection (📖 p.177), Meckel's diverticulum (📖 p.173), Inflammatory bowel diease (📖 p.173)

Table 6.1 Causes of vomiting and diarrhoea in primary care	
Cause	**Notes**
Physiological	• *Breast-fed babies* – loose, often explosive 'mustard grain' stools • *Babies* – may posset part of each feed – 📖 p.65 • *Toddlers* – intermittent loose stools related to diet
Gastrointestinal infection	Diarrhoea and/or vomiting. Consider the possibility of temporary cow's milk intolerance if continuing >2wk. – 📖 p.179
Other infection	e.g. otitis media, UTI, tonsillitis, septicaemia
Acute intra-abdominal disease	• Intussusception – 📖 p.178 • Appendicitis – 📖 p.172 • Acute obstruction – abdominal distention and vomiting – admit • Pyloric stenosis – vomiting only – 📖 p.70
Constipation	Usually overflow of soft stool with soiling ± vomiting
Malabsorption	e.g. coeliac disease – usually only diarrhoea – 📖 p.180
Reflux	Gastro-oesophageal reflux – usually only vomiting – 📖 p.65
Other causes of vomiting	• Raised intracranial pressure – 📖 p.220 • Anorexia/bulimia (purgative abuse may → diarrhoea) – 📖 p.312 • Migraine (📖 p.216) or abdominal migraine (📖 p.173) • Travel/motion sickness • Metabolic causes – ketoacidosis (📖 p.191), uraemia (📖 p.182)

Advice for patients: Looking after a child with vomiting and diarrhoea

- If you are breast-feeding continue to do so. Offer feeds frequently.
- If your child is bottle-fed but not weaned, continue normal feeds unless you are told to do something else by your doctor.
- Otherwise give your child frequent small drinks of clear fluids such as rehydation solution bought from the chemist, fresh water, ice cubes to suck, squash or diluted fruit juice.
- If your child usually drinks from a bottle and refuses the bottle, try using a spoon instead.
- Reintroduce normal feeds or meals after 4–6 hours but stick to bland, non-fatty foods such as dry toast, boiled rice or fruit to start with.

Consult your doctor if:

- Your child refuses to take fluids, vomits fluids back, passes less urine than usual or becomes more unwell – for example develops a high fever, is unusually drowsy or irritable
- There is blood in the diarrhoea or symptoms are not improving.

Gastroenteritis/food poisoningND

Ingestion of viruses, bacteria or their toxins commonly causes diarrhoea and/or vomiting. Rota virus is the most common cause in children and accounts for ~1:5 GP consultations with the under-5s.

Prevention: Hand-washing after using the toilet; longer cooking and rewarming times; prompt consumption of food.

Presentation

- *History:* Severity and duration of symptoms, food eaten and water drunk, time relationship between ingestion and symptoms, other affected contacts, recent foreign travel.
- *Examination:* Usually normal. Dehydration may prompt admission.

Investigation and management: See vomiting and diarrhoea – 📖 p.174. Only give antibiotics if recommended following stool culture (exception is giardia diarrhoea).

Traveller's diarrhoea: 50% travellers experience some diarrhoea. Most cases last 4–5d.; 1–2% last >1mo. In all cases send a fresh stool sample for M,C&S at first presentation, noting on the form areas visited. Consider the usual causes for diarrhoea and gastroenteritis. In addition consider:

CholeraND: Caused by Gram -ve bacterium *Vibrio cholerae*.
- *Spread:* By faeco–oral route.
- *Incubation:* Few hours to 5d.
- *Presentation:* Profuse watery stools, fever, vomiting, rapid dehydration.
- *Management:* Admit. Requires expert treatment with rehydration ± antibiotics.

Giardiasis: Common flagellate protozoan. Infection is suggested by an incubation period ≥2wk.; watery stool with flatus ++ (explosive diarrhoea); no fever. Stool microscopy may be -ve. If suspected treat with metronidazole. Rapid response is diagnostic.

Amoebic dysenteryND: May begin years after infection. Diarrhoea begins slowly, becoming profuse and bloody ± fever ± malaise. Diagnosis is confirmed by microscopy of fresh stool. Take specialist advice on management.

Prevention

- Take care to eat and drink uncontaminated food and water.
- Food should be freshly cooked and hot; avoid salads and cold meats/fish.
- Eat fruit that can be peeled.
- Stick to drinks made with boiling water or bottled drinks and water with intact seal; avoid ice in drinks.
- Use water purification tablets if necessary.

Further information

Health Protection Agency (HPA) Infections: Topics A–Z: Gastrointestinal disease 🖥 www.hpa.org.uk

Table 6.2 Common causes of gastroenteritis in the UK

Organism/ source	Incubation	Symptoms					Food
		D	V	P	F	O	
Staph. aureus	1–6h.	✓	✓	✓		↓BP	Meat
B. cereus	1–5h.	✓	✓				Rice
C. perfringens	6–24h.	✓		✓			Meat
C. botulinum	12–36h.		✓			Paralysis	Canned food
Salmonella species	12–48h	✓	✓	✓	✓		Meat, eggs, poultry
Shigella^ND	48–72h.	✓		✓	✓	Blood in stool	Any food
Campylobacter	48h–5d.	✓		✓	✓	Blood in stool	Milk, water
E. coli	12–72h.	✓		✓	✓	Blood in stool	Food, water
Y. enterocolitica	24–36h.	✓		✓	✓		Milk, water
Giardia lamblia	1–4wk.	✓					Water
Crypto–sporidium	4–12d.	✓		✓	✓		Water
Listeria						Flu-like illness, pneumonia	Milk products, pâtés, raw vegetables
V. parahaemolyticus	12–24h.	✓	✓	✓			Fish
Rotavirus	1–7d.	✓	✓		✓	Malaise	Food, water
Small viruses	36–72h.	✓	✓		✓	Malaise	Any food
Entamoeba histolytica	1–4wk.	✓		✓	✓	Blood in stool	Food, water
Mushrooms	15min.–24h.	✓	✓	✓		Fits, coma, renal/liver failure	
Scrombrotoxin	10–60min.	✓				Flushes, erythema	Fish
Heavy metals e.g. zinc	5min.–2h.		✓	✓			
Red beans	1–3h.	✓	✓				

D = diarrhoea; V = vomiting; P = abdominal pain; F = fever; O = other

GP Notes: Related concerns

- Suspected food poisoning is a notifiable disease – 📖 p.89.
- Some children may become cow's milk intolerant after a bout of gastroenteritis – 📖 p.179.
- Think of haemolytic uraemic syndrome (📖 p.184) in any child with diarrhoea who passes blood in the stool.

Coeliac disease

Gluten sensitivity results in inflammation of the bowel and malabsorption. Coeliac disease is a common disorder (UK prevalence 1:300, ♀:♂≈3:1) though only a minority have clinically recognized disease. Presents at any age but, in children, peak incidence is at ~4y.

Predisposing factors:
- **Genetic:** 1:10 chance if a 1st degree relative is affected.
- **Environmental:** 60–70% concordance in twin studies so other factors (e.g. infection, hormonal status) must intervene.

Presentation: May have minimal or atypical symptoms. Common presentations – Table 6.3.

Investigation:
- Bloods: Depending on presenting features consider FBC, ESR, LFTs, Ca^{2+}, thyroid function tests, endomysial antibodies (only available for GP testing in some areas).
- If presenting with diarrhoea, check a stool sample to exclude infective causes.

Initial management: Refer all suspected cases for specialist investigation to confirm the diagnosis:
- Endomysial antibodies – sensitivity >86% and 100% specificity in the right clinical setting. ❶ Available in the community in some areas
- Small intestinal biopsy – shows villous atrophy.

Ongoing management:

Diet: Refer to a dietician for dietary advice on a gluten-free diet. Prescribe adequate amounts of gluten-free products, marking the prescription 'ACBS'. Add supplements of deficient nutrients e.g. iron, folic acid, calcium until well established on a gluten-free diet.

Pneumococcal vaccination: All patients with coeliac disease have a degree of hyposplenism and are more prone to pneumococcal infection. Advise pneumococcal vaccination.

Follow-up: Patients should be followed up every 6–12mo. in a specialist clinic or by a GP under a shared care arrangement. Routine checks include: symptoms, weight and blood tests (Hb, B_{12}, folate, iron, albumin, Ca^{2+}, antigliadin or anti-endomysial antibodies).

Failure to respond to diet: The commonest reason is continued ingestion of gluten (intentional or inadvertent). Re-refer to dieticians. If symptoms recur after a period of remission, re-refer to a specialist for reassessment of the diagnosis.

Long-term complications: Osteoporosis and malignancy (lymphoma or carcinoma of the small intestine). Both are virtually eliminated by adherence to a strict gluten-free diet.

Further information:

British Society of Gastroenterology Interim guidelines for the management of patients with coeliac disease (2002) ⌨ www.bsg.org.uk

Table 6.3 Presentation of coeliac disease

Presentation aged <2y.	Presentation aged >2y.	Presentation with associated features
Chronic diarrhoea	Loss of appetite	Dermatitis herpetiformis (□ p.247)
Failure to thrive after introduction of cereals	Diarrhoea	Type 1 DM (□ p.190)
Abdominal distension	Constipation	Autoimmune thyroid disease (□ p.198)
Vomiting	Anaemia	
Typically pale and miserable	Short stature	Primary biliary cirrhosis
	Rickets	Sjögren's syndrome
Hair thinning		IgA deficiency
		Epilepsy

Advice for parents about coeliac disease:

- Coeliac disease is intolerance to the protein gluten which is contained in a lot of foods.
- Cutting out *all* gluten from your child's diet will lead to an improvement in your child's symptoms and health.
- Coeliac disease is a lifelong condition. If your child ever starts eating gluten again, all his or her symptoms will return.
- Sticking to a gluten-free diet also helps your child to avoid long-term problems associated with coeliac disease such as osteoporosis (thinning of the bones) or lymphoma (lymph node cancer of the bowel).

Gluten-free diet:

- Gluten is found in wheat, barley and rye cereal products.
- Oats can be eaten (in moderation) but check labels carefully as oat flours and other products may contain other cereals too.
- Most processed foods contain gluten so avoid them.
- Look out for gluten in common cooking ingredients such as stock cubes, baking powder, soy sauce and mustard powder.
- Coeliac UK provides a directory of approved products as well as recipes and tips on keeping to a gluten-free diet.
- Gluten-free products, such as bread, biscuits and pasta, are available on prescription – ask your doctor.

A new European directive has made it obligatory for EU food manufacturers to identify the presence of 12 allergens, including gluten, in foods. All new labels must comply. This should make shopping for children with coeliac disease a lot easier.

Information and support for parents and children:
Coeliac UK ☎ 0870 444 8804 🖳 www.coeliac.co.uk

GMS contract

Pneumococcal vaccination may be offered by GMS practices as a directed enhanced service – □ p.87.

Presentation of renal disease

Renal disease in childhood may present to the GP with:
- Asymptomatic haematuria or proteinuria – refer urgently any child presenting with haematuria[N]
- UTI – 📖 p.186
- Nephrotic syndrome
- Nephritic syndrome
- Renal failure.

In all cases specialist management is required.

Nephrotic syndrome: Proteinuria >3g/24h. causing hypoalbuminaemia and oedema. In children, it is caused by glomerulonephritis (90% by minimal change glomerulonephritis).

Presentation: Swelling of eyelids and face, frothing urine due to high protein content, ascites ± peripheral oedema.

Nephrotic crisis: The child is unwell with oedema, anorexia, vomiting, pleural effusions and muscle wasting.

Management: Admit/refer for same-day assessment.

Complications:
- Thromboembolism
- Infection – particularly pneumococcal – if persistent nephrotic syndrome offer vaccination
- Loss of specific proteins e.g. transferrin (causes hypochromic anaemia which is iron resistant)
- Hypercholesterolaemia
- Hypovolaemia and renal failure

Nephritic syndrome: The central feature of nephritic syndrome is blood in the urine from glomerular bleeding. *Other features:*
- Fluid retention
- ↑BP (rarely results in hypertensive encephalopathy)
- Low urine output
- Rising plasma urea and creatinine

Causes:
- Glomerulonephritis e.g. post-streptococcal glomerulonephritis
- Vasculitis e.g. Henoch-Schönlein purpura (📖 p.116)

Renal failure: Deterioration in renal function which may be acute (↓ in function over hours/days) or chronic (↓ in function over months/years).

Acute renal failure: Admit as a paediatric emergency. The most common cause in primary care is haemolytic uraemic syndrome. Other causes include glomerulonephritis, urinary tract obstruction (e.g. due to congenital abnormality of the renal tract) and septicaemia.

Presentation: Sick child with:
- ↓ urine output
- Anorexia, nausea and/or vomiting
- Fluid retention (oedema, increasing breathlessness) or dehydration

- Confusion
- Symptoms/signs of underlying cause e.g. haemolytic uraemic syndrome.

Chronic renal failure: Often asymptomatic until 60–80% of renal function has been lost, though the child may have symptoms/signs of the underlying cause. Later symptoms include:
- ↓ growth/failure to thrive
- Anorexia and/or nausea
- Nocturia or enuresis
- Hypertension
- Bone pain (due to renal osteodystrophy)
- Tiredness and breathlessness (due to anaemia).

Causes include: Glomerulonephritis; reflux nephropathy; hereditary renal disorders e.g. polycystic kidneys, Alport's syndrome, cystinosis; Henoch-Schönlein purpura (￼ p.116); haemolytic uraemic syndrome

❶ Acute crisis may be precipitated by infection (UTI or elsewhere) or dehydration, causing vomiting and an acute ↓ in glomerular filtration rate and renal function – discuss with the child's specialist.

End-stage renal failure (ESRF): End-stage renal failure is irreversible. Dialysis starts when glomerular filtration rate is <5% normal. In children, haemodialysis is the norm. Dialysis is needed lifelong unless a kidney transplant becomes available. In all cases refer back to the renal unit managing the patient if you have any problems.

Haemodialysis: Blood flows opposite dialysis fluid and substances are cleared along a concentration gradient across a semi-permeable membrane. Possible problems include: pulmonary oedema, infection (HIV, hepatitis, bacteria), U&E imbalance, BP (↓ or ↑), problems with vascular access, dialysis arthropathy (especially shoulders and wrists), aluminium toxicity, inconvenience and expense.

Anaemia and erythropoietin: 2° anaemia due to ↓ kidney erythropoietin production is almost universal amongst people with ESRF. Exclude other causes. Recombinant erythropoietin is given if Hb<8.5g/dL (75% patients).

Kidney transplant: Transplanted kidneys are usually sited in an iliac fossa. Median cadaveric graft survival ≈8y. Closer genetic matches have better survival rates. Problems include: rejection, persistent ↑ BP and ↑ cholesterol, renal artery stenosis at 3–9mo. post-op, obstruction at the ureteric anastamosis, ciclosporin-induced nephropathy, infection and malignancy due to immunosuppression, and/or atherosclerosis.

Advice for patients: Information and support for patients and parents

UK National Kidney Federation ☎ 0845 601 0209
￼ www.kidney.org.uk
Kidney Patient Guide ￼ www.kidneypatientguide.org.uk

GMS contract

Pneumococcal vaccination may be offered by GMS practices as a directed enhanced service – ￼ p.87.

Kidney disease affecting children

Haemolytic uraemic syndrome: Commonest cause of acute renal failure in children. Usually follows a bout of gastroenteritis and is due to *E. coli* toxin. Occasionally occurs in the absence of diarrhoea.

Characteristic features:
- Acute renal failure
- Anaemia
- Thrombocytopenia (may result in skin purpura).

Presentation: Have a high index of suspicion in any child with bloody diarrhoea. *Other features include:*
- Dehydration
- Oliguria (though may be polyuria)
- Proteinuria/haematuria
- CNS symptoms – irritability, drowziness, ataxia, coma
- ↑ BP is associated with non-diarrhoeal disease.

Management: Admit. In all cases specialist management (often including dialysis) is required.

Prognosis:
- Mortality in the acute phase is ~15%.
- For children with disease associated with diarrhoeal illness, if the child survives the acute phase, >80% make full recovery. Poor prognostic indicators are age >5y. at onset and dialysis for >2wk.
- Disease in the absence of diarrhoea has much poorer prognosis with the majority progressing to chronic renal failure.

Glomerulonephritis: Symmetrical glomerular injury as a result of an immune process. May be 1° or 2° to other disease (e.g. connective tissue disease) and characterized by microscopic or macroscopic haematuria and red cell casts in the urine.

Types: Table 6.4.

Management: Urgent and ongoing specialist management is required.

Inherited renal diseases: All need specialist management.
Cystinosis: Autosomal recessive disorder due to intracellular cystine accumulation. Children present aged 1–2y. with polyuria/polydipsia, anorexia, nausea and/or vomiting, failure to thrive, vitamin D-resistant rickets, photophobia, lethargy and irritability. Parents may comment the child's hair has become blond. Treatment is with oral mercaptamine which prevents renal and non-renal complications.

Alport's syndrome: X-linked or autosomal recessive disease. Congenital sensorineural deafness with recurrent pyelonephritis, haematuria and renal failure (due to glomerulonephritis). Associated with lens abnormalities, platelet dysfunction and hyperproteinaemia. Causes death in males by 20–30y. without transplantation. Females have normal life expectancy. Renal failure does not recur after transplantation.

Henoch-Schönlein purpura: 📖 p.116

Table 6.4 Types of glomerulonephritis affecting children

Type	Features
Minimal change	Peak incidence aged 2–4y. Presents with nephrotic syndrome (90% nephrotic syndrome in children <5y.). Prognosis is excellent and progression to chronic renal failure rare. 60% have ≥1 relapse in childhood.
Proliferative	Typically presents with acute nephritic syndrome 2wk. after Streptococcal infection e.g. sore throat. Accounts for 90% of acute glomerulonephritis. Prognosis is excellent and >90% children recover completely.
Membrano-proliferative	50% present as nephrotic syndrome. Accounts for 8% nephrotic syndrome in children. 50% progress to end-stage renal failure.
Focal	*Berger's disease* – cause of 50% of recurrent haematuria in children. Episodes are associated with viral infection and/or flank pain. Good prognosis – only rarely progresses to chronic renal failure in children. *Focal, segmental glomerulosclerosis* – can affect any age group. Always associated with proteinuria (often nephrotic syndrome). 50% progress to chronic renal failure <10y. after diagnosis. May recur in transplanted kidneys.
Rapidly progressive/crescentic	Presents with haematuria, oliguria, ↑BP, acute renal failure. Vigorous treatment can save renal function but prognosis is poor. Associations – anti-glomerular basement membrane antibodies, Henoch-Schönlein purpura, post-streptococcal infection (rare).

🛈 Terminology:

Focal – some glomeruli affected **Segmental** – part of each glomerulus affected
Diffuse – all glomeruli affected **Global** – all of each glomerulus is affected

GP Notes: Vaccination of children with chronic renal disease

In addition to the usual childhood vaccinations, children with:
- Chronic renal disease should be given influenza vaccination
- Chronic renal disease and/or nephrotic syndrome should be given pneumococcal vaccination.

GMS contract

Influenza and pneumococcal vaccination may be offered by GMS practices as a directed enhanced service – 📖 p.87.

Advice for patients: Information and support for patients and parents

UK National Kidney Federation ☎ 0845 601 0209
🖳 www.kidney.org.uk

Urinary tract infection

8% girls and 2% boys have a urinary tract infection (UTI) in childhood – the majority in the 1st year of life. Amongst neonates, boys have more infections than girls. In all other age groups $♀:♂≈10:1$.

Consequences of UTI in childhood

- 5–15% of children with UTI develop renal scarring within 1–2y. of the 1st infection.
- There is a higher incidence in children with renal tract abnormalities and vesicoureteric reflux.
- Infections causing renal scarring are associated with adult pyelonephritis, ↑BP, impaired renal function and renal failure.
- Prognosis is worst for children with recurrent infection, severe reflux and scarring at first presentation.

Causative organisms: Most childhood UTIs are caused by normal bowel flora–E. coli (80%), Klebsiella, Pseudomonas and other gram-negative organisms.

Clinical features of UTI in children

- *Infants and toddlers:* Usually non-specific including vomiting, irritability, fever, abdominal pain, failure to thrive and prolonged jaundice.
- *Older children:* Dysuria, urinary frequency, abdominal pain, haematuria, enuresis.

Investigation: Suspect diagnosis and check urine in any child with urinary symptoms or any infant with fever >38.5°C with no definite cause. Send urine for M,C&S.

Management

- The aim of management is to treat infection and prevent long-term complications.
- Treat symptomatic infection without waiting for the result of the urine specimen with trimethoprim for 7–10d., altering the antibiotic should the responsible organism prove resistant on culture.
- If UTI is confirmed arrange post-treatment urine sample collection to confirm clearance.
- Prophylactic antibiotics (usually trimethoprim od) should be started after the first infection and continued at least until results of imaging are known.
- Prophylactic antibiotics may be required long term if there is reflux or an underlying abnormality to prevent (further) renal scarring.

Follow-up: Local policies vary – consult local guidelines.

- Refer all children to a paediatrician after the 1st proven UTI – arrange USS in the meantime if possible.
- Further imaging depends on age of the child and local protocols:
  - *Infants <1y.* generally need a micturating cystourethrogram (MCUG) to assess for reflux
  - *Older children* may require IVP or DMSA scans.

Further information

NICE Urinary tract infection: diagnosis, treatment and long-term management of urinary tract infection in children (due to publish in July 2007).

Balanitis: Acute inflammation of the glans and foreskin. Common organisms: *Staphylococcus, Streptococcus, Coliforms, Candida*. Balanitis can occur at any age but is most common amongst young boys when it is associated with non-retractile foreskin or phimosis.

Management:
- If a baby has candidal nappy rash and mild balanitis, consider treating with topical antifungal e.g. clotrimazole or nystatin as a fungal cause is most likely.
- Otherwise treat with oral antibiotics e.g. flucloxacillin.
- If recurrent, refer for circumcision, particularly if due to phimosis or non-retractile foreskin.

Associated conditions:
- **Phimosis:** Foreskin obstructs urine flow. Common amongst small children. Time usually obviates need for circumcision. Refer if recurrent balanitis.
- **Non-retractile foreskin:** Usually noted by parents. On examination the foreskin is adherent. Retractility increases with age and local policies on referral for circumcision vary – be aware of local guidance. Refer if recurrent balanitis.

⚠ Attempts to retract a non-retractile foreskin can result in *paraphimosis* (foreskin is retracted then unable to be replaced). Refer as emergency to prevent glandular necrosis.

Epididymo-orchitis: Inflammation of the testis and epididymis due to infection. The commonest viral cause is mumps. The commonest bacterial infections are coliforms. May occur at any age.

Presentation: Acute-onset pain in testis; swelling and tenderness of testis/epididymis; fever ± rigors; may be dysuria and ↑ frequency.

Management: May be difficult to distinguish from torsion of the testis. If in doubt admit for urology/surgical opinion. Otherwise, if not associated with viral illness, treat with trimethoprim.

⚠ **Torsion of the testis:** Presents with sudden-onset severe scrotal pain. May be associated with RIF pain, nausea and vomiting. *Examination:* tender, hard testis riding higher than contralateral testis. Admit as an emergency to a surgical/urology team.

187

GP Notes: Collecting bag specimens of urine

- Urine collection can be problematic in a young child. A clean catch is best but a bag may be necessary.
- When collecting a bag specimen the child should be upright and the bag removed as soon as it has been filled to minimize contamination.
- Special pads are also available and are preferred by parents.
- It is important to indicate what method of collection was used for proper interpretation of results.
- ⓘ Any positive culture obtained via a bag or pad specimen should be checked with a urine sample taken by clean catch, suprapubic aspirate or catheter specimen (rarely needed).

Neuroblastoma and Wilm's tumour

Neuroblastoma: Tumour derived from neural crest tissue. 80 cases/y. are reported in England and Wales – 8% of all paediatric tumours. Neuroblastoma tends to affect children <4y. old (50% <2y.; 90% <9y.). *Sites:* adrenal medulla – 50%; abdominal sympathetic ganglia – 25%; chest – 20%; pelvis – 5%; neck – 5%.

Presentation: Variable and often non-specific – depends on site of the tumour and extent of metastases. ~½ present with metastatic disease.
- *General effects:*
  - Pallor
  - Fever
  - Anorexia and weight ↓
  - Irritability
  - Flushing
  - Ataxia
  - Diarrhoea
  - Failure to thrive
- *Local effects of the tumour:* Abdominal mass (or thoracic mass on CXR); local spread may cause paraplegia or cauda equine syndrome. Infants <6mo. may have rapidly progressive intra-abdominal disease.
- *Effects of metastases:* Lymphatic and haematogenous spread, particularly to liver, lungs and bone, is common. Associated symptoms:
  - Bone pain ± pathological fracture
  - Breathlessness
  - Periorbital bruising (looks like a black eye), proptosis or Horner's syndrome
  - Firm skin nodules (usually babies – 'blueberry muffin' appearance).

Investigate with a FBC if [N]: Persistent or unexplained bone pain (X-ray is also needed); pallor or fatigue; unexplained irritability; unexplained fever; persistent or recurrent URTI; generalized lymphadenopathy and/or unexplained bruising.

If neuroblastoma is suspected: Carry out an abdominal examination (and/or urgent USS), and consider CXR and FBC. If any mass is found, refer urgently.

Specialist management and prognosis: Treatment is with surgery, chemotherapy and/or radiotherapy. *Prognosis:* early-stage disease has a 95% 5y. survival; late-stage disease has 20% 5y. survival. Children with extra-abdominal tumours, and those who are <1y. at diagnosis, have better prognosis.

Wilm's nephroblastoma: 70 cases/y. in England and Wales. Kidney tumour composed of primitive renal tissue. The left kidney is affected more often than the right and it is bilateral in 10%. Usually affects children <5y. old (peak age 2–3y.). ♂>♀. Rarely associated with Beckwith-Wiedemann syndrome, aniridia or hemihypertrophy.

Presentation:
- *General effects:* Fever, anorexia and weight ↓, anaemia
- *Local effects of the tumour:* Unilateral abdominal mass ± pain ± unexplained haematuria
- *Effects of metastases:* 20% have metastases to liver, lungs or bone (rare) at presentation. May present with symptoms/signs of metastases.

Management[N]: If a child presents with abdominal distension, examine the abdomen. *Refer if:* Intrabdominal mass (immediate referral) or unexplained haematuria (urgent referral).

Specialist treatment and prognosis: Treatment is with surgery ± chemotherapy ± radiotherapy depending on histology and stage at diagnosis. Early-stage tumours have 80% 5y. survival; late-stage tumours have 50% 5y. survival.

Referral guidelines[N]:

Refer urgently/immediately: Children with:
- Abdominal mass
- Unexplained petechiae or bruising
- Hepatosplenomegaly
- Skin nodules in a baby which could be metastatic neuroblastoma
- Proptosis
- Leg weakness – refer immediately if gait abnormalities or motor or Sensory signs
- Unexplained back pain (perform FBC as well)
- Unexplained urinary retention
- Unexplained behavioural and/or mood changes or unexplained deteriorating school performance or developmental milestones
- Thoracic mass on CXR
- FBC suggesting malignancy.

Refer urgently: When a child/young person presents several times (≥ 3x) with the same problem, but with no clear diagnosis.

Abdominal distension: Examine the abdomen, particularly if persistent or progressive:
- If a mass is found, refer immediately
- If the child is uncooperative and abdominal examination is not possible, or if examination is difficult, consider referral for urgent abdominal USS.

Consider referral: When there is persistent parental anxiety, even when a benign cause is considered most likely.

GMS contract			
Cancer 1	The practice can produce a record of all cancer patients diagnosed after 1.4.2003	5 points	
Cancer 3	% of patients with cancer diagnosed <18mo. ago who have a patient review recorded as occurring <6mo. after the practice received confirmation of diagnosis	up to 6 points	40–90%
Education 7	The practice has undertaken ≥12 significant event reviews in the past 3y. which could include new cancer diagnoses	Total of 4 points for 12 significant event reviews	

Further information

NICE Referral guidelines for suspected cancer – quick reference guide (2005) 🖳 www.nice.org.uk

Childhood diabetes mellitus

Diabetes mellitus (DM) is the most common endocrine disease of childhood and incidence is increasing, particularly in the under-4s. Peak incidence is aged 12–14y. Children are nearly always affected by type 1 diabetes although, with increasing childhood obesity, type 2 (non-insulin-dependent, maturity-onset) diabetes is no longer as rare as it used to be.

Type 1 diabetes: Also known as insulin-dependent diabetes (IDDM) or juvenile-onset diabetes.
- Autoimmune disease probably triggered by environmental factors.
- Islet cell antibodies may initially be present.
- Associated with other autoimmune disease and certain genotypes (HLA DR3/4 – though identical twin concordance ≈30%).
- Patients are prone to profound weight ↓ and ketoacidosis.
- Insulin is needed from diagnosis.

Presentation
- *Short history* (days/weeks) of polyuria and polydipsia with weight ↓.
- *Non specific-symptoms* e.g tiredness, malaise with history of polydipsia and polyuria only revealed by direct questioning. Always think of DM and check urine for glucose if a child starts wetting the bed again at night after a period of being dry.
- *Acute ketoacidosis* – see opposite.

Diagnosis and initial management: Check BM. Diagnosis is on the basis of history and BM >11. Any child with suspected diabetes should be referred for a same-day hospital assessment[N].

Management of acute ketoacidosis: See opposite.

Specialist management of a new diagnosis of diabetes: The hospital team may initiate treatment without admission if the child is well, and sufficient specialist support is available in the community (should include 24h. telephone advice).

Specialist management involves:
- Stabilization of blood glucose with insulin and diet
- Education about use of insulin, blood sugar monitoring, exercise, diet, intercurrent illness and hypoglycaemia (avoidance, recognition and management).

Subsequent management: The majority of care of children with diabetes is from specialist multidisciplinary teams consisting of a paediatric consultant with special interest in diabetes, a paediatric diabetic nurse specialist, a dietician and psychologist. Usually follow-up is every 3mo., but can be more frequently as needed.

Aims of management:
- To achieve a glycosylated haemoglobin (HbA1c) <7.5 without frequent and disabling hypoglycaemia[N].
- Intensive regimens ↓ microvascular complications but must be weighed against ↑ risk of hypoglycaemia.

Acute ketoacidosis:

Presentation: The child may be a known diabetic or ketoacidosis may be the presenting feature of diabetes in a child not known to be diabetic.

- History of 2–3d. deterioration often precipitated by infection. The younger the child the more rapid the deterioration.
- On examination the child is typically dehydrated with Kussmaul breathing (deep sighing breaths), ketotic (fruity) smelling breath, shock (↓ BP and postural drop, tachycardia) ± coma.

Investigation: BM is usually >20mmol/l and urine (if available) tests +ve for ketones.

Management:

- Arrange to admit as an emergency to hospital.
- If shocked/coma – lie flat, elevate feet and resuscitate:
  - Airway – check airway is clear
  - Breathing – give 100% O_2 if available
  - Circulation – gain IV access if possible and give 10ml/kg 0.9% saline rapidly. Repeat up to 3x as needed.

⚠ Diabetic ketoacidosis can present with vomiting and abdominal pain mimicking acute abdomen – always check for ketotic breath and Kussmaul breathing.

GP Notes: The GP's role in ongoing management of the diabetic child

- Support of child and family including liason with secondary care services as required
- Emergency management of hypoglycaemia
- Management of intercurrent illness
- Vaccination
- Support in adolescence – particularly when transferring from paediatric to adult services.

Advice for patients: Information and support for children and parents

Diabetes UK ☎ 0845 120 2960 🖥 www.diabetes.org.uk

191

Further information

WHO Definition, diagnosis and classification of diabetes mellitus and its complications (2000) 🖥 www.diabetes.org.uk
NICE Diagnosis and management of type 1 diabetes in children and young people (2004) 🖥 www.nice.org.uk

Commonly used insulin regimens:
- Twice daily mix of short- and intermediate-acting insulin.
- Short-acting insulin 3 times a day before meals with intermediate- or long-acting insulin before bed – this allows more flexibility so is the usual regime for adolescents.
- Continuous subcutaneous insulin infusion is an option where a multiple injection regime fails to achieve adequate control[N].

Hypoglycaemia: Blood glucose <4mmol/l. Hypoglycaemia is a particular risk in children with diabetes as:
- They vary their routines (exercise and diet) considerably
- May present atypically *and*
- May have hypoglycaemic unawareness.

Presentation:
- Sweating
- Hunger
- Tremor
- Odd or violent behaviour
- Tachycardia ± ↑ BP
- Coma (📖 p.38) – may or may not have had warning signs.

❗ Younger children may present atypically with behavioural changes or headache.

Management of hypoglycaemia: Check BM.
- If the child is conscious, give simple carbohydrate (e.g. 3 glucose tablets, 100ml of a sugar-containing soft drink e.g. Lucozade® or Hypostop®).
- If unable to take oral carbohydrate due to impaired consciousness, give IM glucagon (children <25kg–0.5mg; children >25kg–1mg). Glucagon may have reduced effect if the child is starved or drunk. An alternative is 2–5ml/kg 10% glucose solution IV. Once the child has regained consciousness, supplement with simple carbohydrate as for the conscious child.
- As symptoms improve give complex carbohydrate e.g. biscuits.
- Repeat glucose testing within 15min.
- Monitor frequent blood sugars hourly over the next 4h. and 4-hourly for the following 24h.
- Review reasons for hypoglycaemia.

Prevention of hypoglycaemia:
- Common reasons for episodes of hypoglycaemia include missed or late meals, increased activity and/or problems with insulin administration.
- Ensure the child/parents always carry a supply of ready glucose e.g. glucose tablets or Hypostop gel®.
- Ensure that the child has a supply of in-date glucagon at home and someone knows when and how to use it.
- Liaise with the specialist team if frequent or severe episodes of hypoglycaemia.

Intercurrent illness: Intercurrent illness often ↑ insulin require-ment. As a result the child may become hyperglycaemic and even develop ketoacidosis even if dietary intake is ↓.

Management:
- Frequent blood monitoring (e.g. 4-hourly).
- Check urine for ketones.
- Give additional short-acting insulin as needed – 10–20% of the child's total dose every 2–4h. as needed to keep the BM <15.
- If BMs are low, insulin dose may need to be decreased – but NEVER stop insulin.
- Suggest easily digested food or sugar-containing fluids to replace meals if the child is not eating normally.

🔔 Remember vomiting can be a sign of ketoacidosis.

Vaccination: In addition to routine childhood vaccinations (📖 p.84), diabetic children should have pneumococcal vaccination and annual influenza vaccination.

GMS contract

Influenza and pneumococcal vaccination may be offered by GMS practices as a directed enhanced service – 📖 p.87.

Advice for patients: Information and support for children and parents

Diabetes UK ☎ 0845 120 2960 🖥 www.diabetes.org.uk

Further information

NICE Diagnosis and management of type 1 diabetes in children and young people (2004) 🖥 www.nice.org.uk

Growth disorders

Take every opportunity to weigh and measure every child. Plot height, weight (and head circumference if <1y.) on centile charts. Always correct the age of the child for prematurity at birth.

Failure to thrive: 📖 p.68

Short stature: Height <3rd centile. Mainly healthy children (80%) but may indicate physical or emotional problems, especially if both parents have heights >3rd centile or serial measurements show growth has fallen below that expected from the centile chart. *Causes*:

- *Genetic:* Achondroplastic dwarfism; familial short stature; Turner's syndrome; familial growth delay – children have delayed pubertal growth spurt but eventually reach normal height
- *Physical:* Low birth weight conditions; endocrine causes e.g. growth hormone deficiency, hypopituitarism, hypothyroidism, DM; chronic illness e.g. severe asthma, heart disease, chronic infection
- *Non-organic:* Poor nutrition; emotional neglect; eating disorders

Assessment:

- Ask how the child eats and problems with feeding the child – appetite, food fads, special diets, quantities and times of the day, snacks etc.
- Ask about other physical problems e.g. breathlessness, diarrhoea.
- Examine the child carefully from top to toe, looking for any physical abnormalities or signs of developmental delay.
- Watch the way the child interacts with you and the parent. Look for evidence of neglect or maltreatment.
- Look to see how large the parents are – 2 small parents will probably have a small child.

Management: Treat any reversible causes. Continue to measure height and weight regularly. Try to use the same scales on each occasion. Refer to paediatrics if no cause for short stature is found; if an abnormality requiring specialist paediatric care is found; or if, despite treatment of a reversible cause, the child fails to grow along his/her growth curve.

Pituitary dwarfism: ↓ function of the anterior pituitary gland causing short stature or failure to thrive. Skeletal maturation, assessed by bone age, is usually >2y. behind chronological age. *Causes*:

- Idiopathic
- Genetic
- Midline defect e.g. cleft palate
- Pituitary tumour e.g. craniopharyngioma

Management: Specialist management is essential. Treatment is with growth hormone and replacement of cortisol and thyroid hormone if needed and/or gonadal sex steroids if normal puberty fails. ⓘ Slipped femoral epiphysis is more common amongst children being treated with growth hormone.

Excessive height: Most children with height >97th centile come from tall families. Pathological causes of excess height are rare and include pituitary adenoma (gigantism), thyrotoxicosis, precocious puberty, Marfan's syndrome and homocystinuria. Refer if a child is much taller than predicted height or deviates from his growth curve.

Head growth: At birth, head circumference is 32–37cm (term infant). The anterior fontanelle measures 2.5x2.5cm at birth, becoming smaller until it closes any time from 6–18mo. Most head growth occurs in infancy. Refer children with head circumference <3rd or >97th centile.

- **Microcephaly:** 📖 p.205
- **Macrocephaly:** Large head circumference. *Causes:* Hydrocephalus (suspect if the head circumference deviates from the normal curve or if there are signs of ↑ intracranial pressure – refer); megalencephaly (usually benign and familial – rarely associated developmental delay)
- **Asymmetrical skull:** *Causes:* Postural effects e.g. children who always sleep on 1 side; craniosynostosis (premature fusion of skull sutures – if suspected refer for prompt neurosurgical opinion)

Disorders of puberty:

Precocious puberty: Puberty before normal age for the population. In the UK, this is <8y. for girls and <9y. for boys. In all cases refer for specialist investigation and advice on management. *Types:*
- **True:** Course and pattern are normal but early. *Causes:* Idiopathic (90% ♀; 50–60% ♂), hypothalamic tumour, other CNS pathology.
- **Pseudo:** Pattern is abnormal – ≥1 element of puberty occurs (e.g. breast development), but other elements do not. *Causes:* Testicular or ovarian tumour, congenital adrenal hyperplasia, hepatoblastoma, adrenal virilizing tumours, Cushing's syndrome.

Delayed puberty: No pubertal changes in a girl aged 13y. or boy aged 13½ y. or failure of progression of puberty over 2y. Affects ~2% of population. In all cases refer to paediatrics for further investigation. Constitutional delay accounts for 90%. *Other causes:* Chromosomal abnormalities e.g. Turner's or Klinefelter's syndromes; GnRH deficiency e.g. pituitary lesions, gonadal failure, hypothyroidism; hypothalamic suppression e.g. anorexia, sportsmen, systemic illness.

Primary amenorrhoea (without delayed puberty): No menstruation by age 16y. when growth and sexual development is normal. Refer to paediatrics or gynaecology for further investigation. *Causes:* Familial; structural abnormality (e.g. imperforate hymen and haematocolpos); 2° causes of amenorrhoea e.g. stress, anorexia, thyroid disorders.

GP Notes: Calculating expected height

Small parents have small children and tall parents have tall children – always calculate expected height of the child before deciding the child has short stature or excessive height.

Expected height = (mother's height + father's height) ÷ 2

Then: add 6cm for a boy or subtract 6cm for a girl
❶ 3% of 'normal' children fall under the 3rd and 3% above the 97th centiles.

Advice for patients: Information and support for children and parents

Height Matters 🖥 www.heightmatters.org.uk

Childhood obesity

Obesity is one of the most important preventable diseases in the UK. About 10% of schoolchildren in the UK are obese and the incidence is increasing. Obesity is set to take over from smoking as the number one preventable cause of disease in the UK.

Classification: BMI (weight in kg ÷ (height in m)^2) can be used to assess obesity in children but child reference tables must be used. Overweight is defined as BMI ≥91st centile and obese as BMI ≥98th centile. BMI charts are available at: ⌨ www.healthforallchildren.co.uk

Health risks of childhood obesity:
- Hypercholesterolaemia
- ↑ BP (25% of children with BMI >95th centile are hypertensive)
- Type 2 DM (4% incidence in children with BMI >95th centile)
- Gallbladder disease
- Sleep apnoea
- Psychological problems (low self-esteem, bullying)
- Orthopaedic problems e.g. slipped femoral epiphysis
- Obesity in adulthood – 75% are obese in adulthood leading to ↑ risks of vascular disease, orthopaedic problems, DM and certain cancers.
- Exacerbation of asthma

Risk factors: Genetic predisposition (accounts for about $^1/_3$ obesity); physical inactivity – particularly television watching; low socio-economic group; maternal smoking cessation.

Prevention
- Begins in infancy – breast-feeding has a protective effect.
- Instilling healthy patterns of exercise and diet from the early years – family perceptions are important as many parents don't recognize their children are obese or overweight.

⓵ There is little evidence to show that dietary advice by GPs or practice nurses is heeded. Most influence on diet comes from national food policy, price of food, advertising, general education and cultural influences.

Assessment
- History – including family history, eating and exercise patterns, psychological factors and motivation to make changes
- Height and weight
- Pubertal assessment where appropriate
- Physical examination – particularly looking for signs of endocrine problems e.g. truncal obesity or striae suggesting Cushing's syndrome; acne and hirsuitism suggesting polycystic ovaries; dysmorphic features; signs of orthopaedic complications
- BP (use appropriate-size cuff)
- Urinanalysis for glucose and protein

Treatment: In children who are still growing, aim for a ↓ rate of weight gain relative to height gain rather than weight loss. For adolescents who have stopped growing, aim for weight loss of ~1lb (0.5kg)/wk.

General principles:
- *Suggest a healthy balanced diet* (Figure 6.1) for the whole family, particularly ↑ fruit/vegetable consumption and wholefoods and ↓ energy-dense food e.g. crisps and sweets.
- *Avoid* snacks between meals (use healthy options e.g. fruit if really necessary), fizzy or sweet drinks (ideally children should drink water, otherwise choose low-calorie options) and serve up smaller portions.
- *Increase exercise levels* – obese children may find sport embarrassing. Make exercise enjoyable and build it into daily routine e.g. walking.
- *Psychosocial issues* – counselling may help if self-esteem is very low. Involve the school if bullying is a problem.
- *Follow-up* on a regular basis is essential to maintain motivation.

Reasons to refer to paediatrics:
- Obesity causing morbidity e.g. sleep apnoea, diabetes, hypertension
- Precocious or delayed puberty
- Short stature (<9th centile, delayed growth velocity or short in relation to other family members)
- Other signs or symptoms of an endocrine or chromosomal cause of obesity
- Significant learning disability
- Severe progressive obesity in a child aged < 2y.

Further information:
NICE Obesity: prevention, identification, assessment and management of overweight and obesity in adults and children (2006) ▣ www.nice.org.uk

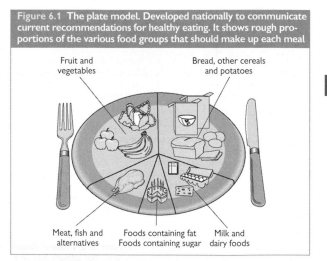

Figure 6.1 The plate model. Developed nationally to communicate current recommendations for healthy eating. It shows rough proportions of the various food groups that should make up each meal

Fruit and vegetables

Bread, other cereals and potatoes

Meat, fish and alternatives

Foods containing fat
Foods containing sugar

Milk and dairy foods

Thyroid and other endocrine problems

Congenital goitre: Enlarged thyroid gland present at birth ± hypo- or hyperthyroidism. Hypothyroid babies are treated with thyroxine; if there is tracheal compression or hyperthyroidism treatment is surgical.

Hypothyroidism:

Neonatal (congenital) hypothyroidism: 📖 p.18

Juvenile (acquired) hypothyroidism: Usually due to autoimmune thyroiditis (Hashimoto's thyroiditis). Often insidious onset with ↑ weight, constipation, dry or coarse hair, and sallow, cool or mottled coarse skin. In children there may also be growth retardation, delayed skeletal maturation ± delayed puberty. TFTs confirm diagnosis. Refer to paediatrics for specialist management. Treatment is with thyroxine replacement.

Hyperthyroidism:

Neonatal hyperthyroidism: Rare but potentially life-threatening. Occurs in infants of mothers with current or prior Graves' disease due to passage of autoantibodies across the placenta. *Presentation:*

- Feeding problems
- ↑ BP
- Irritability
- Tachycardia
- Exophthalmos
- Goitre
- Frontal bossing
- Microcephaly
- Failure to thrive
- Vomiting
- Diarrhoea

Refer for specialist management. Affected infants generally recover in <4mo. Long-term consequences include premature fusion of the cranial sutures (craniosynostosis) and developmental delay.

Juvenile hyperthyroidism: Usually due to Graves' disease – an autoimmune disease in which antibodies to the TSH receptor are produced.

Features due to hyperthyroidism:
- Weight ↓
- Tremor
- Palpitations (may have AF)
- Hyperactivity
- Diffuse goitre ± thyroid bruit

Eye features:
- Double vision
- Eye discomfort ± protrusion (exophthalmos and proptosis)
- Lid lag
- Ophthalmoplegia

TFTs confirm diagnosis. Refer for specialist management. Treatment is with antithyroid medication. Spontaneous resolution in <2y. is the norm.

Congenital adrenal hyperplasia (CAH): Also known as *adrenogenital syndrome* or *adrenal virilism*. Autosomal recessive trait due to absence or deficiency of any of the enzymes needed for synthesis of cortisol. Each enzyme block causes a characteristic deficiency. 2 patterns:
- Androgens accumulate causing virilization of an affected female fetus
- Androgen synthesis is impaired causing inadequate virilization of an affected male fetus (much rarer).

Presentation and management: Ambiguity of the external genitalia. Less severe forms may go unnoticed until puberty. There may be a family history of CAH, ambiguous genitalia or neonatal death. Rarely presents with Addisonian crisis. Refer for specialist management. Treatment is usually with glucocorticoid ± mineralocorticoid replacement.

Addison's disease: Primary adrenocortical insufficiency. In the UK, most cases are due to autoimmune disease. Presents with tiredness, muscle weakness, hypoglycaemia, hyperpigmentation (buccal, palmar creases, new scars) or Addisonian crisis (rare). Refer to a paediatric endocrinologist – treatment involves glucocorticoid ± mineralocorticoid replacement.

Hypoadrenal (Addisonian) crisis: May occur in children on long-term steroids (treatment or replacement) if the steroids are stopped suddenly or not ↑ during intercurrent illness or may be a presenting feature of CAH or Addison's disease. Presents with vomiting, hypotension and shock.

Management: Give IM or IV hydrocortisone: Children >12y.: 100mg; Children 1mo.–12y.: 2–4mg/kg. Admit to hospital for further management.

Prevention: Patients on long-term steroids should carry a steroid card and wear a Medic-Alert bracelet or similar. Advise patients on long-term steroids to double the dose of steroids during pyrexial illness.

Male hypogonadism: ↓ function of the testes. 3 types:
- *Primary:* Damage to the Leydig cells impairs androgen (testosterone) secretion e.g. Klinefelter's syndrome, anorchia (absent testes)
- *Secondary (hypogonadotropic):* Disorders of the hypothalamus or pituitary impair gonadotropin secretion which may result in impotency and/or infertility e.g. panhypopituitarism
- *Resistance to androgen action:* Age of onset dictates presentation:
  - in utero – ambiguity of genitalia or female appearance, small penis, incomplete testicular descent
  - in childhood – delayed or impaired puberty, impaired development of male 2° sexual characteristics ± gynaecomastia
  - in adulthood – ↓ libido, impotence, loss of muscle power, testicular atrophy, fine wrinkling of the skin around eyes and lips, sparse body hair, osteopoenia, gynaecomastia.

Management: Refer for specialist investigation. Treatment depends on the nature of the deficiency.

GP Notes: Dealing with sexual ambiguity detected at the 6-week check
- Be honest – don't guess the gender of the child.
- Explain that there are rare conditions where girls may be virilized or boys undermasculinized, causing girls to look like boys and vice versa.
- Arrange paediatric assessment as soon as possible for further investigations, gender assignment and ongoing management.

GMS contract

Thyroid 1	The practice can produce a register of patients with hypothyroidism	1 point	
Thyroid 2	% of patients with hypothyroidism with thyroid function tests recorded in the past 15mo.	up to 6 points	40–90%

Chapter 7

Musculoskeletal and neurological problems in children

Birth trauma

Head trauma:

Caput succedaneum: Swelling, bruising and oedema of the presenting portion – usually scalp. Unsightly but resolves spontaneously.

Cephalhaematoma: Uncommon. Haemorrhage beneath the periosteum. Unilateral and usually parietal. Presents as a lump – the size of an egg – on the baby's head. Treatment is not required, but anaemia or hyperbilirubinaemia may follow.

Depressed skull fractures: Rare. Most result from forceps pressure; rarely caused by the head resting on a bony prominence *in utero*. May be associated with subdural bleeding, subarachnoid hemorrhage or contusion/laceration of the brain itself. Seen and felt as a depression in the skull. X-ray confirms diagnosis; neurosurgical elevation may be needed.

Intracranial haemorrhage: Rare. Suggested by lack of responsiveness, fits, respiratory distress ± shock. Admit as an emergency.

Nerve injuries:

Cranial nerve trauma: The facial nerve is injured, most often causing facial asymmetry, especially during crying. Usually resolves spontaneously by 2–3mo. of age. Refer to paediatric neurology if not resolving.

Brachial plexus injury: Follows stretching caused by shoulder dystocia, breech extraction or hyperabduction of the neck in cephalic presentations. Often associated with other traumatic injuries e.g. fractured clavicle or humerus.

- *Partial injuries of the brachial plexus:* Most recover but site and type of nerve root injury determine prognosis. If persistent refer to paediatric neurology for further investigation. A biceps deficit lasting >3mo. has poor prognosis and requires surgery. Figure 7.1.
  - Injuries of the upper brachial plexus (C5–6) affect muscles around the shoulder and elbow – *Erb's palsy.*
  - Injuries of the lower plexus (C7–8 and T1) affect primarily muscles of the forearm and hand – *Klumpke's palsy.*
- *Injuries of the entire brachial plexus:* No movement of the arm + sensory loss. Refer immediately for neurological opinion. Prognosis for recovery is poor.

Fractures:

Midclavicular fracture: Most common fracture during birth. Usually occurs due to shoulder dystocia. Refer if suspected. Most clavicular fractures are greenstick and heal rapidly and uneventfully. A large callus forms at the fracture site in <1wk. and remodelling is completed in <1mo. Can be associated with brachial plexus injury and/or pneumothorax.

Long-bone fractures: The humerus and femur may be fractured during difficult deliveries. Refer if suspected. Usually long bones heal rapidly without any residual deformity.

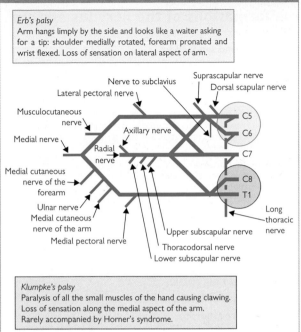

Figure 7.1 Brachial plexus injuries in neonates

Erb's palsy
Arm hangs limply by the side and looks like a waiter asking for a tip: shoulder medially rotated, forearm pronated and wrist flexed. Loss of sensation on lateral aspect of arm.

Klumpke's palsy
Paralysis of all the small muscles of the hand causing clawing. Loss of sensation along the medial aspect of the arm. Rarely accompanied by Horner's syndrome.

Congenital orthopaedic problems and malformations of the nervous system

Polydactyly and syndactyly:

Polydactyly: Extra digits vary from small fleshy tags to complete duplications. Isolated defect or associated with syndromes. Small fleshy tags are removed in the first few months – surgery for more substantial digits is delayed until the child is >1y. Refer to orthopaedics/plastic surgery.

Syndactyly: Digits may be joined by a web of skin or more firmly fused. Webbing is usually mild and treatment is for cosmetic reasons, if at all. Where digits are fused separation and skin grafting is carried out at ~4y. Refer to plastic surgery.

Club foot (talipes): Consists of inversion of the foot, adduction of forefoot relative to hindfoot and equinus (plantar flexion).
- *Positional talipes:* Moulding deformity seen in neonates. The foot can be passively everted and dorsiflexed to the normal position. Treatment is with physiotherapy. Follow up to check the deformity is resolving.
- *True talipes:* The foot *cannot* be passively everted and dorsiflexed to the normal position. Refer to orthopaedics. Treatment is with physiotherapy, splints ± surgery.

Congenital dislocation of the hip (CDH)/developmental dysplasia of the hip (DDH): 📖 p.24

Congenital scoliosis: 📖 p.26

Hypermobility syndrome: Occurs in children or young adults with lax joints. <½ are symptomatic. Those that have symptoms present with recurrent joint pains, mainly affecting the knees. Other symptoms include joint effusion, dislocation, ligamentous injuries, low back pain and premature osteoarthritis. The condition is benign, and joints become stiffer with age. Treatment, when needed, is with physiotherapy. Rarely associated with rare congenital disorders e.g. Ehlers-Danlos syndrome.

Genetic problems:

Cleido-cranial dysostosis: Autosomal dominant inheritance. Part/all of the clavicle is missing and ossification of the skull is delayed – sutures remain open. Associated with short stature. No treatment is needed.

Osteogenesis imperfecta: Autosomal dominant inheritance (rarely recessive). Several types but all have an underlying problem with collagen metabolism, resulting in fragile bones which break easily. Other features include lax joints, thin skin, blue sclerae, hypoplastic teeth and deafness. Presentation varies according to severity. May be obvious at birth or present later. Can be mistaken for non-accidental injury. Treatment is supportive.

Osteopetrosis (marble bone disease): Autosomal dominant form presents in childhood with fractures, osteomyelitis ± facial paralysis. Recessive form is more severe causing bone marrow failure and death. Bone marrow transplantation is of limited success.

Brain malformations: All associated with developmental delay, convulsions ± failure to thrive.

- *Microcephaly:* 1:1000 births. Small head out of proportion with the size of the body. Associated with developmental delay. *Causes:* Genetic, intrauterine infection (e.g. rubella, CMV), chromosome abnormality, fetal alcohol syndrome, hypoxia.
- *Holoprosencephaly:* Failure of development of the forebrain, with associated midface developmental abnormalities. ~½ have trisomy 13. Survival is rare >6mo. Recurrence in subsequent pregnancies is ~5%.
- *Congenital hydrocephalus:* 📖 p.220

Neural tube defects: Most neural tube defects are detected antenatally at routine antenatal screening. Types of defect:
- *Anencephaly:* Absent cerebral cortex and skull vault. Incompatible with life – those infants born alive die within hours of birth.
- *Cranium defects:* Vary from meningocoele (meninges protrude through skull) to encephalocoele (brain tissue protrudes through skull).
- *Spina bifida:* The vertebral arch is incomplete.
  - *Occulta:* Common. The lesion is covered with skin and fascia. Usually asymptomatic but may be mild gait or bladder problems.
  - *Cystica:* Involves herniation of the meninges (meningocoele). Uncommon but treatable usually with minor residual defect.
  - *Whole cord herniation* (myelomeningocoele) is more common and often results in neurological deficit. It is associated with hydrocephalus, and learning and psychological problems.

Primary care management: Support the child and family and ensure receipt of all available benefits. Liaise with the primary health care team and community and specialist services to ensure prompt provision of equipment and services. Tell carers about local facilities, voluntary and self-help organizations.

Advice for patients: Support for parents and children

Steps Support for children with lower limb conditions
☎ 0871 717 0044 🖥 www.steps-charity.org.uk
Hypermobility Syndrome Association (HMSA) ☎ 0845 345 4465
🖥 www.hypermobility.org
Association for Spina Bifida and Hydrocephalus (ASBAH)
☎ 0845 450 7755 🖥 www.asbah.org.uk
Brittle Bone Society ☎ 08000 282 459 🖥 www.brittlebone.org
Osteopetrosis Support Trust 🖥 www.osteopetrosis.org.uk

GP Notes: Folate supplementation in pregnancy

↓ risk of neural tube defect by 72%.
- *If no previous neural tube defects:* 0.4mg od when pregnancy is being planned and for 13wk. after conception.
- *If 1 parent is affected, on anti-epileptic medication or previous child affected:* 5mg od from the time the pregnancy is being planned until 13wk. after conception.

Supplements can be prescribed or are available OTC from chemists and supermarkets.

Musculoskeletal problems in childhood

> **Septic arthritis:** Most common in children <5y. old. Tends to affect the hip or knee. The child is usually systemically unwell and holds the affected joint completely still. The joint may be swollen, hot and tender. This is an emergency – if suspected admit. Treatment is with IV antibiotics and surgical washout of the joint.

Nocturnal musculoskeletal pains (growing pains): Episodic, muscular pains – usually in the legs – lasting ~30min. and waking the child from sleep. Rubbing the limb → rapid relief. There is no pain or disability in the morning. Diagnosis can be made on history if there are no associated symptoms and examination is normal. If in doubt, check ESR/CRP, which should be normal. In most cases reassurance ± analgesia is all that is needed. In resistant cases, physiotherapy may help.

Idiopathic musculoskeletal pain: Pain for which no cause can be found. Can become chronic. Take a history and examine carefully to exclude other causes. Investigate further only if history or examination suggest a pathological cause. Treatment is with analgesia and reassurance. Advise to return for reassessment ± orthopaedic referral if pain worsens, continues >6wk., changes in nature or other symptoms develop.

Osteomyelitis: Infection of bone. May spread from boils, abscesses or follow surgery. Often no primary site is found. More common in those with DM, sickle cell disease, impaired immunity and/or poor living standards. *Organisms involved: S. aureus, Streptococcus, E. coli, Salmonella, Proteus* and *Pseudomonas* species, TB.

Signs: Pain, unwillingness to move affected part, warmth, effusions in neighbouring joints, fever and malaise

Investigation: Blood cultures +ve in 60%, ↑ESR/CRP, ↑WCC

Management: Refer suspected cases for same-day orthopaedic opinion. Diagnosis is confirmed with imaging e.g. MRI or bone scanning (X-ray changes take a few days to appear). Treatment is with IV then po antibiotics (≥6wk.) and surgery to drain abscesses.

Complications: Septic arthritis, pathological fracture, deformity of growing bone, chronic infection

Chronic osteomyelitis: Occurs after delayed/inadequate treatment of acute osteomyelitis. *Signs:* Pain, fever and discharge of pus from sinuses. It follows a relapsing and remitting course over years. Specialist management is needed.

Bone tumours: 1° malignant tumours are all rare – Ewing's sarcoma, osteosarcoma, chondrosarcoma. Presents with aching bone pain and/or swelling. History of injury does not exclude the possibility of sarcoma.

Management: Refer all persistent bone pain/bony swellings for X-ray and specialist management – excision, chemotherapy, radiotherapy and reconstruction.

Box 7.1 Referral guidelines for cancer in children and young people[N]

Consider referral
- When a child or young person presents with persistent back pain – an examination is needed and a FBC and blood film.
- When there is persistent parental anxiety, even when a benign cause is considered most likely.

Refer urgently: When a child/young person presents several times (≥3x) with the same problem, but with no clear diagnosis.

Bone sarcomas (osteosarcoma and Ewing's sarcoma): Refer children or young people with:
- rest pain, back pain and unexplained limp (a discussion with a paediatrician or X-ray should be considered before or as well as referral)
- persistent localized bone pain and/or swelling, and X-ray showing signs of cancer. In this case refer urgently.

Soft tissue sarcoma: Refer urgently a child or young person presenting with an unexplained mass at almost any site that has ≥1 of the following features. The mass is:
- deep to the fascia
- non-tender
- progressively enlarging
- associated with a regional lymph node that is enlarging
- >2cm in diameter in size.

GMS contract			
Cancer 1	The practice can produce a record of all cancer patients diagnosed after 1.4.2003	5 points	
Cancer 3	% of patients with cancer diagnosed <18mo. ago who have a patient review recorded as occurring <6mo. after the practice received confirmation of diagnosis	up to 6 points	40–90%
Education 7	The practice has undertaken a ≥12 significant event reviews in the past 3y. which could include new cancer diagnoses	Total of 4 points for 12 significant event reviews	

Further information
NICE Referral guidelines for suspected cancer – quick reference guide (2005) ▯ www.nice.org.uk

Rickets: Vitamin D deficiency causes rickets in children. The body makes its own vitamin D when sunlight falls on the skin in the summer months but a diet with adequate vitamin D is needed to maintain the supply in the winter.

Clinical features of rickets:
- Bone pain/tenderness: arms, legs, spine, pelvis
- Skeletal deformity: bow legs, pigeon chest (forward projection of the sternum), rachitic rosary (enlarged ends of ribs), asymmetrical/odd-shaped skull due to soft skull bones, spinal deformity (kyphosis, scoliosis), pelvic deformities
- Pathological fracture
- Dental deformities: delayed formation of teeth, holes in enamel, ↑ cavities
- Muscular problems: progressive weakness, ↓ muscle tone, muscle cramps
- Impaired growth → short stature (can be permanent)

Causes and management:

Dietary deficiency (<30nmol/l): is by far the most common cause in children. Children with pigmented skin in Northern climes are particularly at risk. Give vitamin D and Ca^{2+} supplements.

Secondary rickets: Vitamin D deficiency is due to other disease e.g. malabsorption, liver disease, renal tubular disorders or chronic renal failure. Treat underlying cause/supplement Ca^{2+} and vitamin D.

Vitamin D-dependent rickets: Rare autosomal recessive disorder resulting in an enzyme deficit in the metabolism of vitamin D. Refer for specialist care. Treated with vitamin D and Ca^{2+} supplements.

Hypophosphataemic rickets (vitamin D-resistant rickets): X-linked dominant trait resulting in ↓ proximal renal tubular resorption of phosphate. Parathyroid hormone and vitamin D levels are normal. Specialist management is needed. Treatment is with phosphate replacement ± calcitriol.

Foot problems:

Flat feet: All babies and toddlers have flat feet. The arch develops after 2–3y. of walking. Persistent flat feet may be familial or due to joint laxity. If pain free, foot is mobile and the child develops an arch on standing on tiptoe, no action is required. Else refer to orthopaedics.

Osteochondritis: Table 7.1

Sever's disease: Apophysitis of the heel. *Peak age:* 8–13y. Treated with analgesia, raising the heel of the shoe a little, calf-stretching and avoiding strenuous activities for a few weeks.

In-toe and out-toe gait:
- *In-toe:* Originates in the femur (persistent anteversion of the femoral neck), tibia (tibial torsion) or foot (metatarsus varus). Does not cause pain or affect mobility. Usually resolves by age 5–6y.
- *Out-toe:* Common <2y. May be unilateral. Corrects spontaneously.

Table 7.1 Osteochondritis of the foot in children and young adults

	Bone(s) involved	Features	Treatment
Kohler's disease	Navicular bone	*Peak age: 3–5y.* Presents with pain and tenderness over the dorsum of the mid-foot. X-ray – small navicular bone of ↑ density.	Pain usually resolves with simple analgesia and rest.
Freiberg's disease	2nd and 3rd metatarsal heads	Most common in teenagers and young adults. ♀>♂ Presents with pain in the foot on walking. The head of the metatarsal is palpable and tender. X-ray shows a wide, flat metatarsal.	Treatment is usually conservative with cushioning of shoes and simple analgesia. If severe refer to orthopaedics. Excision of the metatarsal head may relieve pain.

GP Notes: Dietary sources of vitamin D and calcium

Vitamin D: Rich sources of vitamin D include margarine, eggs, dairy products and oily fish. Breakfast cereals have vitamin D supplements added.

Calcium: Rich sources of calcium include dairy products, bread, sardines, baked beans and boiled cabbage. Calcium supplements are also added to breakfast cereals.

Advice for patients: Information and support

Steps Support for patients with lower limb conditions and their families ☎ 0871 717 0044 🖥 www.steps-charity.org.uk
Arthritis Research Campaign (ARC) ☎ 0870 850 5000 🖥 www.arc.org.uk

Knee problems

Bow legs and knock knees:

- *Genu varum (bow legs):* Outward curving of the tibia usually associated with internal tibial torsion. Except in severe cases always resolves spontaneously. Severe cases raise the possibility of rickets or other rare developmental disorders – refer for orthopaedic opinion.
- *Genu valgum (knock knees):* Common amongst 2–4y. olds. Innocent if symmetrical and independent of any other abnormality. Severe, progressive cases suggest rickets – refer for X-ray.

Chondromalacia patellae: Common in teenage girls. Pain on walking up or down stairs or on prolonged sitting. *Signs:* Pain on stressing the undersurface of the patella. Arthroscopy (indicated only in severe cases) reveals degenerative cartilage on the posterior surface of the patella.

Management: Analgesia + physiotherapy (vastus medialis strengthening relieves pain in 80%). For persistent cases, exclude spondylarthropathy and refer to orthopaedics for arthroscopy.

Osgood-Schlatter disease: Seen in athletic teenagers. Pain and tenderness ± swelling over the tibial tubercle. X-rays not required.

Management: Avoid aggravating activities. Usually settles over a few months. If not settling refer to orthopaedics or rheumatology for further assessment.

Hip problems

Transient synovitis of the hip (irritable hip): The most common reason for limping in childhood. *Peak age:* 2–10y. ♂>>♀. The child is usually well but complains of pain in the hip or knee and may refuse to weight bear. Often occurs after a viral infection. Cause is unknown. Exclude septic arthritis – refer to orthopaedics. Usually resolves in 7–10d. without treatment.

Perthes' disease: Pain in the hip or knee, limp and limited hip movement developing over ~1mo. Due to avascular necrosis of the femoral head. Bilateral in 10%. *Peak age:* 4–7y. (range 3–11y.). ♂:♀≈4:1.

Management: If suspected refer for X-ray and to orthopaedics. Treatment is with rest, X-ray surveillance, bracing and/or surgery depending on severity.

Prognosis: Usually heals over 2–3y. Joint damage may lead to early arthritis. Young patients do best. Risk factors for poor outcome include:
- ♀
- Onset >8y.
- Involvement of the whole femoral head
- Pronounced metaphyseal rarefaction
- Lateral displacement of the femoral head.

Slipped upper femoral epiphysis: The upper femoral epiphysis slips with respect to the femur, usually in a postero-inferior direction. Bilateral in 20%. *Incidence:* 1:100,000. *Peak age:* 10–15y. ♂:♀≈3:1. Typically affects obese, underdeveloped children or tall, thin boys.

Presentation:
● Pain at rest in the groin, hip, thigh or referred to the knee.
● Limp and/or pain on movement.
● ↓ hip movements – particularly abduction and medial rotation. The affected leg may be externally rotated and shortened.

Management: Confirm diagnosis on X-ray (include lateral views) – shows backwards and downwards slippage of the epiphysis. Refer to orthopaedics – surgical pinning or reconstructive surgery is needed. Monitoring of the other hip is essential.

Complications: Avascular necrosis; coxa vara; early arthritis; slipped epiphysis on the contralateral side.

Congenital dislocation (or developmental dysplasia) of the hip: 📖 p.24

Scoliosis: 📖 p.26

Pulled elbow: Common in children <5y. Traction injury to elbow causes subluxation of radial head. Often occurs when the child is pulled up suddenly by the hand. Child will not use the arm. No clinical signs. ♂>♀. Left arm > right. X-rays are unhelpful.

Management: Apply anterior pressure with the thumb on the radial head whilst supinating and extending the forearm. Immediate recovery is seen after reduction.

Advice for patients: Information and support

Steps Support for patients with lower limb conditions and their families ☎ 0871 717 0044 🖥 www.steps-charity.org.uk
Arthritis Research Campaign (ARC) ☎ 0870 850 5000
🖥 www.arc.org.uk

GP Notes: The limping child

● If a child is limping, take it seriously and look for a problem.
● Children find it difficult to localize pain and pain can be referred from the hip to the knee, so examine the whole limb carefully.
● Other causes of referred pain include: spinal pathology, psoas spasm from GI pathology (e.g. appendicitis).
● Limping without pain is uncommon and may be due to undiagnosed congenital hip dislocation – 📖 p.24.

Arthritis in children

Joint and limb pains are common in children. Arthritis is rare.

Presentation of arthritis in children:

Older children: Usually presents with well-localized joint pains ± hot, tender, swollen joints.

Babies and young children: May present with immobility of a joint or a limp, but the diagnosis can be extremely difficult.

Differential diagnosis of joint pains in children:

- Juvenile chronic arthritis (JCA)
- Infections e.g. TB, rubella
- Rheumatic fever
- Henoch-Schönlein purpura
- Traumatic arthritis
- Hypermobility syndrome
- Leukaemia
- Sickle cell disease
- SLE & connective tissue disorders
- Transient synovitis of the hip (irritable hip)
- Septic arthritis
- Perthes' disease
- Slipped femoral epiphysis

Septic arthritis: 📖 p.206

Types of childhood arthritis: Table 7.2

Management of children with arthritis

- If suspected, refer urgently to paediatrics for confirmation of diagnosis.
- Once confirmed, ensure the child is referred to a specialist paediatric rheumatology unit to avoid long-term disability. These units have multidisciplinary facilities for rehabilitation, education and surgical intervention (if necessary) and support both the family and the child.
- NSAIDs and paracetamol help pain and stiffness, but corticosteroids and immunosuppressants (e.g. methotrexate) are often required for systemic disease.
- Ensure families apply for any benefits that might be available to them.
- Tell families about self-help and support groups.
- Support families in any applications made to adapt the home or school environment for the child's condition.

Advice for patients: Information and support

Arthritis Research Campaign (ARC) ☎ 0870 850 5000
🖳 www.arc.org.uk

Table 7.2 Childhood arthritis

Type of arthritis	Features
Oligoarthritis or pauciarticular onset arthritis	
Persistent:	Most common form of JCA (50–60%) but still rare.
	Peak age: 3y. ♀>>♂.
	Affects ≤4 joints, especially wrists, knees and ankles. Often asymmetrical.
	Associated with uveitis (often with +ve anti-nuclear antibody) which requires regular screening by slit-lamp examination – rarely causes blindness.
	Generally prognosis is good, with remission in 4–5 y.
Extended:	Chronic arthritis with an oligoarticular onset of the disease, which progresses to involve >4 joints. Joints tend to be stiff rather than hot and swollen.
Still's disease	10% of JCA.
	Affects boys and girls equally up to 5y., then girls are more commonly affected.
	Presentation:
	• Fever – high, swinging, early-evening temperature
	• Rash – pink maculopapular rash
	• Musculoskeletal pain – arthralgia, arthritis, myalgia
	• Generalized lymphadenopathy
	• Hepatosplenomegaly
	• Pericarditis ± pleurisy (uncommon)
	Investigations: Blood – ↑ ESR/CRP; FBC – ↑ neutrophils, ↑ platelets. Autoantibodies are -ve.
	⚠ *Differential diagnosis:* Malignancy – particularly leukaemia or neuroblastoma; infection.
Polyarticular onset JCA	Develops with or without a preceding systemic illness at any age >1y.
	Usually occurs in teenagers, producing widespread joint destruction.
	There is symmetrical arthritis of hands, wrists, PIP joints ± DIP joints.
	Rheumatoid factor is usually -ve (+ve in 3% – often teenage girls).
Juvenile spondylo-arthropathy	Affects teenage and younger boys, producing an asymmetrical arthritis of lower-limb joints.
	Associated with HLA-B27 and acute anterior uveitis.
	Represents the childhood equivalent of adult ankylosing spondylitis. ~60% of childhood sufferers develop ankylosing spondylitis later in life.
Psoriatic arthritis	Polyarthritis affecting large and small joints including fingers and toes. The arthritis can be very erosive.
	Psoriasis may be present in the child or a first-degree relative. 📖 p.252

Headache in children

Recurrent headache with no obvious cause is common in children and a source of much parental anxiety with parents particularly fearing brain tumours. Exclude other causes of headache before making a diagnosis of functional headache.

History

- Site and character are variable – most commonly frontal.
- Accompanying symptoms (e.g. neurological symptoms, headache worse in the early morning) make an organic cause more likely.
- Increasing severity of headache with time requires further investigation.
- Aura preceding the headache may suggest classical migraine.
- Other behavioural or psychological problems (e.g. school refusal, irrational fears) make a functional diagnosis more likely.
- Nausea and vomiting may accompany any type of headache.

Examination

- In acute, severe headache, check no fever and examine for photophobia, purpuric skin rash and neck stiffness.
- Neurological examination – including gait, cranial nerves, fundi for papilloedema and visual acuity in both eyes (a young child can lose vision in 1 eye without noticing).
- Neck and face – looking for local tenderness e.g. from a tooth abscess or sinusitis.
- If the pain is functional, examination will be normal.

Investigation

- In young children, measure head circumference and plot on a centile chart.
- Suggest parents have the child's eyes tested (free <16y.).
- No further investigations are needed if the examination is normal and there are no symptoms suggesting organic disease.
- If there is fever, the child is obviously not well, purpuric rash, neck stiffness and/or photophobia, admit as a paediatric emergency to rule out meningitis.
- If there are any symptoms suggesting an intracranial cause, refer to paediatrics – as an emergency if neurological signs or papilloedema.

Management of functional headache

- Acknowledge the pain is real and the worries of both parents and child. Reassure them that there is no serious underlying cause like a brain tumour.
- Encourage adequate fluid intake.
- Reserve paracetamol for episodes of more severe pain than usual.
- Stress that if the pain should change or be unusually severe the child should be reassessed by a doctor.
- Most children recover spontaneously with time.

⚠ If, despite reassurance, there is still significant parental worry, refer to paediatrics. Urgency depends on clinical state of the child and level of concern[N].

Table 7.3 Differential diagnosis of headache in children

	Cause	Features	Management
Acute new headache	Meningitis	Fever, photophobia, stiff neck, rash, photophobia	IV or IM penicillin V and immediate admission – 📖 p.48
	Encephalitis	Fever, confusion, ↓ conscious level	Immediate admission – 📖 p.48
	Subarachnoid haemorrhage	'Thunder-clap' or very sudden onset headache ± stiff neck	Immediate admission – 📖 p.219
	Head injury	Bruising/injury; ↓ conscious level, amnesia	Consider admission – 📖 p.50
	Acute febrile illness	Fever and symptoms of underlying cause e.g. URTI, tonsillitis	Treat underlying cause
	Sinusitis	Tender over sinuses ± history of URTI	Treat with steam, analgesia ± antibiotics – 📖 p.278
	Dental caries	Facial pain ± tenderness	Treat with analgesia ± antibiotics – refer to dentist
	Tropical illness	History of travel, fever	Refer to paediatrics for urgent investigation
Acute recurrent headache	Migraine	Aura, visual disturbance, nausea/vomiting, triggers	Treat with analgesia. Consider prophylaxis if frequent or disabling attacks – 📖 p.216
	Recurrent functional headache	See opposite	See opposite
Chronic headache	Medication overuse headache	Rebound headache on stopping analgesics	Aim to ↓ consumption of analgesics until taken <15d./mo. – 📖 p.218
	↑ intracranial pressure	Worse on waking/sneezing, neurological signs, ↑ BP, ↓ pulse rate	Same-day paediatric assessment – 📖 p.220

Migraine and other headaches

There is considerable overlap between migraine and recurrent functional headache or tension-type headache in children. There may also be a link between childhood migraine and *cyclical vomiting* (attacks of vomiting, pallor and lethargy lasting 1h.–5d.), *abdominal migraine* (episodic central abdominal pain lasting 1–72h. associated with sweating, pallor, anorexia, nausea ± vomiting) and **benign paroxysmal vertigo of childhood** (recurrent brief attacks of vertigo in otherwise well children).

History, examination and differential diagnosis: 📖 p.214

Migraine: Migraine affects 10% of UK schoolchildren. ♂:♀≈1:2. It is more than just a headache. Attacks can force the child to abandon everyday activities – affected children miss an average 4 school days/y. due to migraine. Even when symptom free, children may live in fear of the next attack.

Cause: Disturbance of cerebral blood flow under the influence of 5-HT.

Clinical picture: 2 common types in children:
- **Classical migraine:** Aura lasting 10–30min. followed by unilateral throbbing headache ± nausea or vomiting ± photo/phonophobia. The aura can take the form of visual chaos (e.g. zig-zag lines, jumbling of print, dots), hemianopia, hemiparesis, dysphasia, dyspraxia, dysarthria or ataxia (basilar migraine)
- **Episodic migraine (common migraine):** Unilateral throbbing headache ± nausea or vomiting ± photo/phonophobia but without aura – often premenstrual in teenagers. In younger children headache may be relatively short-lived (as short as 1h.) and is often bilateral or felt in the middle of the head.

ⓘ Aura alone with no headache is rare in children – refer for consideration of alternative diagnoses.

Trigger factors: ½ have a trigger for their headaches. Consider:
- **Psychological factors:** Stress/relief of stress; anxiety/depression; extreme emotions e.g. anger or grief
- **Food factors:** Lack of food/infrequent meals; foods containing monosodium glutamate, caffeine and tyramine; specific foods e.g. chocolate, citrus fruits, cheese
- **Sleep:** Overtiredness (physical/ mental); changes in sleep patterns (e.g. late nights, weekend lie-in, holidays); long-distance travel
- **Environmental factors:** Loud noise; bright/flickering lights; strong perfume; stuffy atmosphere; VDUs; strong winds; extreme heat/cold
- **Health factors:** Hormonal changes (e.g. monthly periods, COC pill); unaccustomed physical activity.

Assessing severity: Assessment scales such as the MIDAS scale (see opposite) can be useful for older children in assessing impact of symptoms on daily life and monitoring response to treatment.

Management: 📖 p.218

Migraine disability assessment score (MIDAS): Used to assess the impact of migraine symptoms on lifestyle.

Instructions: Please answer the following questions about ALL the headaches you have had over the last 3mo. If you did not do the activity in the last 3 mo., write 0.

1. On how many days in the last 3mo. did you miss work or school because of your headache?	☐ days
2. How many days in the last 3mo. was your productivity at work or school ↓ by ≥½ because of your headaches? (*Do not include days you counted in question 1 where you missed work or school*)	☐ days
3. On how many days in the last 3mo. did you not do household work* because of your headache?	☐ days
4. How many days in the last 3mo. was your productivity in household work ↓ by ≥½ because of your headaches? (*Do not include days you counted in question 3 where you did not do household work*)	☐ days
5. On how many days in the last 3mo. did you miss family, social or leisure activities because of your headaches?	☐ days

MIDAS score TOTAL ☐ days

A. On how many days in the last 3mo. did you have a headache? (*If a headache lasted more than 1 day, count each day*)	☐ days
B. On a scale of 0–10, on average how painful were these headaches? (*Where 0 = no pain at all and 10 = pain as bad as it can be*)	☐ days

Questions A and B measure the frequency of the migraine and the severity of pain. They are not used to reach the MIDAS score, but provide extra information helpful for making treatment decisions.

Interpreting the MIDAS score

I	Score: 0–5	Minimal/infrequent disability	Tend to have little or no treatment needs. Can often manage with OTC medication. If infrequent severe attacks may require triptan.
II	Score: 6–10	Mild/infrequent disability	May require medication for acute attacks e.g. NSAID ± anti-emetic or triptan.
III	Score: 11–20	Moderate disability	Will need medication for acute attacks. Consider prophylaxis. Consider other causes for headaches e.g. TTH.
IV	Score: ≥21	Severe disability	

* Unpaid work such as housework, shopping and caring for children and others.
The migraine disability assessment score is reproduced with permission of British Association for the Study of Headache.

Management: Aims to control symptoms and minimize their impact on the patient's life.

Management of an acute attack
- *Advise to rest* in a quiet, dark place and sleep if possible.
- *Analgesia:* Ibuprofen or paracetamol at 1st signs of an attack ± anti-emetic e.g. domperidone. If vomiting consider pr administration. Avoid using metoclopramide or prochlorperazine in children as may cause acute dystonic reactions.
- *Severe attacks:* For children >12y., in addition consider $5HT_1$ agonists e.g. sumatriptan po, nasal spray or s/cut (not effective if taken before the headache develops – stops 70–85% attacks – start with lowest dose and ↑ as needed).

Treatment of recurrence within the same attack: Repeat symptomatic treatments within their dose limitations – pre-emptively if recurrence is usual/expected. If using triptans, a 2nd dose may be effective, but repeated dosing can cause rebound headache.

Management of chronic migraine
- Reassure about the benign nature of migraine.
- Instruct patients and/or parents about management of an acute attack.
- Ask the patient/parent to keep a diary to identify possible trigger factors, assess headache frequency, severity and response to treatment.
- Avoid trigger factors where possible.
- Stop the COC pill if migraine starts or worsens when the pill is started, especially if focal symptoms develop.
- Consider prophylaxis if frequent or very severe attacks.

Prophylaxis: Consider if ≥4 attacks/mo. or very severe attacks. Evidence of effectiveness is weak in children. Try a drug for 2mo. before deciding it is ineffective. If effective, continue for 4–6mo. then ↓ dose slowly before stopping.
- *β-blockers:* e.g. propranolol. Contraindicated in children with asthma.
- *Pizotifen:* Licenced for children >2y. If tolerance develops ↑ dose. Side effects are common and include sleepiness and ↑ weight.
- *Amitriptyline and sodium valproate:* Unlicensed – only use under consultant direction.

Alternative therapies: Feverfew – some evidence of effectiveness after 6wk. use[c] but only one trial included children (all >9y.). Feverfew may interact with NSAIDs. Acupuncture may be helpful.

Medication overuse (analgesic) headache: Persistent headache may develop in patients with other causes of headache e.g. functional headache or migraine if they overuse the medication used to treat those conditions. Implicated drugs include: triptans, aspirin, paracetamol and NSAIDs. ♀:♂≈3:1. Ask any patient complaining of chronic daily headache to give a detailed account of medication use (including OTC) – a diary can be helpful. *Management:* Aim to ↓ consumption of analgesics until taken <15d./mo.

Subarachnoid haemorrhage (SAH): Spontaneous bleeding into the subarachnoid space. Rare in childhood and usually due to A-V malformation. Typically presents as a sudden devastating headache– 'thunder-clap headache'– often occipital. Rarely (6%) preceded by a 'sentinel headache' representing a small leak ahead of a larger bleed. Vomiting and collapse with loss of consciousness ± fitting ± focal neurology follow.

Examination: May be normal initially. Neck stiffness takes 6h. to develop. In later stages:
- Papilloedema
- Retinal/intraocular haemorrhages
- Focal neurology
- ↓ level of consciousness

Action: If suspected admit immediately. 1:4 admitted with suspected SAH turn out to have one. In most no cause for headache is found.

Trigeminal neuralgia: Paroxysms of intense stabbing, burning or 'electric shock'-type pain lasting seconds to minutes in the trigeminal (V) nerve distribution. 96% unilateral. Mandibular/maxillary > ophthalmic division. Between attacks there are no symptoms. Frequency of attacks is highly variable. Pain is often provoked by movement of the face (talking, eating, laughing) or by touching the skin (shaving, washing). Rare in children. Refer for specialist advice.

Advice for patients: about managing migraine

- Migraine headaches, although painful and unpleasant, are not caused by any serious problem within the brain.
- Keep a diary of the attacks as this will help identify factors which might trigger off an attack as well as keeping a record of how often you get your migraine, how bad the attacks are and whether treatment makes any difference.
- Avoid things that might trigger your attacks where possible. Common triggers include caffeine-containing drinks like tea and coffee, certain foods such as chocolate, citrus fruits or cheese, tiredness, stress (or even relief of stress), loud noises, bright or flickering lights, or change in sleep or eating pattern.
- Learn to relax, and try to keep to regular bedtimes and meals.
- At the first sign of an attack give medication as advised or prescribed by your doctor. Rest or sleep in a dark room helps many sufferers.
- If the headache comes back or you know from experience that it is likely to, take another dose of medication as long as this is not sooner than recommended on the dose instructions.

Further information and support for parents and children:

Migraine Action ☎ 0870 050 5898 🖳 www.migraine.org.uk
Migraine Trust ☎ 020 7436 1336 🖳 www.migrainetrust.org

Further information

British Association for the Study of Headache Guidelines for all doctors in the diagnosis and management of migraine and tension-type headache (2nd edition – 2003) 🖳 www.bash.org.uk
DTB Managing migraine in children (2004) **42** pp.25–8

Raised intracranial pressure

Raised intracranial pressure: Presents with increasing headache (particularly on waking or causing early morning waking) associated with drowsiness, listlessness, vomiting, focal neurology and/or seizures. If suspected admit as an acute paediatric emergency.

Examination
- Drowsiness ± ↓ conscious level
- Irritability
- Focal neurological signs including VI nerve palsy
- Papilloedema
- Dropping pulse and rising BP
- Pupil changes – constriction first then dilatation

Causes
- Head injury (📖 p.50)
- Intracranial haemorrhage
- Hydrocephalus
- Brain abscess
- 1° or 2° brain tumours (see below)
- Meningitis or encephalitis (📖 p.48)
- Cerebral oedema (2° to tumour, trauma, infection, ischaemia)

Hydrocephalus: Characterized by dilatation of the cerebral ventricles and accumulation of CSF. May be:
- *Communicating:* Due to ↓ reabsorption of CSF. *Causes:* Post-meningitis; SAH (80% develop some degree of hydrocephalus); trauma; neoplastic infiltration in the subarachnoid space
- *Non-communicating:* CSF flow is blocked due to an obstruction within the ventricles. Due to congenital malformations, tumour, brain abscesss, SAH, meningeal scarring due to meningitis, or cranial trauma.

Presentation:
- *Macrocephaly:* May obstruct labour. Usually progressive with ↑ head circumference out of proportion with the growth of the body. Cranial sutures separate and anterior fontanelle becomes large and tense.
- *Setting sun sign:* Eyelids are retracted, eyes are depressed forwards and downwards, and upward gaze is impaired.
- *Convulsions, developmental delay and/or peripheral spasticity* ± hypopituitarism.

Management: Refer for urgent neurological assessment. ❶ All patients with a CSF shunt should have pneumococcal vaccination.

Brain tumours: ~300 children/y. in the UK are diagnosed with brain tumours (peak age 3–8y.). Medulloblastoma of the posterior fossa is the most common type of tumour in children (20% tumours).

Risk factors: Genetic conditions (e.g. neurofibromatosis, tuberous sclerosis, Li-Fraumeni syndrome, von Hippel-Lindau syndrome); past history of head irradiation.

Presentation and referral: Box 7.2

Differential diagnosis: Other causes of raised intracranial pressure; degenerative brain disease; metabolic or electrolyte disturbance.

Further information:
NICE Referral guidelines for suspected cancer (2005)
🖥 www.nice.org.uk

Box 7.2 Referral for suspected brain tumour[N]

Refer immediately

Children with:
• ↓ conscious level
• Headache and vomiting that cause early morning waking or occur on waking as these are classic signs of ↑ intracranial pressure.
   ❶ <1% of patients presenting with headache have a brain tumour

Children <2y. with:
• New-onset seizures
• Bulging fontanelle
• Extensor attacks
• Persistent vomiting

Refer urgently or immediately children with

• New-onset seizures
• Cranial nerve abnormalities
• Visual disturbances
• Gait abnormalities
• Motor or sensory signs
• Unexplained deteriorating school performance or developmental milestones
• Unexplained behavioural and/or mood changes

Refer urgently

• When a child presents several times (≥3x) with the same problem, but with no clear diagnosis
• Children aged ≥2y. with persistent headache where you cannot carry out an adequate neurological examination in primary care
• Children aged <2y. with:
  • abnormal ↑ in head size
  • arrest/regression of motor development and/or altered behaviour
  • abnormal eye movements and/or lack of visual following
  • poor feeding/failure to thrive
  • squint – urgency depends on other factors

❶ Persistent parental anxiety is sufficient reason for referral, even where a benign cause is considered most likely.

GMS contract			
Cancer 1	Practice can produce a record of all cancer patients diagnosed after 1.4.2003	5 points	
Cancer 3	% of patients with cancer, diagnosed <18mo. ago, who have a patient review recorded as occurring <6mo. after the practice received confirmation of diagnosis	up to 6 points	40–90%
Education 7	Practice has undertaken ≥12 significant event reviews in the past 3y. which could include new cancer diagnoses	Total of 4 points for 12 significant event reviews	

Advice for patients: Support for patients and carers

Association for Spina Bifida and Hydrocephalus (ASBAH)
☎ 0845 450 7755 🖳 www.asbah.org.uk
Brain and Spine Foundation ☎ 0808 808 1000
🖳 www.brainandspine.org.uk
Brain Tumour UK ☎ 0845 4500 386 🖳 www.braintumouruk.org.uk

Funny turns in small children

Small children are often brought to the GP by their parents because they have had a funny turn. As in adults, the major questions are:
- Was the episode a fit?
- If so, what caused it?
- If not, then is there another serious underlying cause e.g. heart disease?

History: A good history from a witness is essential. Ask:
- What happened? When and where?
- Were there any precipitating events or warning signs something was going to happen? e.g. Does the child have a viral illness? Did s/he have a fever? Was the child angry or upset when the funny turn happened? Did s/he hit his/her head?
- Did the child lose consciousness?
- Did the child jerk his/her limbs? If so, was the jerking generalized or restricted to one area of the body?
- What did the child look like during the attack? e.g. colour, floppiness
- How long did the attack last?
- Did anything else happen during the attack? e.g. tongue biting
- What happened after the attack? Was the child conscious straight away? Was there disorientation or drowsiness?

Also check
- General history – is the child well? Does the child have any ongoing medical problems?
- Birth history – problems in pregnancy, birth trauma
- Past medical history – serious illness, neurological and/or developmental problems, heart problems
- Family history – epilepsy

Examination: Complete general and neurological examination. Remember to check developmental milestones and plot head circumference and weight on centile chart.

Differential diagnosis
- Epileptic attacks – febrile convulsion (📖 p.224) or childhood epilepsy (📖 p.228)
- Non-epileptic attacks

Non-epileptic attacks: Usually self-limiting and harmless but can be very frightening for parents/carers. Parental education about the likely duration and cause of attacks and reassurance that the child will come to no harm are important.

Simple blue breath-holding attacks: Onset usually >6mo. of age. Common. Provoked by frustration or upset. *Signs:* +ve valsalva manoeuvre, cynanosis, stiffening and coma. No treatment needed – spontaneous recovery. Most children 'grow out' of the attacks by 3y.

White reflex asystolic (anoxic) attacks: May start before 6mo. but most common from 6mo.–2y. Usually triggered by minor injury or anxiety. *Signs:* Vagal asystole, pallor, rapid coma, stiffening, upward eye movement ± urinary incontinence. No treatment needed – spontaneous recovery.

Reflex syncope or vasovagal attacks ('faints'): Common. Peripheral vasodilatation, bradycardia and venous pooling → postural hypotension. Often cause is unclear though ♀>♂. *Known precipitants:* Fright (e.g. during venesection) or emotion. *Features:*
- *Prodrome:* Dizziness, visual disturbance, nausea, sweating, ringing in the ears, a sinking feeling and yawning
- *Faint:* Extreme pallor, momentary unconsciousness (with fall to the floor if standing ± tonic-clonic jerks if held upright)
- *Rapid recovery*

No treatment is needed – reassure.

Others causes are rare in children but include:
- Cardiac arrhythmias – the NSF for Coronary Heart Disease recommends all children with recurrent loss of consciousness or collapse on exertion are referred for paediatric cardiology assessment
- Hyperventilation
- Benign monoclonus of infancy
- Benign paroxysmal vertigo
- Sleep phenomena
- Hypoglycaemia
- Munchausen syndrome by proxy

Further information
NICE The epilepsies: the diagnosis and management of the epilepsies in adults and children in primary and secondary care (2004) ⊞ www.nice.org.uk
NSF for Coronary Heart Disease (2005) ⊞ www.dh.gov.uk

Febrile convulsions

A febrile convulsion is a seizure occurring in a child aged 6mo.–5y. (peak age 18mo.), associated with fever arising from infection or inflammation outside the central nervous system in a child who is otherwise neurologically normal.[1] 2–4% of all children have a febrile convulsion.

Classification

- *Simple febrile convulsions:* Isolated, generalized, tonic–clonic seizures lasting <10–15min.
- *Complex febrile convulsions:* last 15–30min., or are focal, or recur during the febrile illness, or are not followed by full consciousness within 1h.

Causes: In ↓ order of frequency:
- Viral infections
- Otitis media
- Tonsillitis
- UTI
- Gastroenteritis
- Lower respiratory tract infection
- Meningitis
- Post-immunization.

Assessment: By the time the GP arrives, the febrile convulsion is usually over, so diagnosis is based on a history of short, generalized tonic–clonic seizure in a febrile child.

Examination and investigation: The main concern when assessing children who have had a febrile convulsion is to detect and manage bacterial meningitis (📖 p.48). Check temperature, assess level of consciousness and examine for a source of infection (see causes above). If there is no obvious cause and the child is not being admitted, check an MSU for urinary tract infection.

> ⚠ Complex are more likely than simple febrile convulsions to be provoked by a serious condition. Suspect serious pathology if a child has:
> - had a prolonged febrile convulsion
> - had a focal febrile convulsion *or*
> - not recovered within an hour of a febrile convulsion.

Differential diagnosis
- *Epilepsy*
- *Any other cause of convulsion:*
  - Meningitis or encephalitis
  - Cerebral palsy with intercurrent infection
  - Hypoglycaemia
  - Neurodegenerative disorders
  - Poisoning (e.g. inadvertent drug ingestion)
  - NAI (📖 p.322)

Management of the fitting patient: 📖 p.52
Management of febrile convulsions: 📖 p.226

GP Notes: Frequently asked questions about febrile convulsions

What is the risk of recurrence after a febrile convulsion?
Febrile convulsions recur in subsequent febrile illnesses in ~30% of children – 9% have >3 seizures. Recurrence is most common in the year following the first febrile convulsion. Recurrence is more likely if:
- First febrile convulsion aged <15mo.
- First febrile convulsion is complex
- Family history of febrile convulsions or epilepsy in a 1st degree relative
- Child attends day nursery (↑ frequency of febrile illnesses).

Is there an increased risk of epilepsy after febrile convulsion?
Rarely – 1% of children having a febrile convulsion go on to develop epilepsy (compared to 0.4% children who have not had a febrile convulsion). Risk ↑ if any of the following features are present:
- Neurological abnormalities or developmental delay before the onset of febrile convulsions
- Atypical seizures
- Family history of epilepsy
- Complex convulsions.

Are there long-term complications after febrile convulsions?
Long-term adverse effects are rare. There is no evidence of subsequent impaired intelligence or poorer academic achievement but there is a slightly increased risk of epilepsy.

Is immunization contraindicated after febrile convulsion?
There is evidence to suggest immunizations do not ↑ risk of recurrent febrile convulsions.[1] Immunization is not contraindicated.

1 Offringa and Moyer (2001) *BMJ* 323(7321) pp.1111–14

Management: Most children do not need admission.
Admit if:
- The child was drowsy before the seizure
- The child is irritable, systemically unwell or 'toxic' and/or the cause of the fever is unclear
- Petechial rash
- Symptoms/signs of meningitis – 📖 p.48
- Recent/current treatment with antibiotics (may mask symptoms/signs of meningitis)
- Age <18mo. (meningitis may present with non-specific signs)
- The cause of the fever requires hospital management in its own right
- Complex convulsion
- Early review by a doctor not possible
- Inadequate home circumstances
- Carer anxious or unable to cope

For children not being admitted:
- Reassure parents/carers that febrile convulsions do not harm the child.
- Advise on controlling fever in the future: an antipyretic e.g. paracetamol or ibuprofen syrup, cool clothing. If not managing to lower temperature with these measures, fan the child or sponge with lukewarm water.
- Teach parents to manage a recurrent convulsion: recovery position, nothing forced into mouth.
- Recommend that immunization schedules be completed.
- Advise the parents/carers to seek urgent medical help if the child deteriorates in any way, fits again or they are worried.
- Arrange early review e.g. later the same day or the following morning.

Consider referral to paediatrics or paediatric neurology if:
- Diagnosis of febrile convulsion is in doubt.
- Febrile convulsions have been frequent, severe and/or complex and prophylactic treatment might be indicated.
- The child is at ↑ risk of epilepsy e.g. coexistent neurological or developmental conditions; history of epilepsy in 1st degree relative.
- The parents/carers are still anxious despite reassurance or request a specialist opinion.

Prophylactic measures: Prescribe under consultant direction only.
- *Rectal diazepam:* May prevent febrile convulsions in subsequent illness if given at the onset of a febrile episode. Rectal diazepam is safe for home use provided parents are properly educated about its use.
- *Continuous prophylaxis:* Use of anticonvulsants on a regular basis to prevent febrile convulsions is controversial. In general benefits are outweighed by risks.

Advice for patients: Information for parents about febrile convulsions

What are febrile convulsions?

A febrile convulsion or fit happens when normal brain activity is disturbed when a child has a fever. It usually occurs without warning. During the fit your child may:
- Become stiff or floppy
- Become unconscious or unaware of their surroundings
- Display jerking or twitching movements
- Have difficulty breathing.

Febrile convulsions are frightening to watch, but they are not harmful to your child, don't cause brain damage and will not cause your child to die.

What happens after a febrile convulsion?

Your child will become tired for up to an hour after the fit. If your child remains sleepy or is difficult to rouse after sleep, seek medical attention.

Will my child have another febrile convulsion?

Possibly – febrile convulsions may recur. About 1 in 3 children who have had a febrile convulsion will have another. The risk of another febrile convulsion decreases with time as the child gets older. Immunization is still advised after a febrile convulsion, even if, as rarely happens, the febrile convulsion followed an immunization.

Are febrile convulsions the same as epilepsy?

No – febrile convulsions are not epilepsy. Rarely, in about 1 in 100 children who have had more than one febrile convulsion, epilepsy can develop later.

How can I prevent fevers which cause convulsions?

Controlling fever eases symptoms. It does not prevent febrile convulsions. A high temperature can be reduced by:
- Giving paracetamol or ibuprofen – read the instructions on the packet carefully and only give your child the recommended dose for his age
- Removing excessive clothing or bedding – in the home this usually means stripping your child down to underwear or nappy.

What should I do if my child has another convulsion?

Remember, most fits stop within a couple of minutes without treatment.
- Stay calm.
- Look at your watch or a clock and time the convulsion.
- Don't try to restrain your child or put anything in his mouth.
- Stay with your child and lie him on his side.
- Loosen tight clothing from around his neck and move objects away that may cause injury.
- Ring your GP or NHS direct after the convulsion has stopped.

Call an ambulance if:
- The fit lasts for more than 5 minutes
- Another fit starts up after the first one stops
- Your child has difficulty breathing or looks particularly unwell

Childhood epilepsy

Childhood epilepsy is a susceptibility to continuing seizures. Prevalence ↑ with age from ~4/1000 children at 7y. to ~5/1000 children at 16y. 60% of adult epilepsy starts in childhood.

Risk factors:
- Neurological abnormalities or developmental delay – ~$\frac{1}{2}$ institutionalized people with multiple disabilities and ~$\frac{1}{3}$ people with a severe learning difficulty have epilepsy
- Family history
- Past history of febrile convulsions – 1% go on to develop epilepsy

Diagnosis: Seizures, faints and funny turns can be difficult to distinguish and diagnose – ☐ p.222. A reliable eyewitness account is the key.

⚠ Refer to a specialist paediatrician with training and expertise in epilepsy for diagnosis. All children who have had a first non-febrile seizure should be seen in <2wk.[N]

Classification: As in adults, seizures can be:
- *Partial:* The seizure begins in one area of the brain only. Termed 'simple' if no impairment of consciousness, and 'complex' if consciousness is impaired. Partial seizures may become generalized
- *Generalized:* The whole brain is involved. Consciousness is usually but not always impaired. Includes absence, myoclonic and tonic–clonic seizures (limbs stiffen and jerk with loss of consciousness).

Epileptic syndromes: In children, epilepsy is considered in terms of the 'epileptic syndrome'. Identifying a syndrome enables predictions about cause, severity and prognosis. Epileptic syndromes are characterized by a set pattern of seizure type(s) ± other features:
- Physical appearance
- Child's age at onset
- Family history
- Associated learning disability and/or developmental delay
- Associated neurological findings
- EEG (should be undertaken in any child with a history of ≥2 epileptic seizures).

ⓘ It is not possible to identify a syndrome in 30% – and symptoms/signs may take months to evolve until diagnosis can be made in others.

There are a large number of childhood epileptic syndromes. Table 7.4 lists some of the more common ones. Broadly they divide into:
- *Benign syndromes:* Children are often mildly affected, easily controlled and/or mature out of epilepsy
- *Malignant syndromes:* Result in treatment-resistant epilepsy with severe or progressive motor and/or intellectual disability.

Features of epileptic syndromes: ☐ p.230

Management of the fitting patient: ☐ p.52

Long-term management of epilepsy: ☐ p.232

Table 7.4 Epileptic syndromes

Benign syndromes	Malignant syndromes
Febrile convulsions (📖 p.224)	Infantile spasms
Benign rolandic epilepsy	Severe myoclonic epilepsy
Benign occipital epilepsy	Lennox-Gastaut syndrome
Panayiotopoulos syndrome	Partial seizures 2° to structural brain disease
Early myoclonic epilepsy	Landau-Kleffner syndrome
Absence seizures	

The most common epileptic syndromes seen in the UK are:

- *Benign childhood epilepsy with centrotemporal spikes* (benign rolandic epilepsy) – 15–20% childhood epilepsy
- *Juvenile myoclonic epilepsy* – 4–12% childhood epilepsy
- *Childhood absence epilepsy* – 10–12% childhood epilepsy
- *Localization-related epilepsies* categorized as symptomatic (known underlying cause) or cryptogenic (symptomatic cause suspected but not found) – up to 30% childhood epilepsy.

Advice for patients: Information and support for patients and parents

Epilepsy Action ☎ 0808 800 5050 🖫 www.epilepsy.org.uk

Further information

NICE 🖫 www.nice.org.uk

- The epilepsies: the diagnosis and management of the epilepsies in adults and children in primary and secondary care (2004)
- Newer drugs for epilepsy in children (2004)
- Referral guidelines for suspected cancer – quick reference guide (2005)

Benign rolandic epilepsy: Also known as *childhood epilepsy with centrotemporal spikes.*

- Clonic, partial sensorimotor attacks affect the face, tongue, pharynx, hand and arm. Most common on falling asleep (>½ have seizures only during sleep) or soon after waking. Secondary generalization to tonic–clonic seizures may occur. EEG is characteristic.
- Starts in children aged 2–12y. (peak age 7–10y.) – usually stops by 13y. Frequently there is a family history.
- Use of drug treatment depends on frequency and severity of seizures.

Juvenile myoclonic epilepsy (JME):

- Sudden, brief, bilaterally symmetrical and synchronous involuntary muscle contractions. Upper body > lower body. May cause the patient to throw objects or fall. Consciousness is often maintained. Frequently occurs soon after waking. Triggers may include light (1:2), tiredness, emotion. EEG is characteristic.
- Age of onset 8–24y. (peak age 10–16y.) – 50% have FH of epilepsy.
- Generalized tonic–clonic seizures – often starting with a series of myoclonic jerks – appear <4y. after onset of myoclonic seizures in ~90%.
- Absence seizures also occur in 15–30% patients with JME.
- Usually treated with sodium valproate – fits may not be well controlled with medication.
- JME does not remit spontaneously. Lifelong medication is needed – relapse rate is ~90% on withdrawal of anti-epileptic medication.

Lennox-Gastaut syndrome: Severe early-onset form of myoclonic epilepsy – starts age 2–6y. – with intractable seizures and a typical EEG.

Absence seizures (petit mal):

- The child stops what he is doing and may stare into middle-space for a period of seconds (mean 4–20sec.). Can occur 50–100x/d. EEG is characteristic.
- Age at onset 4–10y. (peak 5–7y.); ♀>♂; ~15% have a family history.
- Deterioration in school performance may be the first sign. Separating absence attacks from daydreaming can be difficult.
- ~15% go on to develop JME.
- ~10% (without other adverse factors) have absence or tonic–clonic seizures in adult life.
- 80% become seizure free with sodium valproate.

Localization-related epilepsies: Partial (focal) seizures. May be symptomatic (known underlying cause) or cryptogenic (symptomatic cause suspected but not found). Clinical features, disabilities and prognosis depend on cause and location of the brain abnormality.

Infantile spasms (West's syndrome):

- Starts in the first year of life (peak age: 4mo.).
- Runs of tonic spasms – usually flexion spasms ('salaam' spasms) – occur every 5–10sec. There is a typical EEG.
- Associated with loss of vision and social interaction.
- Treatment is with steroids and anti-epileptics (usually vigabatrin).
- Poor prognosis. 30–50% have cerebral palsy; 85% have a cognitive disability. 20% death rate.

Advice for patients: Epilepsy

Experiences of epilepsy:

Mother's description of her son's myoclonic seizure

'In the morning when he wakes up he has myoclonic-type seizures where his head goes to the left and his arms raised and his, He can have about 5 or 10 minutes of these. Sometimes these can carry on until he has the major seizure.'

Experiences of an absence attack

'I was once babysitting with my friend, I think I was about 15 or 16 at the time, and she asked me a question and apparently it was five minutes before I answered her. I didn't realize it was five minutes, but that's what she said. So basically she'd been sitting there, I hadn't answered her and she'd been sitting there and then suddenly I answered this question and because my answer just sounded so random she was like, "What?"'

'I was away with my brother.... And I used to sort of look up to the left a bit, you know. And I was just sort of in a trance I suppose, for a little. And then I would be all right. And he, my brother, just played the ball to me and, you know, I didn't do anything. And then seconds later I came round and he said, "Are you all right?" I said, 'Yeah, I think so," you know, "Yeah, I'm all right." And I had not realized that I'd had it and he mentioned this to my dad.'

Experience of loss of independence caused by epilepsy

'It was as I got older that it became a problem because I think independence is the main thing that you are restricted with, if you have got uncontrolled epilepsy. It is that restriction, it's a nuisance. So for example when I was in my teens and after a very caring, overprotective mother not wanting me to go and ride on friends' motorbikes or go to discos or do anything like that, I tended to think well I've got to struggle to show I can do it and I can do it safely, whereas my little sister gets it handed to her on a plate because she's safe.'

Information and support for patients and parents:

Epilepsy Action ☎ 0808 800 5050 ▣ www.epilepsy.org.uk
West's Syndrome Support Group ▣ www.wssg.org.uk

231

Further information

NICE ▣ www.nice.org.uk
- The epilepsies: the diagnosis and management of the epilepsies in adults and children in primary and secondary care (2004)
- Newer drugs for epilepsy in children (2004)
- Referral guidelines for suspected cancer – quick reference guide (2005)

Management of the fitting patient: 📖 p.52

Long-term management of epilepsy in primary care

> ⚠ Refer all children with a first suspected non-febrile seizure for urgent (within 2wk.) assessment by a specialist paediatrician with training and expertise in epilepsy[N].

A paediatrician or a paediatric neurologist, under shared care protocols with primary care, should oversee ongoing management – including starting and stopping medication.

Education:
- Epilepsy is a diagnosis that can cause great alarm and fear. Education is very important. Good leaflets are available from Epilepsy Action.
- Parents and patients need clear information on:
  - What to expect
  - What to do during an attack
  - Avoiding risks e.g. swimming or cycling alone – but not being overprotective
  - Importance of compliance with medication – especially difficult with teenagers
  - When drug withdrawal may be considered if fit free.

Drug treatment
- Drug treatment is the mainstay of epilepsy management. For children, anti-epileptic treatment is less well supported by clinical trial data than for adults, and drugs are more likely to be used off-licence.
- There is controversy about when to treat – after the 1st, 2nd or 3rd seizure. NICE recommends after 2nd except in specific circumstances.
- The drug chosen is matched to the individual patient and type of epilepsy – this is a specialist decision. Often the most suitable drug can only be established by trial and error.
- Review treatment at regular intervals to ensure children are not maintained on treatment that is ineffective or poorly tolerated, and that concordance with prescribed medication is maintained.

Surgery: Increasingly being used for childhood epilepsy (e.g. lesionectomy). It is useful for intractable partial seizures, hemi-epilepsy and epilepsy with focal EEG and/or radiological features.

Ketogenic diet: Effective in some children with refractory epilepsy – take specialist advice.

Mortality: ↑ x2–3 that of the general population in all people with epilepsy, especially in children with symptomatic epilepsy and those with learning or physical disabilities. Some deaths are related to an underlying condition, accidents or status epilepticus. Sudden unexplained death in epilepsy (SUDEP) is probably due to central respiratory arrest during a seizure.

- Developmental problems are common in some children with early-onset seizures, such as infantile spasms (West's syndrome) and Lennox-Gastaut syndrome.
- 25% of children with epilepsy have special educational needs, and >20% have moderate or severe learning difficulties.
- Specific cognitive difficulties (e.g. with reading or arithmetic) can occur and may have a serious impact on a child's education if not recognized.
- Social stigmatization (perceived or experienced) – children may have problems making friends and with their peers at school because they are not allowed to do everything the other children do or have funny turns and are considered 'odd'.
- Psychosocial problems are common including lack of confidence, poor self-esteem, behavioural problems (e.g. conduct disorder, school refusal), dependence on others, anxiety and depression.
- Adverse effects of anti-epileptic drugs are a significant problem for many children.
- Physical trauma may occur as a result of having a seizure.

Primary care management
- Support the child and family. Ensure receipt of all available benefits.
- Liaise with the primary health care team, community, educational and specialist services to ensure prompt provision of equipment, support and services.
- Tell carers about local facilities, voluntary and self-help organizations.
- Make referrals for new problems promptly.
- Liaise with specialist services to provide ongoing care.

Advice for patients: Information and support for patients and parents

Epilepsy Action ☎ 0808 800 5050 🖥 www.epilepsy.org.uk

233

Further information
NICE 🖥 www.nice.org.uk
- The epilepsies: the diagnosis and management of the epilepsies in adults and children in primary and secondary care (2004)
- Newer drugs for epilepsy in children (2004)
- Referral guidelines for suspected cancer – quick reference guide (2005)

Cerebral palsy

The term cerebral palsy identifies children with non-progressive spasticity, ataxia or involuntary movements. It affects 0.1–0.2% of children (~1% of premature babies/babies small for dates).

Causes
- Prematurity
- *In utero* disorders
- Neonatal jaundice
- Birth trauma
- Perinatal asphyxia
- CNS trauma
- Severe systemic disease during early childhood (e.g. meningitis, sepsis)

Associated disorders
- Fits (25%)
- Squint and other visual problems
- Deafness
- Learning disability – though intelligence is often normal
- Short attention span
- Hyperactivity

Classification: 3 main categories – but mixed forms are common.

Spastic syndromes: 70%. Upper motor neuron involvement.
- Affects motor function and may → hemiplegia, paraplegia, quadriplegia or diplegia.
- Affected limbs are underdeveloped and have ↑ tone, weakness and a tendency toward contractures.
- A scissors gait and toe walking are characteristic.
- In mildly affected children, impairment may occur only during certain activities (e.g. running).
- With quadriplegia dysarthria is common.

Athetoid and dyskinetic syndromes: 20%. Basal ganglia involvement.
- Characterized by slow, writhing, involuntary movements affecting the extremities (athetoid) or proximal parts of the limbs/trunk (dystonic).
- Abrupt, jerky, distal movements (choreiform) may also occur.
- Movements ↑ with emotional tension and stop during sleep.
- Dysarthria is often severe.

Ataxic syndromes: 10%. Involvement of the cerebellum. Weakness, incoordination and intention tremor produce unsteadiness, wide-based gait and difficulty with rapid and fine movements.

Diagnosis: Diagnosis is rarely made in infancy with certainty though often abnormalities in tone, reflexes and posture are noted during routine developmental screening. Refer for paediatric assessment if suspected. Formal diagnosis is usually made by 2y.

Management
- The goal is for children to develop maximal independence within the limits of their handicap.
- A multidisciplinary, coordinated team approach involving physiotherapists, occupational therapists, speech therapists, social workers, teachers, community paediatricians and the primary health care team in liaison with the child and his parents is essential.
- As with all chronically disabled children, the child and parents also need assistance in understanding the disability, setting realistic goals and relieving their own feelings.

Advice for patients: Information and support for parents and children

SCOPE (cerebral palsy) ☎ 0808 800 3333 🖥 www.scope.org.uk

Neurofibromatosis and muscle disorders

Von Recklinghausen disease (type 1 neurofibromatosis):
Autosomal dominant trait. Criteria for diagnosis: ≥2 of:
- ≥6 café-au-lait patches (flat, coffee-coloured patches of skin seen in 1st year of life, increasing in number and size with age) >5mm (prepubertal) or >15mm (postpubertal)
- ≥2 neurofibromas (dermal or nodular)
- Freckling in axilla, groin, neck base and submammary area (women). Present by age 10y.
- ≥2 Lisch nodules – nodules of the iris only visible with a slit lamp
- Distinctive boney abnormality specific to NF1 e.g. sphenoid dysplasia
- 1st degree relative with NF1.

Management: Ongoing specialist management is essential. Complications affect 1:3 patients:
- Mild learning disability
- Short stature
- Macrocephaly
- Nerve root compression
- GI bleeding or obstruction
- Cystic bone lesion
- Scoliosis
- Pseudoarthrosis
- ↑BP (6%) – due to renal artery stenosis or phaechromocytoma
- Malignancy (5%) – optic glioma or sarcomatous change of neurofibroma
- Epilepsy (slight ↑)

Type 2: Much rarer than type 1. Autosomal dominant inheritance. Diagnosis is on the basis of presence of a:
- Bilateral vestibular schwannoma (acoustic neuroma)
- 1st degree relative with NF2 *and either* a unilateral vestibular schwannoma *or* ≥1 neurofibroma, meningioma, glioma, Schwannoma or juvenile cataract.

Management: Screen at-risk patients with annual hearing tests. Once diagnosis made, specialist neurosurgical management is needed.

Complications: Schwannomas of other nerves; meningioma (45%); other gliomas (less common).

⚠ Refer all cases of unilateral or asymmetrical deafness to ENT for MRI to exclude an acoustic neuroma.

Muscular dystrophies: Group of genetic disorders characterized by progressive degeneration and weakness of some muscle groups.

Duchenne muscular dystrophy: Sex-linked recessive inheritance means almost always confined to boys. 30% of cases are due to spontaneous mutation. *Presentation:*
- Late walking in absence of other developmental delay.
- At ~4y. with progressively clumsy walking, difficulty keeping up with others and stairs.
- Gower's sign 'climbing up legs with hands' when getting up from floor.
- Psuedohypertrophy of calf muscles.
- Investigation shows markedly ↑ CK (>40x normal).

Management: Refer for confirmation of diagnosis and ongoing specialist support. Progressive muscular weakness leads to loss of walking between 7–10y. and few survive to >20y. old. Genetic counselling is important. Antenatal diagnosis is possible.

Less severe forms of muscular dystrophy include Becker and facio-scapular humeral dystrophy.

Myotonic disorders: Characterized by myotonia – delayed muscular contraction after relaxation e.g. on shaking hands.

Dystrophia myotonica: Most common myotonic disorder. Inherited as an autosomal dominant trait with variable penetrance. May present as a floppy infant, with talipes and/or as a droopy-faced child. May be associated with learning disability. Treatment is supportive. Genetic counselling is important.

Myaesthenia gravis: Autoimmune disease in which antibodies to the acetylcholine receptor cause a deficit of receptors at the neuromuscular junction → muscle weakness. Antibodies are detectable in 90% of patients. ♀:♂≈2:1. Associated with thymic tumours and other autoimmune diseases e.g. RA, SLE, hyperthyroidism. Generally follows a relapsing or slowly progressive course. If thymoma present, 5y. survival ≈30%.

Presentation: Teenagers with easy fatigability of muscles. Commonly affected muscles are the:
- orbital muscles causing ptosis and diplopia *and*
- bulbar muscles causing slurring of speech – ask to count to 50.

Weakness is exacerbated by infection, drugs (e.g. β-blockers, opiates, tetracycline, quinine), climate change, emotion and exercise.

Management: If suspected refer for confirmation of diagnosis and specialist treatment by a neurologist. Treated with:
- anticholinesterase e.g. pyridostigmine
- immunosuppression with prednisolone, methotrexate or azathioprine
- thymectomy → remission in 30% and benefit in another 40%
- plasmapheresis.

Advice for patients: Information and support for patients

Neurofibromatosis Association UK ☎ 020 8439 1234
🖳 www.nfauk.org
Muscular Dystrophy Campaign ☎ 020 7720 8055
🖳 www.muscular-dystrophy.org
The Dystonia Society ☎ 0845 458 6322 🖳 www.dystonia.org.uk
Myaesthenia Gravis Association ☎ 0800 919 922
🖳 www.mgauk.org

Chapter 8

Dermatology, ophthalmology and ENT

Birthmarks

Strawberry naevus (capillary haemangioma): Figure 8.1
- Affects up to 10% of infants.
- Not usually present at birth.
- Occurs anywhere on the skin surface.
- Starts as a small, red patch then grows rapidly over a few months into a bright-red vascular lump.
- After initial growth, the naevus stays the same size for 6–12mo., then involutes and disappears by 5–7y.
- No treatment is required but parents may need considerable reassurance.
- If interfering with feeding, breathing or vision – refer for treatment with intralesional steroids or laser.

Port wine stain (naevus flammeus): Figure 8.2
- Present at birth.
- Irregular red/purple macule which often affects 1 side of the face.
- Permanent – may become darker and lumpy in middle age.
- May be associated with other abnormalities e.g. intracranial vascular malformation (Sturge-Weber syndrome).

Salmon patch (stork mark): Figure 8.3
- The most common vascular naevus (~50% neonates).
- Small, telangiectatic lesion forming a pink macule – most commonly at the nape of the neck or on the upper face.
- Facial lesions resolve spontaneously – those on the neck may persist. No treatment is needed.

Mongolian blue spot: Figure 8.4
- Bluish discolouration of the skin, usually over buttocks and lower back in dark-skinned babies.
- Of no clinical significance but may occasionally be mistaken for bruising and non-accidental injury.
- Usually disappear by 1y.

Congenital melanocytic naevus: ~1.5% of neonates.
- Noted at birth as raised nodules or plaques of black or brown.
- May be hairy, irregular and single or multiple.
- Classified by size: <1.5cm – small; 1.5–20cm – medium; >20cm – large.
- There is a risk of malignant change to melanoma – the larger the naevus the greater the risk.
- Laser therapy can improve cosmetic appearance.

Accessory nipples:
- Commonly seen on the milk line in both male and female infants.
- Usually small and inconspicuous.
- No treatment is required.

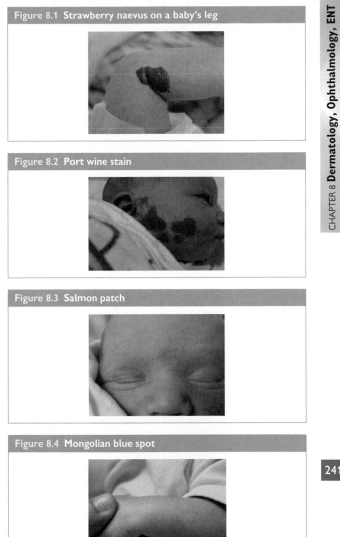

Figure 8.1 **Strawberry naevus on a baby's leg**

Figure 8.2 **Port wine stain**

Figure 8.3 **Salmon patch**

Figure 8.4 **Mongolian blue spot**

Figures 8.1, 8.2, 8.3 and 8.4 are reproduced with permission from the Auckland Board of Health
🖳 www.adhb.govt.nz

Atopic eczema

Affects 15–20% of schoolchildren – usually starts <6mo. of age and by 1y. 60% of those likely to develop eczema will have done so. Associated with other atopic conditions e.g. asthma, hayfever. Remission occurs by 15y. of age in 75%, though some relapse later.

Presentation: Waxing and waning itchy condition:

- *Infants:* Itchy vesicular exudative eczema on face ± hands, often with $2°$ infection. May cause sleep disturbance due to itch. $>\frac{1}{2}$ are free of eczema by 18mo.
- *Children >18mo.:* Involves antecubital and popliteal fossae, neck, wrists and ankles. Lichenification, excoriation and dry skin are common. Face may be erythematous and have typical infraorbital folds. Loss of self-esteem, behavioural and sleep problems are common.

Diagnosis: Itchy skin PLUS ≥3 of:

- History of itching around the skin creases (elbows, knees, wrists) or neck (or cheeks if <4y.). For a young child a report of scratching or rubbing in these areas is sufficient
- Visible flexural eczema (or eczema affecting cheeks, forehead and/or outer limbs in children <4y.)
- History of asthma or hayfever (for children <4y. a history of asthma or hayfever in a first-degree relative is sufficient)
- Generally dry skin
- Onset in the first 2y. of life.

Differential diagnosis: Scabies; ringworm; rare syndromes e.g. Wiskott-Aldrich syndrome, dermatitis herpetiformis

Assessment: Ask:

- Is there a personal or family history of atopy or eczema? $\frac{2}{3}$ of children with a new diagnosis of eczema have a family history.
- How did the symptoms start?
- What areas of the body are affected? Look and see – assessing extent, severity. Exudate or crusting suggests secondary bacterial infection.
- Does anything make the eczema worse or better? Consider pets, irritants e.g. bubble bath or soap, swimming, stress.
- Do the symptoms interfere with sleep?
- Do the symptoms interfere with school or home life?
- What has the child tried before? Ask about specialist referral, prescribed medication (both for eczema and other conditions), over-the-counter medications, complementary therapies, special diets.
- What does the child and family understand about eczema and what are their expectations of treatment?

Management of eczema:

- Acknowledge parents' concerns. Explain the condition and generally good prognosis.
- Advise – loose cotton clothing, gloves in bed. Avoid wool (exacerbates eczema), excessive heat, biological washing powders. Keep nails short.

Figure 8.5 Features of atopic eczema in a child

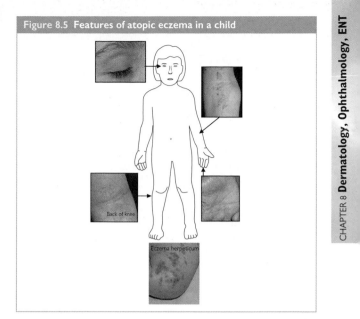

Back of knee

Eczema herpeticum

Complications of eczema:

- *Skin thickening and scaling*
- *Bacterial infection:* 2° infection (usually with *S. aureus*) commonly causes exacerbations (and may not be seen as obvious infection). Bacterial infection is suggested by presence of crusting or weeping, or sudden deterioration of eczema.
- *Viral infection:* ↑ susceptibility to infection e.g. with viral warts and molluscum contagiosum. ⚠ *Eczema herpeticum* – propensity to develop widespread lesions with HSV and VZ – may require admission and IV aciclovir.
- *Cataracts:* Rarely occur in young adults with very severe eczema.
- *Growth retardation:* Children with severe eczema, cause unknown. A growth chart should be kept for children with chronic severe eczema.

Drug treatment of eczema:

Emollients: e.g. aqueous cream, bath emollients
- Use regularly on skin and as soap substitutes. Several different products might need to be tried before one that suits the child is found. In general greasy ointments are best for dry skin or at night and creams are preferable for inflamed areas and during the day.
- Ideally applied 3–4x/d. – best applied to moist skin. Ensure you prescribe enough emollient to last the interval between prescriptions.
- Addition of an antipruritic substance e.g. lauromacrogol to the emollient may help break the scratch–itch cycle.
- Addition of an antiseptic to bath emollient may ↓ bacterial infection.

Topical steroids:
- Prescribe the least potent strength that is effective (e.g. start with hydrocortisone 1%). Apply once daily or twice daily depending on severity and response. Emphasize steroid creams are for short-term intermittent use and to avoid application near the eyes.
- Ointments are preferable on dry, scaly eczema; creams on wet, exudative eczema.
- Emollients – especially if applied just prior to steroid creams – ↓ steroid requirement.

❗ Doctors' and parents' fears about side effects of topical steroid treatment can lead to chronic under-treatment – a short course of a more potent steroid may be necessary to gain control.

Antibiotics: For infected eczema – can be topical (alone or in combination with a steroid e.g. Fucidin H) or oral (e.g. flucloxacillin or erythromycin qds for 2wk.). Take swabs for M,C&S if adequate antibiotic treatment is ineffective.

Antihistamines: Sedative antihistamines given nocte ↓ desire to itch and may improve sleep e.g. promethazine, hydroxyzine.

Oral steroids: Rescue therapy while waiting for an urgent consultant opinion. Only use short courses e.g prednisolone 20–30mg od for 5d.

Topical immunosuppressants e.g. tacrolimus – on consultant advice only.

Other treatments:

- *Bandages:* Excoriated or lichenified eczema. Tar bandages (Tarband, Coltapaste) are most effective and messiest; Ichthammol (Icthband) or zinc and calamine (Calaband) may be more acceptable. Bandages can be applied at night on top of steroid ointment. Refer to dermatology.
- *Wet wrapping:* Can be used for exudative eczema – Tubigrip bandage or tubular gauze soaked in emollient ± weak topical steroid is applied and covered with a dry bandage. Refer to dermatology.
- *Dietary manipulation:* A few (<10%) benefit. Egg and milk are the most common allergens. If undertaken at all, advise dietician supervision to avoid malnutrition.
- *Allergen avoidance:* Some parents identify specific allergens (e.g. house dust mite, pets) and avoid them. Evidence of effectiveness in relieving symptoms is lacking.

GP Notes: When should I refer a child with eczema?

- Infection with disseminated HSV (eczema herpeticum) – to paediatrics or dermatology E
- Severe eczema resistant to treatment. Additional secondary care treatments include phototherapy and immunosuppressive agents U
- Infection which cannot be cleared in primary care U
- Severe social/psychological problems due to eczema S
- Treatment requires excessive amounts of topical steroids S
- Failure to control symptoms in primary care S/R
- Patient/family might benefit from additional advice on application of treatments (e.g. bandaging techniques) R
- Patch testing required if contact dermatitis suspected R
- Dietary factors are suspected (refer direct to dietician) R

E= Emergency admission; U=Urgent; S= Soon; R=Routine

Advice for patients: Eczema

Information for parents about treatment of eczema:

- About ¾ of all children with eczema grow out of it by their teens.
- Until then their eczema will come and go. Treatment can't cure eczema but will improve the symptoms.
- Emollients help replace the moisture in dry skin which occurs in eczema. Apply your child's emollient as often as needed and at least 3–4 times a day.
- Frequent use of emollients is hard work, particularly if your child is young or uncooperative, but worthwhile as using emollients will reduce the amount of steroid creams your child will need.
- At bathtime, use bath emollient instead of soap. Make sure the bath water isn't too hot as hot water makes the itching of eczema worse. Staying in the bath for 15–20 minutes lets the skin absorb the moisturizer. Apply your child's emollient cream after a bath.
- At other times use your child's emollient cream as a soap substitute.
- Your child will probably need intermittent courses of steroid cream in addition to emollients. Intermittent use is not harmful long term.
- Keep using emollients even when the skin is free of eczema to prevent flare-ups.

Information and support for children and parents:
National Eczema Society ☎ 0870 241 3604 🖳 www.eczema.org

245

Further information

BMJ 🖳 www.bmj.com
- Barnetson & Rogers *Childhood atopic eczema* (2002) 324 pp.1376–9
- Santer et al *Childhood eczema* (2005) 331 p.497

NICE Atopic eczema: Management in children from birth up to the age of 12 years. 🖳 www.nice.org.uk

Other eczema-like conditions

Contact dermatitis[G]**:** Precipitated by an exogenous agent which is:
- *Irritant* (e.g. water, abrasives, chemicals, detergent) *or*
- *Allergen* (e.g. nickel – 10% ♀, 1% ♂; chrome; rubber).

More common in older children with a past history of atopic eczema.

Differential diagnosis: Atopic eczema, psoriasis, fungal infection

Presentation: Affects any part of the body – site and knowledge of occupation, hobbies, sports etc. help elucidate cause.
- *Acute:* Itchy erythema and skin oedema ± papules, vesicles or blisters
- *Chronic:* Lichenification, scaling and fissuring

Management:
- *Identification of the allergen or irritant:* Consider referral for patch testing (📖 p.108).
- *Exclusion of the offending allergen or irritant from the environment:* Though may be impossible. There is some evidence that nickel avoidance diets can help patients with nickel sensitivity[G]. Nickel testing kits are available from dermatology departments.
- *Emollients:* Help skin to recover – apply frequently.
- *Topical steroids:* Help but are secondary to avoidance measures.

Nappy rash: Commonest type of nappy eruption. Usually seen in young infants – rare >12mo. Irritant dermatitis due to skin contact with urine or faeces.

Presentation: Glazed erythema in the nappy area, sparing skin folds. Secondary bacterial or fungal infection is common.

Differential diagnosis:
- Seborrhoeic eczema
- Candidiasis
- Napkin psoriasis

Management:
- Advice on keeping nappy area clean, dry and well moisturized.
- Topical treatment with an antifungal combined with hydrocortisone (e.g. clotrimazole + hydrocortisone cream) is effective if the nappy rash is not clearing.

Juvenile plantar dermatosis:
- Presents with red, dry, fissured and glazed skin principally over the forefeet. Sometimes involves the whole sole.
- Usually starts in primary school years and resolves spontaneously in mid-teens.
- Due to wearing socks and/or shoes made from synthetic materials.
- Emollients help but topical steroids are ineffective. Advise cotton socks and leather shoes.

Seborrhoeic dermatitis: Chronic scaly eruption affecting scalp, face and/or chest. *Differential diagnosis:* Psoriasis, contact dermatitis, fungal infection

Treatment:
- *Facial, truncal and flexural involvement:* Imidazole + hydrocortisone (e.g. clotrimazole + hydrocortisone cream).
- *Scalp lesions*: Ketoconazole or coal tar shampoo.
- Recurrence requiring repeated treatment is common.

Infantile seborrhoeic eczema:
- Starts in the first few weeks of life.
- Affects body folds – axilla, groins, behind ears, neck ± face and scalp ('*cradle cap*').
- Flexural lesions present as moist, shiny, well-demarcated scaly erythema.
- On the scalp, neck and behind the ears, a yellowish crust is usual.
- Treat flexural lesions with emollients and 1% hydrocortisone ointment or with clotrimazole and hydrocortisone.
- Scalp lesions respond to OTC cradle cap preparations or 2% salicyclic acid in aqueous cream applied od and washed out with baby shampoo.

Dandruff: Is exaggerated physiological exfoliation of fine scales from an otherwise normal scalp. More severe forms merge with seborrhoeic dermatitis and treatment is the same.

Other rare conditions:
- *Actinic prurigo:* Starts in childhood. Papules and excoriations on sun exposed sites. Refer to dermatology if suspected. Management is with sunscreens and avoidance.
- *Dermatitis herpetiformis:* Closely related to coeliac disease (💷 p.181 – 2–5% patients with coeliac disease have dermatitis herpetiformis). ♂>♀ (2:1). Itchy, vesicular rash on elbows (extensor surface), knees, buttocks and scalp. Refer to dermatology for confirmation of diagnosis. Responds to withdrawal of gluten.

Advice for patients: Advice for parents on preventing and relieving nappy rash

- Keep the nappy area dry – superabsorbant disposal nappies or nappy liners help.
- Give your baby as much time as possible with the nappy off.
- Apply aqueous cream as a moisturiser and soap substitute.
- Apply a barrier cream (e.g. Sudocrem®) between nappy changes, though this may interfere with the action of some modern nappies

---

Further information
British Association of Dermatologists Guidelines for the management of contact dermatitis (2001) 🖥 www.bad.org.uk

Urticaria (hives) and angio-oedema

Urticaria is common. Most children with urticaria do not have systemic reactions but, very rarely, urticaria may progress to anaphylaxis. Conversely, urticaria is often a feature of anaphylactic reactions.

Features:
- Superficial, itchy swellings of the skin known as *weals*.
- Deeper swellings of the skin and alimentary tract are called *angio-oedema*. These may be painful rather than itchy and last longer.
- Weals and angio-oedema often coexist but either may occur alone.

Anaphylaxis: 📖 p.42

Urticaria: Weals ± angio-oedema. May be acute (≤6wk. continuous activity) or chronic (>6wk. activity). Typically individual weals last 1–24h. then disappear without trace.

Causes: Often no cause is found. If chronic then termed *chronic idiopathic urticaria.*
- *Systemic allergic reaction:* Sudden onset of urticaria ± angio-oedema. The offending allergen can often be identified e.g. food (peanuts, shellfish, egg are common culprits), drugs (e.g. penicillin), insect sting. Symptoms last hours to days.
- *Childhood viral infection:* Appears less suddenly than an allergic reaction. The child may or may not have other symptoms of viral infection. Disappears in <1wk.
- *Contact:* Urticaria is provoked by contact with a substance. Can be an allergic response or due to a physical irritant (e.g. nettle rash). Usually self-limiting in <2h. if the cause is removed.
- *Physical:* A physical stimulus which is usually harmless consistently provokes an urticarial response. Common examples are dermatographism (pressure on the skin provokes urticaria – affects 5% of the population), sunlight (solar urticaria), water, sweat and heat or cold. Usually short-lived (<1h.), with the exception of delayed pressure urticaria which is slower to develop and fade.
- *Other systemic disease:* Lymphoma, thyrotoxicosis, parasitic infestations can all present with urticaria which may be chronic.

Differential diagnosis: Erythema multiforme, erythema toxicum (in small babies), skin infection, measles

Management: Treat with antihistamines as needed (e.g. chlor-phenamine). If recurrent or chronic and an allergen or trigger can't be identified, refer to dermatology or for allergy testing.

Urticaria pigmentosa (cutaneous mastocytosis): Appears in infancy (usually <2wk. old). Dark freckle-like lesions on the face, limbs or trunk become urticarial when the skin is rubbed. No treatment is needed – clears spontaneously in childhood.

Hereditary angio-oedema:

- Due to deficiency of C_1 esterase inhibitor which allows complement activation to go unchecked.
- Autosomal dominant – usually presents in childhood with episodes of angio-oedema without weals. May affect the larynx → respiratory depression, or GI tract → abdominal pain.
- Emergency treatment is with hospital admission for fresh frozen plasma or C_1 inhibitor concentrate infusion. Maintenance therapy (usually with anabolic steroids – consultant supervision only) is necessary only for patients with symptomatic recurring angio-oedema or related abdominal pain.

Figure 8.6 Typical urticarial rash

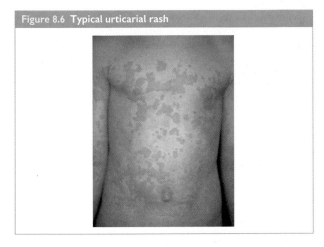

Further information

British Association of Dermatologists. Guidelines for the management of urticaria and angio-oedema (2001) 🖳 www.bad.org.uk

Acne

Acne vulgaris is a chronic inflammatory condition characterized by comedones, papules, pustules, cysts and scars. Acne is common and affects >80% teenagers. Peak age: 18y.; ♂=♀. Severity of acne is often overestimated by the patient and minimized by the doctor.

Cause: Complex – androgen secretion results in:
- ↑ sebum excretion
- pilosebaceous duct blockage (producing comedones)
- colonization of the duct with *Propionibacterium acnes* bacteria
- release of inflammatory mediators.

Inflammatory acne is the result of the host response to the follicular *Propionibacterium* acne.

Rarer causes:
- Endocrine – polycystic ovaries, Cushings, virilizing tumours
- Infantile – faces of male infants – cause unknown
- Squeezing – acne excoriée
- Cosmetics
- Drugs – systemic steroids, androgens, topical steroids
- Physical occlusion e.g. under a violinist's chin

Presentation: Spots on face, neck ± back and chest. Examination:
- Blackheads (dilated pores with black plug of keratin = comedones) and whiteheads (small cream-coloured dome-shaped papules)
- Red papules, pustules ± cysts.

There may be scarring from old lesions and scars can become keloidal. Burrowing abscesses and sinuses with scarring (conglobate acne) are signs of severe acne.

Differential diagnosis: Bacterial folliculitis (may coexist – 📖 p.254).

Classification: Table 8.1

Management: *Aims to:* ↓ number of lesions; prevent scarring; ↓ the psychological impact of the condition. Treatment – Table 8.1. Reassess every 2–3mo. and continue treatment until new lesions stop developing.

Reasons for dermatology referral:
- Acne fulminans – seen in adolescent males, severe acne is associated with fever, arthritis and vasculitis U
- Severe acne or painful, deep nodules or cysts and could benefit from oral isotretinoin - S
- Severe social/psychological sequelae S
- At risk of/developing scarring despite primary care remedies R
- Poor treatment response R
- Suspected underlying cause for acne (e.g polycystic ovaries) R

U=Urgent; S= Soon; R=Routine

Perioral dermatitis: Papules and pustules which appear around the mouth and chin of a girl who has used topical steroids. Treat with oral tetracycline as for acne.

	Description	Management
Table 8.1	**Treatment of acne (*BNF* 13.6)**	
Mild acne	Open and closed comedones and some papules	Topical treatment applied to the whole area (not just the spots): *Benzoyl peroxide* applied bd – start at lowest strength and build up as needed. *Topical retinoids* (e.g. isotretinoin) – apply low-strength preparation every 2–3 nights initially and build up strength and frequency as tolerated. Warn patients they should avoid the sun. Retinoids cause erythema and scaling in most patients which settles with time and acne may worsen for the first few weeks of treatment. *Topical antibiotics* (e.g. Dalacin T) – resistance is increasing, use only in combination with benzoyl peroxide or if benzoyl peroxide has failed. Avoid if using oral antibiotics.
Moderate acne	More frequent papules and pustules with mild scarring	Try topical treatment first. If not working after 4–8wk. try either long-term oral antibiotics (e.g. tetracycline) for a minimum of 8wk. Topical preparations may be used simultaneously with systemic therapy.
Severe acne	Nodular abscesses → more widespread scarring	As for moderate acne. If ineffective or relapses rapidly after antibiotics are stopped, refer to a dermatologist for consideration of oral retinoid treatment (e.g. Roaccutane). ⚠ Oral retinoids are teratogenic.

GP Notes: The full impact of acne

Acne is not a trivial disease – it causes scars (skin and emotional) lasting a lifetime. Anxiety, social isolation and ↓ in self-confidence are common.

Advice for patients: Information about acne

- Acne is not due to poor hygiene. Blackheads are normal skin products and are not dirty.
- Acne is not due to your diet and what you eat doesn't affect it.
- Wash your skin with soap and water twice a day. Apply a moisturizer (e.g. aqueous cream) after washing.
- If that doesn't help, try an acne lotion from the chemist or see a doctor. Treatment for acne won't work overnight. Don't consider your treatment has failed until you have been using it for at least 3 months.
- If your treatment works, you will need to continue it for a period of months or even years.

Further information and support
Acne Support Group ☎ 0870 870 2263 🖳 www.stopspots.org

Further information
BMJ Webster GF Acne vulgaris (2002) 325 pp.475–9 🖳 www.bmj.com

Psoriasis

Psoriasis is a chronic, non-infectious inflammatory skin condition characterized by well-demarcated, erythematous plaques topped by silvery scales. Epidermal cell proliferation rate is ↑ x20 and turnover time ↓ from 28d. to 4d. Affects ~2% Caucasian population (less in other races) but rare <8y. ♂=♀.

Presentation: Table 8.2

Cause: Genetic (polygenic inheritance; 35% have a family history; there is a 25% probability that a child with 1 parent with psoriasis will be affected–60% chance with 2). Environmental factors trigger disease.

Precipitating factors:
- Trauma (Koebner phenomenon)
- Sunlight – aggravates psoriasis in 10%
- Drugs e.g. β-blockers, NSAIDs, chloroquine
- Infection
- Alcohol
- Psychological stress

Management: Social or psychological problems are common. Be supportive. Explain the condition and treatment. Advise on self-help.

Treatment options (BNF 13.5): Frequent emollients ±
- **Coal tar** – anti-inflammatory and anti-scaling properties. The thicker the patch the stronger the preparation required. Available as topical pastes, oinments, bath additives and shampoos.
- **Dithranol** – plaque psoriasis – apply to lesion only. Stains.
- **Vitamin D analogue** e.g. calcipotriol – plaque and scalp psoriasis – no unpleasant smell/staining of clothing. Calcipotriol is licenced for children >6y.. Maximum dose: 6–12y. –50g/wk.; >12y. –75g/wk.
- **Mild topical steroids** – can be used for flexural, facial or scalp psoriasis.
- **Salicyclic acid** – ↓ surface scale. Available as Lassar's paste (apply bd), or together with dithranol (Psorin® scalp gel or oinment) or together with coal tar (e.g. Sebco® scalp oinment).

🚫 Plaques can become inflamed and/or aggravated on starting topical treatments, after prolonged use of topical steroids or if steroids are stopped suddenly.

Reasons for referral to dermatology: Additional 2° care treatment options include phototherapy and PUVA, oral retinoids, cytotoxic and immunosuppressive therapy and specialist nursing services. Refer if:
- Generalized pustular or erythrodermic psoriasis E
- Widespread guttate psoriasis (to benefit from early phototherapy) U
- The child's psoriasis is acutely unstable U
- Severe social or psychological sequelae S
- Rash is so extensive as to make self-management impractical S
- Rash is in a sensitive area (e.g. face, hands, feet, genitalia) and the symptoms troublesome S
- Time off school is interfering with education S
- For management of associated arthropathy (rare in children) S
- Rash fails to respond to primary care management R

E=Emergency; U=Urgent; S=Soon; R=Routine

Table 8.2 Patterns of psoriasis

Pattern	Features
Erythroderma	Inflammatory dermatosis affecting >90% skin surface. Admit.
Generalized pustular	Rare but serious. Unwell with fever and malaise. Sheets of small sterile yellowish pustules develop on an erythematous background and spread rapidly. Admit.
Guttate	Acute symmetrical raindrop lesions on trunk/limbs. Most common presentation in children – may follow strep- tococcal throat infection. Treat tonsillitis with penicillin V if still ongoing. Often resolves within a few weeks with no treatment or emollient ± mild steroid. Refer severe cases urgently for consideration of UVB phototherapy. Recurrent guttate psoriasis associated with recurrent throat infection is an indication for tonsillectomy. *Differential diagnosis:* pityriasis rosea
Plaque	Commonest form overall. Well-defined disc-shaped plaques involving the knees, elbows, scalp, hair margin or sacrum. Plaques are usually red and covered with waxy white scales which may leave bleeding points if detached. Plaques may be itchy.
Scalp psoriasis	May be confused with dandruff but generally better demarcated and thicker scales.
Flexural	Affects axillae, groin and genital/perianal areas. Plaques are smooth and often glazed. Fairly common in children. *Differential diagnosis:* flexural candidiasis
Napkin psoriasis	Well-defined eruption in nappy area of infants.
Nail	Uncommon in children. If it occurs it is usually only minor pitting. Onycholysis is rare but may be the only manifestation of psoriasis.
Palmoplantar pustulosis	Yellow/brown-coloured sterile pustules on palms or soles. Very rare in children.

Figure 8.7 Typical rash of guttate psoriasis

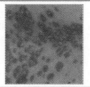

Advice for patients: Information and support

Psoriasis Association ☎ 0845 676 0076
🖥 www.psoriasis-association.org.uk

Further information

British Association of Dermatologists Recommendations for the initial management of psoriasis (2003) 🖥 www.bad.org.uk

Figure 8.7 is reproduced with permission from 🖥 psoriasisguide.ca courtesy of Dr Lyn Guenther

Bacterial skin infection

Impetigo: Figure 8.8
- Superficial skin infection due to *Staphylococcus aureus*.
- A thin-walled blister ruptures easily to leave a yellow crusted lesion.
- May occur anywhere – commonest on face. Lesions spread rapidly and are contagious. Avoid spreading to other children – no sharing of towels etc.; some schools prohibit attendance until lesions are cleared.
- Localized cases – treat with topical antibiotics (e.g. Fucidin H). Widespread infection – treat with oral flucloxacillin or erythromycin.
- *Differential diagnosis:* HSV, fungal infection e.g. ringworm.

Scalded skin syndrome: Acute toxic illness usually of infants. Characterized by shedding of sheets of skin. May follow impetigo. *Management:* Emergency paediatric admission. Requires IV antibiotics.

Folliculitis, boils and carbuncles: Infection of hair follicles is usually with *Staphylococcus aureus*. Predisposing factors include DM (evidence mixed), obesity and immunosuppression.

Folliculitis: Presents as pustules with surrouding erythema. Treat with topical antiseptics. Treat resistant lesions with topical antibiotics – reserve systemic antibiotics (flucloxacillin or erythromycin qds) for severe or refractory infections.

Deeper infection:
- *Boil:* Hard, tender, red nodule surrounding a hair follicle becoming larger and fluctuant after several days. May discharge pus before healing and leave a scar.
- *Carbuncle:* Swollen, painful area discharging pus from several points. Occurs when a group of hair follicles become deeply infected. May be associated with fever ± malaise.

Management:
- Apply moist heat to relieve discomfort, help localize the infection and promote drainage.
- If there is associated fever, surrounding cellulitis or the lesion is on the face, treat with oral antibiotics e.g. flucloxacillin or erythromycin qds.
- If the lesion is large, painful and fluctuant, consider admission for incision and drainage (young child, uncooperative child, boil in a sensitive area e.g. genital region, face, neck, axilla, breast area in older girls). Do not attempt incision and drainage in the surgery if you are not confident. After incision and drainage treat with oral antibiotics until inflammation resolves.
- If the lesion is not settling with primary care treatment, admit.

Recurrent infection:
- Exclude DM and consider referral to exclude an immune deficiency syndrome.
- Take swabs for culture from lesions and carrier sites (nose, axilla, groin). Treat carrier sites with topical antibiotics (e.g. Naseptin cream) or antiseptics (e.g. chlorhexidine in the bath). If not settling refer for consultant advice

Acute paronychia: Infection of the skin and soft tissue of nail fold, most commonly caused by *Staphylococcus aureus*. Often originates from a break in the skin as a result of minor trauma, e.g. nail biting. Skin and soft tissue of the nail fold are red, hot and tender; nail may appear discoloured/distorted. Treat in the same way as a boil (see opposite).

Staphylococcal whitlow (felon): Infection involving the bulbous distal pulp of the finger following trauma or extension from an acute paronychia. Rapid onset of erythema, swelling and exquisite tenderness of the finger bulb. *Diffferential diagnosis:* Herpetic whitlow – 📖 p.256. *Management:* Admit for drainage and antibiotics.

Erysipelas and cellulitis: Acute infection of the dermis usually affecting the face or lower leg.

Presentation:
- May be preceded by fever ± 'flu-like' symptoms.
- Presents with a painful, reddened area with a well-defined edge ± local swelling ± blistering.
- There may be an obvious entry wound.

Management: Oral penicillin V or erythromycin qds for 7–14d. Severe infections may require hospital admission for IV antibiotics. Recurrent infections (>2 episodes at 1 site) require prophylactic long-term penicillin (e.g. penicillin V od or bd) and attention to potential entry portals (e.g. tinea pedis).

Complications: Lymphangitis ± permanent damage to lymph drainage; glomerulonephritis (📖 p.185) or guttate psoriasis (📖 p.253).

Figure 8.8 Impetigo on the chin of a child

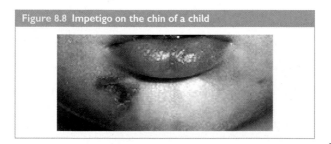

Viral skin infection

Viral warts: Common and benign. Due to infection of epidermal cells with human papilloma virus (HPV)—>50 types identified. Certain types are associated with infection at different sites: common hand warts – type 2; plantar warts – types 1 and 4; genital warts – types 6, 11, 16 and 18. The virus is transmitted by direct contact. Immunosuppressed patients are particularly vulnerable.

Presentation:
- *Common warts:* Dome-shaped papules with papilliferous surface. Usually >1. Commonest on hands but may affect other areas. In children 30–50% disappear spontaneously in <6mo.
- *Plantar warts (verrucas):* On soles of feet (Figure 8.9). Common in children. Pressure makes them grow into the dermis. Often painful. Characterized by dark punctate spots on the surface (may need to pare callus off to see). Warts group together to form mosaics.
- *Plane warts:* Smooth, flat-topped papules, often slightly brown in colour. Commonest on face and backs of hands. Usually >1. Manage as for common/plantar warts. Eventually resolve spontaneously. May show Koebner phenomenon.

Treatment: Table 8.3

Table 8.3 Treatment of viral warts in general practice		
Treatment option	**Examples**	**Notes**
Topical salicylic acid	Salactol, Duofilm, Bazuka	Avoid using on the face or for patients with atopic eczema. Ensure dead skin is pared off daily before reapplication.
Cryotherapy	Liquid nitrogen	May cause blistering and be painful several days after treatment.
Curettage/cautery		Useful for solitary warts on face. Warts may recur.
⚠ Refer immunosuppressed patients for specialist advice on management.		

Molluscum contagiosum: Most common in pre-school children.
- Caused by a DNA pox virus and spread by contact (including towels). Presents as discrete, pearly-pink umbilicated papules, 1–3mm diameter (Figure 8.10).
- If squeezed papules release a cheesy material.
- Lesions are multiple and grouped – usually on the trunk, face or neck.
- Untreated lesions resolve spontaneously after several months.
- In the older child, removal by expressing the contents with forceps, curettage or cryotherapy is possible but usually unnecessary.

Cold sore: 📖 p.92

Herpetic whitlow: Swollen, painful and erythematous lesion of the distal phalanx, results from inoculation of HSV through a skin break or abrasion.

Systemic viral infections with skin manifestations: 📖 pp.90–5

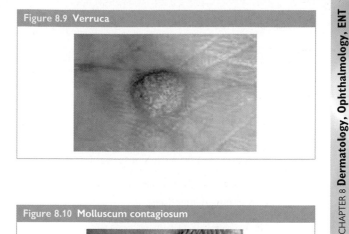

Figure 8.9 **Verruca**

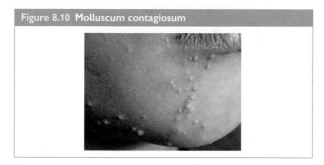

Figure 8.10 **Molluscum contagiosum**

GP Notes: Cryotherapy and cautery for warts in children

Cryotherapy and cautery are painful. Cryotherapy may also cause scarring. Only consider:
- If the wart/verruca is not resolving spontaneously after >3mo. of topical treatment *and*
- If the child (not parent) really wants treatment and is old enough to understand the nature and side effects of treatment.

Further information

British Association of Dermatologists Guidelines for the management of cutaneous warts (2001) 🖳 www.bad.org.uk

Figure 8.10 is reproduced with permission of the UK Clinical Virology Network
🖳 www.clinical-virology.org

Fungal skin infection

There are 2 major groups of fungal skin infections seen in the UK.

Candidiasis: A virtually uniform commensal of the mouth and GI tract which produces opportunistic infection. *Risk factors:* Moist, opposing skin folds; obesity; DM; neonates; poor hygiene; humid environment; use of broad-spectrum antibiotic. Presentation – see Table 8.4.

Dermatophyte infection: Tinea denotes fungal infection. Common. Affects skin, hair or nails. Skin scrapings or nail clippings may confirm diagnosis. Presentation – see Table 8.5.

General measures for prevention of fungal infections: Keep body folds separated and dry (e.g. with dusting powder) and minimize hot and humid conditions (e.g. advise open footwear).

Management of fungal infections:

Topical treatment:

- **Nail infections:** If confined to 1 or 2 nails, consider using a lacquer or paint e.g. amorolfine lacquer 1–2x/wk for durations in the *BNF(5.2)*.
- **Skin lesions:** Imidazole cream, spray, powder; terbinafine cream.
- **Mouth lesions:** Remove tongue deposits with a soft toothbrush by brushing 2x/d. Oral pastilles, suspensions or gels (e.g. nystatin, miconazole).

Systemic treatment: Griseofulvin is the only systemic antifungal licenced for use in children, though terbinafine is commonly used. Use for recurrent, extensive, systemic or resistant infection and nail or scalp infection under consultant supervision.

Further information

BMJ Fuller et al Diagnosis and management of scalp ringworm (2003) 326 p.539 ▭ www.bmj.com

Presentation	Symptoms	Differential diagnosis
Oral	Sore mouth; poor feeding in infants. Commonest in babies and children with poor oral hygiene. White plaques are visible on buccal musosa which can be wiped off ± angular stomatitis.	Aphthous mouth ulcers Hand, foot and mouth
Nappy candidiasis	Babies – in the nappy area.	Nappy rash Napkin psoriasis
Infected infantile seborrhoeic eczema	Erythema, scaling and pustules involve the flexures. There may be associated satellite lesions.	Other forms of eczema
Systemic candidiasis	Occurs in immunosuppressed individuals (e.g. HIV, malignancy). Red nodules may appear on the skin.	

Table 8.4 Presentation of candidiasis

Tinea	Affects	Presentation	Differential diagnosis
Corporis *Ringworm*	Trunk or limbs	Single/multiple plaques with scaling and erythema, especially at the edges. Lesions enlarge slowly and clear centrally (hence 'ringworm').	Discoid eczema Psoriasis Pityriasis rosea
Pedis *Athlete's foot*	Feet ♂>♀	Itchy maceration between toes. *Risk factors:* swimming; occlusive footwear; hot weather.	Contact dermatitis Psoriasis Pompholyx
Capitis*	Hair and scalp Incidence is increasing, particularly amongst inner city children	• Diffuse scale-like dandruff *or* • Boggy swelling (kerion) *or* • Pustular scalp lesions *or* • Defined, inflamed scaly areas ± alopecia with broken hair shafts	Alopecia areata Psoriasis Seborrhoeic eczema
Unguium	Nails Rare in children Toenails > fingernails	Begins at distal nail edge and progresses proximally to involve the whole nail. Tinea pedis often co-exists.	Psoriasis Trauma Candidiasis

Table 8.5 **Dermatophyte infections**

*Always confirm diagnosis with mycological analysis of scalp scales/hairs. Systemic treatment is needed to clear infection as creams don't penetrate hairs.

Pityriasis (tinea) versicolor: Chronic, often asymptomatic, fungal infection of the skin (*Pityrosporum orbiculare*). Common in humid/tropical conditions. In the UK often affects teenagers.

Presentation: On untanned white skin appears as pinkish-brown, oval or round patches with a fine superficial scale. In tanned or darker skin patchy hypopigmentation occurs. Involves trunk ± proximal limbs.

Differential diagnosis: Vitiligo; pityriasis rosea; tinea corporis

Management: Treat with a topical imidazole antifungal (e.g. clotrimazole cream) *or* topical selenium sulphide shampoo to all affected areas at night, washed off the following morning (repeated ×2 at weekly intervals). Recurrences are common and hypopigmentation may take some time to clear.

Figure 8.11 **Ringworm**

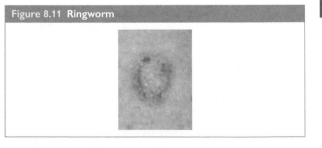

Infestations

Scabies: The scabies mite (*Sarcoptes scabei*) is ~½ mm long and spread by direct physical contact. Average infection consists of 12 mites. Symptoms appear 4–6 wk. after infection.

Presentation: Intense itching. Examination reveals burrows (irregular, tortuous and slightly scaly <1cm long). In young children tends to affect head, neck, palms and soles. Itching results in excoriations. Untreated infection becomes chronic.

Differential diagnosis: Dermatitis herpetiformis; papular urticaria; eczema

Management: Treat with scabicide e.g. permethrin 5% cream. Apply to the whole body except head and neck including scalp, neck, face and ears. Make sure finger/toe webs are covered and brush lotion under the ends of finger/toe nails. Reapply after 1wk. All close contacts need treatment. Advise parents to launder all worn clothing and bedding after application. Itching may persist for some time after elimination of infection – use oral antihistamines for symptomatic relief.

Complications: 2° infection (treat with topical or systemic antibiotics).

Headlice: Most common in children age 4–11y. (♀>♂) but may occur in anyone. Contrary to popular belief lice infest clean as often as dirty hair. Adult lice are about the size of a sesame seed, brownish grey in colour and wiggle their legs – Figure 8.12. Only adults are contagious. *Spread:* Only by close head to head contact. Lice don't jump/fly and don't stay viable away from a host.

Symptoms/signs: Normally asymptomatic. Detected by contact tracing of other cases or routine inspection at home or school. Occasionally presents as itchy scalp. Presence of 'nits' (egg shells – white dots attached to hair), eggs or dead lice indicate past infection – a moving louse must be found to confirm active infection.

Detection: After washing hair, apply conditioner and comb with a fine-tooth detector comb (available from pharmacy). In at-risk groups e.g. schoolchildren repeat weekly. Lice are removed by the comb and seen trapped in its teeth.

Management:
• *Prophylactic preparations* – no evidence of effectiveness.

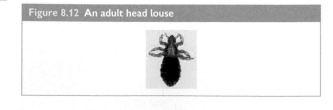

Figure 8.12 An adult head louse

- *Insecticides* – effective. 3 types (no evidence which performs best): malathion, phenothrin and permethrin are available OTC but are expensive and NHS prescriptions are often sought. Carbaryl is available on prescription only. Malathion and phenothrin/permethrin are used as 1st and 2nd line; carbaryl reserved for 3rd line. Apply according to manufacturer's instructions asking patients to use 2 applications, 7d. apart. 2–3d. after the final application check hair with detector comb to ensure lice have cleared. Supply enough for 2 applications. Shampoos are not effective – use lotions, liquids or cream rinses.
- *Mechanical clearance* – wet-comb conditioned hair with a fine-tooth comb until all lice are removed and repeat at 3–4d intervals for 2wk. Alternative to insecticides but requires motivation.
- *Other methods of treatment* – electric combs, aromatherapy (tea tree oil), herbal treatments. No evidence supporting use.
- *Contact tracing* – all cases. Trace those in close contact over the previous month.

Reinfestation/resistance to treatment: If lice have not cleared there are 3 possible reasons:
- *Reinfestation* – lice found are large adults only. Ask patient to check close contacts again. Re-treat with a different insecticide
- *Incorrect use of insecticide/mechanical clearance* – lice at mixed stages of development will be seen. Check procedure with the patient and make sure instructions are understood. Repeat treatment with a different insecticide
- *Resistance to insecticide* – lice are seen at all stages of development. Re-treat with another product.

Threadworms: Common in the UK, especially amongst children. *Enterobius vermicularis* causes anal itch as it leaves the bowel to lay eggs on the perineum. Often seen as silvery thread-like worms at the anus of children. *Treatment*: Mebendazole (child >2y.–100mg as a single dose – available OTC). Treat household contacts as well as the index case.

GP Notes: Scabies

- Itching in several family members at the same time suggests scabies.
- Use aqueous preparations as alcoholic ones sting.
- Some children live in 2 households – treat ALL close contacts.
- Treatment failure can occur when children suck their fingers.

Advice for patients: Information about threadworms

Threadworms live in the gut and lay their eggs on the skin around the bottom. This causes itching. These eggs can easily be picked up under fingernails and transferred to the mouth, causing reinfection.

To break this cycle, as well as medication for the whole family, it is important to make sure:
- Hands are washed (including scrubbing nails) after visiting the toilet and before meals
- Nails are cut short
- Your child has a morning bath to wash off eggs laid during the night
- Wash bedding/nightclothes after treatment.

Other skin diseases affecting children

Inherited skin disease:

- *Epidermolysis bullosa:* A group of genetically inherited diseases characterized by blistering on minimal trauma. Range from being mild and trivial to being incompatible with life. Commonest type is *simple epidermolysis bullosa* (autosomal dominant) – blistering is caused by friction, is mild and limited to hands and feet. Patients are advised to avoid trauma.

- *Albinism:* Rare genetic syndrome (autosomal recessive – prevalence 1:20,000) in which the melanocytes are unable to produce skin, hair or eye pigment. Patients have white hair, pale skin, pink eyes, poor sight, photophobia and nystagmus. Several different varieties exist. *Management:* Strict sun avoidance, sunglasses, sunscreens. Refer any skin lesions for biopsy (↑ risk squamous cell carcinoma).

- *Ichthyosis:* A group of inherited disorders characterized by dry, scaly skin. Vary from mild to severe. Commonest form is *ichthyosis vulgaris* – prevalence 1:300; autosomal dominant; small branny scales on extensor aspects of limbs and back – mild and often undiagnosed. *Management:* Topical emollients ± bath additives. Severe cases require expert dermatology advice.

- *Keratoderma:* Hyperkeratosis of palms and soles – may be inherited or acquired. *Tylosis* is diffuse hyperkeratosis of the palms and soles. It is usually inherited (autosomal dominant). *Management:* Keratolytics e.g. 5–10% salicylic acid ointment or 10% urea cream.

- *Keratosis pilaris:* Common, sometimes inherited condition. Small horny plugs are found on upper thigh, upper arm and face. Associated with icthyosis vulgaris. Keratolytics e.g. Lassar's paste or 10% urea cream improve symptoms.

Vitiligo:

- Affects 1% of the population. ♂=♀. *Peak age of onset:* 10–30y.
- *Cause:* Autoimmune; 30% have a family history. *Associations:* Pernicious anaemia, Addison's and thyroid disease.
- *Presentation:* May be precipitated by injury or sunburn. Presents as sharply defined white macules which contain no melanocytes. Often symmetrical distribution. *Commonest sites:* Hands, wrists, knees, neck, face around eyes and mouth.
- *Management:* Prognosis is variable – some develop a few lesions which remain static, some progress to larger depigmented areas, some even repigment. There is no cure. Advise use of sunscreens for affected areas (ACBS prescription); camouflage cosmetics (refer to Red Cross for advice on application, ACBS prescription). In severe cases refer for dermatology opinion – high-dose steroids or PUVA may help.

Alopecia areata: Chronic inflammatory disease affecting the hair follicles ± nails (~10%). Presents as patches of hair loss usually on the scalp but can affect any hair-bearing skin. 20% have a family history. Investigation is usually unnecessary. Treatment depends on severity of hair loss. Mild cases – reassure and monitor hair loss; more severe cases – refer to dermatology.

Milia: Small white raised spots (1–2mm diameter) usually on the face (upper cheeks and eyelids). Commonest in children but can occur at any age. *Management:* No treatment required.

Figure 8.13 Vitiligo on the forearms

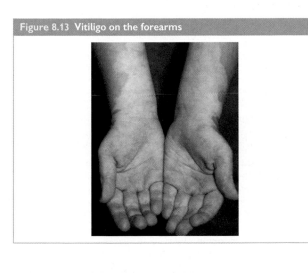

Figure 8.14 Milia on the lower eyelid

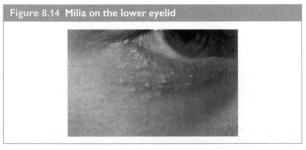

Advice for patients: Information and support for patients and families of children with ichthyosis

Ichthyosis Support Group 🖳 www.ichthyosis.co.uk

Figure 8.13 permission sought from 🖳 www.dermis.net

Pityriasis rosea:

- Acute self-limiting disorder of unknown cause most commonly affecting teenagers.
- Generalized eruption is preceded by the herald patch – a single or a couple of large, oval lesion(s) 2–5cm diameter – Figure 8.15.
- Several days later the rash appears consisting of many smaller lesions mainly on trunk but also upper arms and thighs.
- Lesions are oval, pink and have a delicate "collarette" of scale. May be asymptomatic or cause mild → moderate itch.

Differential diagnosis: Guttate psoriasis; pityriasis versicolor

Management: Treatment does not speed clearance. Topical steroid may relieve itch. Fades spontaneously in 4–8wk.

Pityriasis alba: Finely scaled white patches on face or arms. Affects children predominantly. Associated with atopy.

Management: Usually no treatment is required. Resolves spontaneously over months or years. If severe refer to dermatology for confirmation of diagnosis. Treatment for severe cases is with topical steroids and/or PUVA.

Erythema multiforme: Figure 8.16. Immune mediated disease characterized by target lesions on hands and feet. Causes:

- *Idiopathic* (50%)
- *Infective* – streptococcal, HSV, hepatitis B, mycoplasma
- *Drugs* – penicillin, barbiturates
- *Other* – SLE, malignancy.

Presentation: Target lesions (red rings with central pale or purple area) on hands and feet. New lesions appear for 2–3wk. Frequently oral, conjunctival and genital mucosa is affected – if severe termed Stevens-Johnson syndrome.

Management: Identification and removal of the underlying cause. Mild cases resolve spontaneously and require symptomatic measures only. Admit if extensive involvement.

Erythema nodosum: Figure 8.17. Tender erythematous nodules (1–5cm diameter) on extensor surfaces of limbs (especially shins) ± ankle and wrist arthritis ± fever. ♀:♂≈3:1. Resolves in <8wk., non-scarring. No treatment needed.

Associations: 20% of cases are idiopathic with no associations.

- Acute sarcoidosis
- Drugs e.g. oral contraceptives
- Inflammatory bowel disease—UC, Crohn's
- Malignancy
- TB
- Streptococcal infection

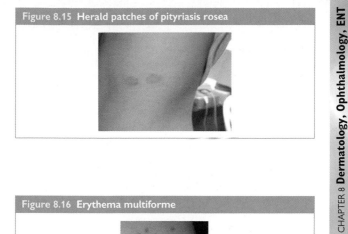

Figure 8.15 Herald patches of pityriasis rosea

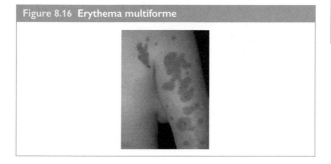

Figure 8.16 Erythema multiforme

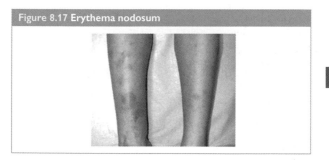

Figure 8.17 Erythema nodosum

Congenital ENT and eye problems

Accessory auricle: *Incidence:* 1.5:100 live births. Small skin lesions consisting of skin or skin and cartilage are present in front of the ear. No treatment is necessary but accessory auricles are often removed for cosmetic reasons.

Bat ears: Common congenital abnormality in which a fold of the pinna is absent. The child is noted to have protruding ears. Runs in families. Referral for surgery is indicated if the condition is causing psychosocial problems.

Congenital deafness: *Causes:*

- Genetic (50%)
- Intrauterine infection e.g. rubella
- Drugs given to the mother in pregnancy e.g. streptomycin
- Birth asphyxia
- Meningitis
- Severe neonatal jaundice

Presentation:

- Neonatal screening is now available to all babies born in the UK. December 2005 - 📖 p.22.
- Otherwise diagnosis is made when a parent notices abnormal responses from the child, during routine child health surveillance or when speech fails to develop.

Management: 📖 p.282

Cleft lip and palate: *Incidence:* 1:600 live births – ½ have other abnormalities too (e.g. hypoplastic mandible). Due to failure of fusion of the processes contributing to facial development (Figure 8.18). Often, though not always, detected at routine antenatal USS. The cleft may be unilateral or bilateral and involve lip and/or palate. Cleft lips are usually repaired in the 1st few days of life; cleft palates at ~3mo. depending on the weight of the baby.

Problems associated with cleft lip and/or palate:

- Feeding difficulties with associated poor weight gain.
- Aspiration pneumonia.
- Hearing problems, particularly glue ear. In some areas children with cleft palate are routinely given grommets at ~18mo. Treat otitis media promptly. Audiology review is important.
- Speech problems – refer for speech therapy.
- Dental problems – universal with cleft palate. Orthodontic treatment is always required.

Congenital squint: 📖 p.20

Microphthalmos: 1:1000 live births. Small eyes. Associated with Down's syndrome and other genetic abnormalities.

Cataract in children: Presents with squint, white pupil, nystagmus or loss of binocular vision. Examination reveals a shadow in the red reflex/absent red reflex with difficulty visualizing the fundus. May be hereditary or associated with Down's syndrome, galactossaemia or congenital rubella. In all cases refer urgently to ophthalmology.

Congenital glaucoma: 1:10,000 live births. ♂>♀. Usually bilateral. Presents with irritation of the eye (watering, rubbing), photophobia, large eyes with large, fixed pupils ± cloudy cornea. Refer urgently for paediatric ophthalmic opinion. Surgery is needed to prevent blindness.

Congenital ptosis: Ptosis describes drooping of the upper eyelid. Unilateral/bilateral weakness of the levator muscle is present from birth. Children may compensate by tilting their heads upwards to see better. ~½ have associated superior rectus muscle weakness. Refer for surgical correction if obstructing vision as may cause amblyopia if left untreated.

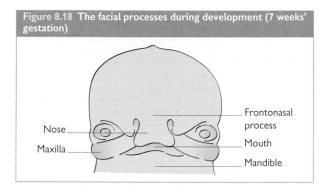

Figure 8.18 The facial processes during development (7 weeks' gestation)

Nose
Maxilla
Frontonasal process
Mouth
Mandible

Advice for patients: Information and support for parents

Cleft Lip and Palate Association (CLAPA) ☎ 020 7833 4883
🖳 www.clapa.com
Eye Care Trust Information on anophthalmia and microphthalmia
☎ 0845 129 5001 🖳 www.eye-care.org.uk
Micro- and Anophthalmic Children's Society (MACS)
☎ 0800 169 8088 🖳 www.macs.org.uk

Blindness and refractive errors

Screening for visual abnormalities: 📖 p.20

Blindness: Is defined as inability to perform any work for which eyesight is essential (not the total absence of sight). In practice this means <3/60 vision (may be >3/60 if patient has severe visual field defect e.g. glaucoma). Partial-sightedness does not have a standard definition but usually implies vision in the range 3/60–6/60. Blindness is rare amongst children in developed countries (prevalence ~3:10,000), but much more common in less affluent countries.

Causes of blindness in infants and children: Congenital infection e.g. rubella; congenital ocular or cerebral abnormality e.g. cataract, glaucoma; retinopathy of prematurity; trauma; retinoblastoma; acquired infection e.g. ophthalmia neonatorum (if untreated), onchocerciasis (in Africa); vitamin A deficiency (poorer countries).

Registration of blindness and partial sight: Voluntary in England. Refer patients with low vision for assessment. Application is made by a consultant ophthalmologist to social services. Registration makes a child eligible for additional benefits e.g. disability living allowance, assessment of special educational needs, training in Braille, disabled parking badge, ↓TV licence fee, some travel concessions, access to talking books and large-print libraries, special visual aids.

Support: Many patients benefit from links with national support organizations who provide information, and active local organizations who support the blind and partially sighted with drivers and guides.

Congenital colour blindness: Inherited as a sex-linked characteristic (♂:♀≈20:1). Patients may request to be tested. This is done using a standard set of cards (Ishihara test). Each card consists of a number in coloured dots against a contrasting background of more coloured dots. Coloured dots are paired to detect different patterns of colour blindness. Lack of red/green discrimination is most common. Colour blindness prohibits certain types of employment (e.g. airline pilot, train driver).

Amblyopia (lazy eye): Squint, ptosis, cataract, unequal refractive errors or astigmatism can cause the image from one eye to be disregarded. This neglect leads to amblyopia (poor vision in the absence of a visual disorder). Treatment is with glasses ± patching, and squint surgery if necessary. Becomes irreversible if persists to >7–8y. of age.

Refractive errors:

Hypermetropia (long sight): Most common refractive error. Close objects are out of focus. Common in infants and ↓ with age. Often associated with convergent squint. Other symptoms include eye tiredness and headache. Convex (magnifying '+') lenses are used for correction.

Myopia (short sight): Close objects can be focused on the retina but distant objects are out of focus. Uncommon <6y. and worsens to mid-teens. Often +ve family history. Concave lenses (minifying) and/or contact lenses are used to correct the defect.

Astigmatism: The degree of curvature across the cornea or lens differs in the vertical and horizontal planes. Thus objects are distorted longitudinally or vertically. Lenses can be used to correct this defect.

Retinitis pigmentosa: Familial disorder causing retinal degeneration.
- *Symptoms:* Night blindness, loss of visual field, difficulty in light adaptation, gradual loss of central vision.
- *Signs:* Black pigment flecks in the retina, optic atrophy, attenuated blood vessels.
Usually first noticed in adolescence and progresses to blindness.

Retinoblastoma: Rare tumour of the eye. 30 cases/y. in England and Wales. Usually affects children <1y. old – most are <5y. old. May be familial (6% – dominant inheritance) when the tumour is usually bilateral. Sporadic tumours are usually unilateral.

Presentation:
- Usually detected by a white pupillary reflex found at routine developmental screening.
- Alternatively may present with squint or inflammation of the eye.

Management: Refer any suspected cases for urgent ophthalmology opinion. Treatment of unilateral tumours is surgical. Bilateral tumours are treated by enucleation or laser ablation of the worst affected eye and radiotherapy to the other eye.

Prognosis: 80% patients with unilateral tumours survive long term. Bilateral tumours have a poorer prognosis with 40% surviving long term.

NICE guidance on referral for suspected retinoblastoma[N]:
Refer urgently children with:
- A white pupillary reflex (leukocoria). Pay attention to parents reporting an odd appearance in their child's eye
- A new squint or change in visual acuity if cancer is suspected. (Refer non-urgently if cancer is not suspected)
- A family history of retinoblastoma and visual problems. (Screening should be offered soon after birth)

Advice for patients: Information and support for patients and their carers

Royal National Institute for the Blind Information and talking book service ☎ 0845 766 9999 🖳 www.rnib.org.uk
LOOK (for families of blind/visually impaired children) ☎ 0121 428 5038
British Retinitis Pigmentosa Society ☎ 0845 123 2354 🖳 www.brps.org.uk
Childhood Eye Cancer Trust (CHECT) ☎ 0121 708 0583 🖳 www.chect.org.uk

Further information
NICE Referral guidelines for suspected cancer – quick reference guide (2005) 🖳 www.nice.org.uk

The red or swollen eye

> **⚠ Signs of a potentially dangerous red eye:**
> - ↓ visual acuity
> - Pain deep in the eye (not surface irritation as with conjunctivitis)
> - Absent or sluggish pupil response
> - Corneal damage on fluorescein staining
> - History of trauma
>
> Get the patient seen by a specialist the same day if in doubt – particularly post-op.

Conjunctivitis: Inflammation of the conjunctiva is the commonest eye problem seen in general practice – 1:8 children have an episode of acute infective conjunctivitis every year.

Presentation:
- Red, sore eye
- Eye discharge – clear, mucoid or muco-purulent
- Sticking of the eyelids – especially on waking
- No change in visual acuity

Examination may reveal enlarged papillae ('cobblestones' – associated with allergic conjunctivitis) under the upper eyelid and/or pre-auricular lymph node enlargement.

Infective conjunctivitis: Clinically difficult to distinguish viral and bacterial causes – doctors get it right only ~50% of the time. Both may occur in association with viral URTI.

Management:
- Recent evidence shows that in ~85% of cases, acute infective conjunctivitis clears in <7d. with or without treatment.[1]
- Advise patients to bathe the affected eye(s) with boiled, cooled water morning and night.
- If symptoms are not improving in >5d., take a swab for M,C&S (± chlamydia if neonate) and treat empirically with chloramphenicol qds or fucithalmic bd for 5d.
- If still not clearing, then act on swab results or consider alternative diagnosis e.g. allergy. If chlamydia is confirmed on swab result, seek urgent specialist advice.

⚠ Advise patients to see a doctor if: ↓ visual acuity, eye becomes painful rather than sore/gritty, or symptoms are not improving in 5d.

❶ Chloramphenicol eye drops are available over the counter.

Ophthalmia neonatorum: Caused by *N. gonorrhoea.* Presents as a purulent discharge from the eyes of an infant <21d. old. Send swabs for M,C&S. Treat with hourly ofloxacin eye drops. Refer for urgent ophthalmology opinion as cornea may perforate.

---

1 *Lancet* Rose PW et al Chloramphenicol treatment for acute infective conjunctivitis in children in primary care: a randomised double-blind placebo-controlled trial (2005) 366(9479) pp.6–7

Allergic conjunctivitis: Bilateral symptoms appear seasonally (e.g. hay fever) or on contact with an allergen (e.g. animal fur). Presents with red, watery, itchy eyes ± photophobia ± family/personal history of atopy.

Management: Treat with topical or systemic antihistamines (e.g. sodium cromoglycate eye drops qds). Avoid topical steroids due to long-term complications (cataract, glaucoma, fungal infection). Consider cold compress and washout with cold water during acute exacerbations. Refer if symptoms are persistent despite treatment, or if vision is affected.

Infantile dacryocystitis ('blocked tear duct'): Delay in canalization/obstruction of the lacrimal duct → persistent watering or sticky eyes in 20% babies. Vision is normal and there is no conjunctival inflammation. If the lower lid conjunctiva is reddened, swab to exclude chlamydia (special swab needed).

Management: Advise parents to bathe the lids with cooled boiled water. Avoid antibiotic eye drops unless there is clear infection. Spontaneous resolution is the norm. 4% fail to clear by 1y. – refer to a paediatric ophthalmologist. Treatment is by probing the duct to clear it.

Acute dacryocystitis: Acute infection of the tear sac, can spread to surrounding tissues. Treat immediately with antibiotics e.g. flucloxacillin. Abscess can form – if it does surgical drainage is required, so refer.

Subconjunctival haemorrhage: Spontaneous painless localized haemorrhage (Figure 8.19). May occur in coughing bouts of pertusis. Looks alarming but clears spontaneously in 1–2wk. Consider referral if it follows trauma, especially if the posterior edge of the haemorrhage can't be seen (may be associated with orbital haematoma, penetrating injury or orbital fracture).

Figure 8.19 Subconjunctival haemorrhage: a lesion of uniform colour, with slight conjunctival elevation, limited by the cornea

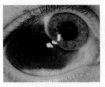

271

Advice for patients: Information

Eye Care Trust: Patient information on conjunctivitis and tear duct disorders ▣ www.eye-care.org.uk
Good Hope NHS Hospital Trust: Patient information on blocked lacrimal duct in children ▣ www.goodhope.org.uk/departments/eyedept
BBC pollen index ▣ www.bbc.co.uk/weather/pollen
Allergy UK ☎ 01322 619898 ▣ www.allergyuk.org

Figure 8.19 permission sought from Dunn & Rawlinson *Surgical diagnosis and management* Blackwell Scientific Publishing ISBN: 0632011653.

Watering eyes (epiphoria): Due to overproduction of tears or outflow obstruction. Caused by emotion, corneal irritation (e.g. blepharitis, corneal abrasion, foreign body, conjunctivitis, entropion), iritis, acute glaucoma, ectropion, blocked tear duct.

Swelling around the eyes: Oedema around the eyes gives the face a bloated appearance. Swollen eyelids may partially close the eyes. In severe cases the whole face becomes oedematous. It is associated with nephrotic syndrome, allergic reactions (e.g. pollen, dust or insect bites), angioneurotic oedema and periorbital cellulitis (below).

Orbital inflammation:

Preseptal cellulitis: Infections of the upper lid may cause significant swelling and redness around the eye. Typically affects children following mild trauma. The eye is unaffected – infection is localized to skin and superficial tissues. Treat as localized cellulitis with oral antibiotics (e.g. flucloxacillin). Monitor carefully as can progress to orbital cellulitis.

Orbital cellulitis: Typically due to spread of infection from the paranasal sinuses. Usually presents with pain, double/blurred vision and general malaise. *Signs:* Fever, eyelid swelling, proptosis and inability to move the eye. Severe cases can lead to septicaemia, meningitis and cavernous sinus thromboses. If suspected, refer immediately to ophthalmology for IV antibiotics/surgical drainage.

Ophthalmic shingles: Zoster (📖 p.92) in the ophthalmic branch of the oculomotor (IIIrd) nerve. Pain, tingling or numbness around the eye precedes a blistering rash and inflammation. In 50% the eye is affected with conjunctivitis, scleritis, episcleritis, keratitis, iritis, visual loss and/or oculmotor nerve palsy. Nose tip involvement makes eye involvement likely (nerve supply is the same as the globe). Refer as an emergency to ophthalmology.

Iritis (anterior uveitis): Acute-onset pain, photophobia, blurred vision, watering, circumcorneal redness, small or irregular pupil ± hypopyon (anterior chamber pus). Pain ↑ as eyes converge and pupils constrict. Associated with arthritis. Refer urgently. Steroid drops ↓ inflammation and mydriatics dilate the pupil and prevent adhesions.

Stye: Common eyelid infection. 2 forms:

Internal stye (hordeolum internum): Abscess of a meibomiam gland. Often causes less swelling than external stye. May point inwards onto the conjunctiva (seen as red patch with yellow centre before it bursts) or outwards through the skin. Treat with hot compresses and topical antibiotics (e.g. chloramphenicol ointment qds).

Chalazion/meibomiam cyst: Following an internal stye, the meibomiam gland may become blocked forming a cyst. Cysts may resolve spontaneously but often become infected (treat with topical antibiotics) and/or chronic. If recurrent infection or chronic cyst refer to ophthalmology for incision and curettage. ❶ Refer early if <7y. as large cysts can affect refraction and generate amblyopia.

External stye (hordeolum externum): Most common form of stye. Due to infection of a lash follicle, or associated sweat or sebum gland. Confined to the skin and always points outwards. Treat with hot compresses and topical antibiotics (e.g. chloramphenicol ointment qds).

Marginal cyst: Non-infected swellings of the glands of Zeis/Moll. No treatment needed unless troublesome, when refer.

Blepharitis: Chronic, low-grade inflammation of meibomian glands and lid margins. Presents with long history of irritable, burning, dry, red eyes. Eyelids have red margins ± scales on the eyelashes – on elevation of the upper lid, look for inflamed meibomian glands.

Management: Prolonged treatment is often needed:
- Removal of scales and crusts from the lid margins (see below)
- Exacerbations – treat with fucithalmic ointment rubbed into the lid margins. Steroid ointment may occasionally be useful (only use on specialist advice and for ≤2wk.). Systemic tetracycline may be necessary in severe cases.

Advice for patients: Blepharitis eye care instructions

- Place a warm, moist face flannel over the eyes for 10–20 minutes morning and night.
- Afterwards, mix a solution of half baby shampoo and half warm water in the cap from a bottle of the baby shampoo. Put the solution on a wet wash cloth or cotton wool bud, and gently scrub from side to side on the upper eyelids and lashes for 15–20 seconds.
- Pull the lower lid down and away from the eyeball and gently scrub side to side along the edge of the lower eyelid and lashes for 15–20 seconds. Avoid scrubbing the eyeball.
- Rinse the cloth and clean any remaining shampoo from the lids with clear, warm water.
- When instructed, place a 1cm strip of fucithalmic ointment under the lower lids at bedtime and rub the excess onto the lid edges.
- If you have a problem with dandruff of the scalp and eyebrows, shampooing frequently with a shampoo containing selenium sulphide or pyrithione zinc (such as Head & Shoulders) will be helpful.
- Continue this treatment for 2–3 months or until the problem is controlled. After an initial treatment period, it will probably be necessary to continue to use lid scrubs from time to time to keep the lid scales under control.

Alternatives to baby shampoo include bicarbonate of soda solution or sterile, impregnated Lid-Care® wipes.

Information for patients
Eye Care Trust Patient information on blepharitis and eyelid disorders ☎ 0845 129 5001 ⌨ www.eye-care.org.uk
Good Hope NHS Hospital Trust Patient information on blepharitis and watery eyes ⌨ www.goodhope.org.uk/departments/eyedept

Sore throat and stridor

Sore throat: Each GP sees ≈120 patients with sore throat every year – mostly children and young adults. 70% sore throats are viral in origin, the rest bacterial (mostly Group A β-haemolytic streptococci). Viral and bacterial infections are indistinguishable clinically but association with coryza, and cough, may point to a viral aetiology

Clinical picture: Pain on swallowing; fever; headache; tonsillar exudates (Figure 8.20); nausea and vomiting; abdominal pain – especially children due to abdominal lymphadenopathy

Differential diagnosis: Glandular fever, especially in teenagers with persistent sore throat.

Investigation: Not usually undertaken.
- Throat swabs cannot distinguish commensal organisms (40% carry Group A β-haemolytic streptococci) from clinical infection, are expensive and do not give instant results so are rarely used.
- Rapid antigen tests give immediate results but have low sensitivity, limiting usefulness.

Management: 90% patients recover within 1 week without treatment. Complications are rare. Advise analgesia and antipyretics (e.g. paracetamol and/or ibuprofen), ↑ fluid intake and salt-water gargles.

Use of antibiotics: Antibiotic prescription can probably be avoided in most patients but educating patients about the reasons for not prescribing is vital to maintain a good doctor–patient relationship.
- *Benefits of taking antibiotics:* Modest benefit in symptom relief (8h. less symptoms); may confer slight protection against some complications (e.g. quinsy and otitis media). ❶ There is no evidence antibiotics protect against rheumatic fever or acute glomerulonephritis.
- *Risks of taking antibiotics:* Possibility of side effects with antibiotic use; ↑ in community antibiotic resistance; 'medicalizing' a self-limiting condition – prescribing ↑ faith in antibiotics and encourages re-attendance with future sore throats.

Before prescribing, weigh risks against benefits. If you decide to prescribe antibiotics, use penicillin V or erythromycin qds for 5–10d. Avoid amoxicillin as this causes a rash in those with glandular fever. An alternative strategy is to issue a 'delayed prescription' – for patients to collect if no better in 2–3d. (70% don't collect the script).

Complications of sore throat: All rare:
- *Quinsy (peritonsillar abscess):* Usually occurs in adults. *Signs:* Unilateral peritonsillar swelling, difficulty swallowing (even saliva) and trismus (difficulty opening jaw). Refer for IV antibiotics ± incision and drainage.
- *Retropharyngeal abscess:* Occurs in children. *Signs:* Inability to swallow, fever. Refer for IV antibiotics ± incision and drainage.
- *Rheumatic fever*
- *Glomerulonephritis*

Figure 8.20 Acute tonsillitis

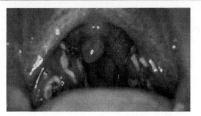

GP Notes: Indications for referral to ENT for tonsillectomy

- *Recurrent acute tonsillitis:* Young children have a lot of throat infections and most will 'grow out' of the problem without the need for surgery. Tonsillectomy is only considered if children miss a lot of school: e.g. >5 attacks causing school absence/y. for 2y.
- *Airway obstruction:* Very large tonsils causing sleep apnoea
- *Chronic tonsillitis:* >3mo. + halitosis
- *Recurrent quinsy*
- *Recurrent guttate psoriasis following tonsillitis*

⚠ Tonsillectomy carries a small risk of severe haemorrhage. Readmit any patient with bleeding post-op for observation.

Advice for patients: (or parents of children) with sore throat

- Sore throat is common and may be caused by viruses or bacteria. Both usually get better without antibiotics.
- You may have other symptoms as well such as cough, fever, tiredness, headache, pain on swallowing and/or swollen glands in your neck.
- Drink plenty of fluids.
- Take paracetamol and/or ibuprofen – taking regular doses works better than just taking doses when you feel you need them.
- Gargles can sometimes sooth the discomfort as well.
- Most sore throats get worse for a few days and then improve and are better within a week.

Further information

Patient UK Information leaflets on sore throat. UTRI, laryngitis, tonsillitis, tonsils and adenoids, and glandular fever 🖥 www.patient.co.uk
ENT UK Patient information on sore throat and tonsillectomy 🖥 www.entuk.org

Further information

SIGN Management of sore throat and indications for tonsillectomy (1999) 🖥 www.sign.ac.uk

Stridor: Noise created on inspiration due to narrowing of the larynx or trachea. Much more common amongst children than adults.

> **⚠ Signs of severe airway narrowing:**
> - Distress
> - ↑ respiratory rate
> - Pallor and cyanosis
> - Use of accessory muscles and tracheal tug

Causes: Congenital abnormalities of the larynx; epiglottis; croup (laryngotracheobronchitis); inhaled foreign body; trauma; laryngeal paralysis

Acute epiglottitis: Bacterial infection causing a swollen epiglottis. Much rarer since introduction of routine Hib immunization.

Presentation: Look for stridor, drooling, fever, upright leaning forward posture. ⚠ If suspected DON'T examine the child's throat as this can precipitate complete obstruction of the airway.

Management: Refer as an emergency but try to maintain a calm atmosphere to avoid distressing the child. *Treatment:* IV antibiotics.

Laryngomalacia (congenital laryngeal stridor): Common amongst small babies. Due to floppy aryatic folds and the small size of the airway in young children. Stridor becomes more noticeable during sleep, excitement, crying and with concurrent URTIs. Normally resolves without treatment but parental concern may necessitate referral.

Subglottic stenosis: Can occur as complicaton of prolonged ventilation and has a similar presentation to laryngomalacia.

Inhaled foreign body: Refer to ENT for assessment.

Laryngitis: Hoarseness, malaise ± fever and/or pain on using voice. Usually viral and self-limiting (1–2wk.) but occasionally 2° bacterial infection occurs. Advise OTC analgesia e.g. paracetamol and/or ibuprofen, try steam inhalations. Consider antibiotics if bacterial infection is suspected e.g. penicillin for 1wk.

Croup (laryngotracheobronchitis): Viral infection occurring in epidemics in autumn and spring.
- Starts with mild fever and runny nose.
- In younger children (<4y.), oedema and secretions in the larynx and trachea cause a barking cough and inspiratory stridor. The cough typically starts at night and is exacerbated by crying and parental anxiety.
- Some children have recurrent attacks associated with viral URTI.

Management: Steam helps (though beware of scalding children). Nebulized steroids or oral dexamethasone can be helpful but most GPs don't carry them. Admit as a paediatric emergency if there is intercostal recession, cyanosis or parents/carers are unable to cope. A significant number of children end up being admitted to hospital for observation – often only for 24h.

🔵 Suspect asthma if a child has recurrent bouts of croup.

Glandular fever (infectious mononucleosis): Consider in teenagers or young adults presenting with sore throat lasting >1wk. Caused by Epstein-Barr virus (EBV). Spread by droplet infection and direct contact ('kissing disease') and has a 4–14d. incubation period.

Symptoms/signs: Sore throat malaise fatigue lymphadenopathy enlarged spleen palatal petechiae rash (10–20%)

Investigation: Send blood for FBC (atypical lymphocytes) and glandular fever antibodies (Monospot or Paul-Bunnell).

Management: Advise rest, fluids and regular paracetamol; try salt-water gargles; consider a short course of prednisolone for severe symptoms; treat 2° infection with antibiotics; counsel re the possibility of prolonged symptoms (up to several months).

⚠ DON'T prescribe amoxicillin as it causes a severe rash.

Complications: 2° infections; rash with amoxicillin; hepatitis; jaundice; pneumonitis; neurological disturbances (rare)

Sleep apnoea in children: Common aged 2–7y. in association with tonsil enlargement during URTI. Sleep disruption can cause daytime sleepiness, hyperactivity, poor attention span and bad behaviour. If tonsils and/or adenoids are big enough to produce sleep apnoea in the absence of current infection, refer to ENT for consideration of tonsillectomy.

Advice for carers of children with croup

- Croup can be very frightening for both you and your child.
- Symptoms may worsen for up to 3 days and then improve over the next week. Young children often become worse late at night.
- *Stay calm.* Reassure your child. Showing anxiety can frighten your child and cause him or her to become upset and cry – which in turn can make breathing more difficult.
- *Sit your child upright.*
- *Keep your child cool.* Remove your child's clothes and give paracetamol and/or ibuprofen.
- *Try a steamy environment* e.g. sit in the bathroom with the door and window closed and the hot tap running (but keep your child away from the hot water). Alternatively try taking your child outside into the fresh air.

Call a doctor/NHS Direct for advice if:
- Your child is struggling for breath – difficulty rather than noise is what is important
- Your child's breathing becomes more rapid
- Your child becomes very restless
- Your child is drooling or unable to swallow
- Your child's colour changes from pink to being very pale or tinged blue

---

Further information and support for parents
Patient UK Information leaflet on croup 🖳 www.patient.co.uk

Nasal problems

Nasal obstruction: Common symptom in children. Usually obstruction is bilateral – think of a foreign body in the nose if unilateral.

Causes of nasal obstruction:
- *Mucosal swelling:* Coryza, rhinitis (📖 p.280), nasal polyps (rare).
- *Septal deviation:* Usually congenital in children e.g. 2° to cleft lip.
- *Other:* Enlarged adenoids (associated with glue ear and deafness), foreign body (📖 p.54).

Nose bleed/epistaxis: Common (9% of 11–14y. olds in one study). Usually from ruptured blood vessels on the nasal septum.

Causes: Nose picking, inflammation (coryza, allergic rhinitis), rarely blood dyscrasias.

Management: Most nose bleeds in children are managed at home – only the most serious present to the GP. Check if the child is taking NSAIDs or anticoagulants and ask about bleeding problems.

Most bleeds can be stopped by:
- Pinching the soft tip of the nose for ≥10min. (avoid looking to see if it has stopped during that time)
- If available, applying an ice pack to the bridge of the nose
- Leaning the child forward to prevent bleeding into the post-nasal space.

⚠ If shocked or bleeding can't be stopped after 30 min, refer to A&E.

🔔 For older children, if the bleeding is not settling and an anterior bleeding point is visualized, it is sometimes possible to cauterize the bleeding point with a silver nitrate stick after application of lidocaine on a piece of cotton wool. Prescribe antiseptic cream e.g. naseptin bd for 1wk. afterwards. DON'T attempt this with small or uncooperative children.

Recurrent nose bleeds: Treatment with antibiotic cream (e.g. naseptin bd for 1wk.) may help. Usually recurrent nose bleeds resolve with time. Consider referral to ENT if persistent/significant parental anxiety.

Acute sinusitis: Infection of ≥1 paranasal sinuses (maxillary, frontal, ethmoid or sphenoid). Usually follows viral URTI though 10% are due to tooth infection.

🔔 Maxillary sinuses pneumatize at ~2y. of age, frontal at 6y. and ethmoid and sphenoid later – sinusititis is not a cause of headache/facial pain in very young children.

Presentation: Frontal headache/facial pain (may be difficult to distinguish from toothache) – typically worse on movement/bending ± purulent nasal discharge ± fever. Often preceded by URTI.

Management: Most sinusitis resolves spontaneously in 7–10d. Treatment options:
- Advise analgesia (paracetamol ± ibuprofen) and fluids for all patients
- Steam inhalation may help

- Short courses of decongestants may help but there is very little evidence of effectiveness
- Steroid nasal sprays (e.g. beclometasone nasal spray, 2 puffs to each nostril bd) may help – evidence of effectiveness is limited
- Reserve antibiotics for patients with severe symptoms or symptoms persisting >7d. – there is limited evidence of benefit[C]. If prescribing, use amoxicillin tds or erythromycin qds for 7d.

Nasal polyps: Rare in children – if present, consider CF.

Symptoms: Nasal blockage; watery discharge; post-nasal drip; loss of smell and/or taste disturbance

Signs: Polyps are smooth and pale, usually bilateral and commonly arise from the middle meatus and middle turbinates. They may completely block the nasal passage.

Management: Steroid nasal sprays may ease symptoms. Refer to paediatrics/ENT for advice on further management.

Adenoidal hypertrophy: The adenoids ↑ in size after birth to reach their maximum size at age 3–7y. Adenoids can obstruct the nasopharyngeal airway.

Common symptoms:
- Nasal symptoms – blocked nose, nasal speech
- Ear symptoms – Eustacian tube dysfunction, glue ear and deafness
- Other symptoms – obstructive sleep apnoea

Management: Where possible adopt a 'wait and see' approach – adenoidal hypertrophy usually resolves with age as the nasopharynx grows and the adenoids regress. If severe symptoms (e.g. glue ear causing deafness, sleep apnoea), refer to ENT for adenoidectomy.

GP Notes: Advice for children with sinusitis

- Sinusitis is common. It is caused by inflammation of the air spaces inside the cheek bones or forehead. It often follows a cold.
- Common symptoms are pain in your face which may be worse on bending, a blocked or runny nose, headache, fever and feeling tired.
- Most cases are caused by a virus and settle without treatment. Antibiotics have no effect on viruses.
- Take paracetamol and/or ibuprofen to help ease the pain.
- Decongestants and inhaling steam may help. Do not use decongestants for longer than 7 days.
- Antibiotics are used for severe or prolonged cases of sinusitis.

Advice for patients: Information

ENT UK Information on sinusitis 🖥 www.entuk.org
Patient UK Information leaflet on sinusitis and nose bleeds
🖥 www.patient.co.uk

Further information
Cochrane: Williams J et al *Antibiotics for acute maxillary sinusitis* (2000)

Rhinitis

Allergic rhinitis: Common disorder. May be seasonal or perennial.
Symptoms: Bilateral intermittent nasal blockage; itchy nose, eyes, palate and throat; sneezing; watery nasal discharge

Signs: Swollen inferior turbinates; ↓ nasal airway; pale or mauve mucosa; nasal discharge; 'allergic crease' on bridge of nose from persistent rubbing (especially in children). Ask about potential allergens e.g. pollen, feathers, house dust mite, moulds and animals.

Investigation: If symptoms are intrusive and difficult to control, refer to allergy clinic for skin prick testing or RAST (radio-allergosorbent) testing. Blood tests for IgE may help identify allergens.

Management:
Allergen avoidance:
- *House dust mite:* Evidence that ↓ house dust mite results in clinical improvement is poor[C]. Advice for committed families – 📖 p.145.
- *Pets:* Removing pets from a home improves symptoms in some cases. If unable to give up the pet then keep it out of living areas and especially the bedroom. Advise regular vacuuming.

Inhalation of steam ± menthol may give some temporary relief from the discomfort of nasal blockage and can be repeated every 2h.

Medication: Table 8.6

Desensitization: Risk of anaphylaxis is high so, in the UK, provision is limited to specialist centres with full resuscitation facilities. Refer via an allergy clinic.

Hayfever: Rhinitis and/or conjunctivitis and/or wheeze due to an allergic reaction to pollen. Occurs at different times in the year depending on which pollen is involved (Table 8.7). In the UK, most hay fever is caused by grass pollen (60%) and silver birch pollen (25%).

Management: Treat with systemic antihistamine (e.g. loratadine, >6y. – 10mg od; 2–5y. – 5mg od) and/or topical steroid nasal spray e.g. beclometasone, 2 puffs bd to each nostril, and/or eye drops e.g. sodium cromoglycate, 1 drop to each eye qds. Start treatment 2–3wk. before the pollen season starts.

When the pollen count is high: Keep windows shut (including car windows – consider pollen filter for the car); wear sunglasses; avoid grassy spaces and mowing lawns.

Vasomotor rhinitis: May be difficult to distinguish from allergic rhinitis. Symptoms and signs are similar though vasomotor rhinitis is associated with less itching. Both are common and may coexist. Symptoms may be exacerbated by tobacco, change in air temperature and perfumes.

Management: Try measures used for allergic rhinitis as appropriate – often less successful. Short-term use of decongestant tablets e.g. pseudoephedrine may help.

Table 8.6 Drug treatment of allergic rhinitis: BNF 12.2.1 &12.2.2

Category	Example	Notes
Intranasal steroid sprays	Beclometasone 2 puffs bd to each nostril	Effective and can be used safely long term. Takes >1wk. to show benefit – try regular use for >2mo. before abandoning.
Topical anti-histamines	Azelastine 1 puff bd to each nostril (children >5y.)	Can be used as an alternative to topical steroids – faster acting (effect within 15min).
Topical decongestants	Ephedrine 1–2 drops to each nostril tds/qds prn	Short term (e.g. 5–7d.) for nasal blockage. Of dubious value. Longer-term use may cause a vicious circle – rhinitis medicamentosa: vasoconstriction → mucosal damage → rebound engorgement and oedema → more decongestant use.
Other nasal sprays	Sodium cromogly-cate 1 puff to each nostril bd/tds or qds	Less effective than topical steroids but can be useful, particularly in children, to give some relief.
Oral antihistamine	Loratidine >6y. 10mg od 2–5y. 5mg od	Can be helpful used alone or in addition to nasal preparations.
Oral steroids	Prednisolone 10–30mg od	May be used occasionally for short-term control of severe symptoms e.g. at exam times. A last option.

Table 8.7 Predominant pollen types

Jan	Feb	Mar	Apr	May	Jun	Jul	Aug	Sep	Oct	Nov	Dec
Alder Hazel		Elm Willow Ash	Silver birch	Oak	Weed pollen						
					Grass pollen			Fungal spores			

GP Notes: When should I refer?

- Children not responding to maximal management in general practice (refer to ENT or allergy clinic)
- Children on prolonged courses of intranasal steroids who have slow growth (refer to paediatrics)

Advice for patients: Information for patients and parents

BBC pollen index 🖳 www.bbc.co.uk/weather/pollen
Allergy UK ☎ 01322 619898 🖳 www.allergyuk.org
Patient UK Information on rhinitis and nose sprays
🖳 www.patient.co.uk

Further information

British Society for Allergy and Clinical Immunology (BSACI) Rhinitis management guidelines (2000) 🖳 www.bsaci.org

Conditions affecting the ear

Earache: Ear pain is a common presenting symptom in general practice. It is often a sign of an ear infection but if the ears are normal on examination you should look for a cause of referred pain e.g. from dental abscess, tonsillitis, sinusitis.

Discharge from the ear: Major causes are:
- Otitis media: discharge is often bloodstained, profuse and mucoid at first and later thickens and becomes yellow – 📖 p.284
- Otitis externa
- Cholesteatoma: 📖 p.286

> ⚠ Always exclude a perforated drum in discharging ears – beware of cholesteatoma. If you can't visualize the drum, review the patient.

Childhood deafness: Temporary deafness is common due to middle ear infections but permanent deafness rare (1–2/1000). ↓ hearing is often noticed by parents or teachers – take concerns seriously and refer for assessment. Deafness causes long-term speech, language ± behavioural problems and early intervention makes a difference.

Management: History, examination, assess hearing as appropriate for age (📖 p.22). Assess development (including speech and language). Treat or refer according to cause:
- *If no earache consider:* Bilateral glue ear (📖 p.286); impacted wax; hereditary cause; past meningitis; head injury or birth complications
- *If earache consider:* Acute otitis media (📖 p.284); impacted wax.

Otitis externa: Pain, discharge from the ear ± hearing loss ± associated lymphadenopathy. Moving the pinna is often painful. If discharging, take a swab and send for M,C&S. Treat with topical antibiotic ± steroid ear drops. Advise simple analgesia. Consider oral treatment with flucloxacillin or erythromycin if no response to topical treatment, severe symptoms, drum can not be visualized, or is perforated and/or uncooperative child. If not settling, refer to ENT.

Barotrauma: Due to changes in atmospheric pressure (e.g. air travel, diving, direct trauma to the ear) in those with poor eustachian tube function. Presents with a sensation of pressure/pain in one or both ears, hearing loss ± vertigo. *Examination* reveals fluid behind the drum and haemorrhagic areas in the drum, or perforation; conductive hearing loss.

Management: Generally there is spontaneous resolution within 2–3wk. Oral/nasal decongestants and antibiotics to prevent infection are of no proven benefit. If perforation has not healed in <1mo. refer to ENT.

Prevention:
- Valsalva manoeuvre, giving an infant a feed, yawning or sucking boiled sweets during flight – particularly during take off and landing – encourages the eustacian tube to open to allow pressure to equalize.
- Decongestants e.g. pseudoephedrine prior to flight.
- Patients with otitis media should not fly.

Foreign bodies in the ear: 📖 p.54

GP Notes: Hearing aids and cochlear implants

Hearing aids: can help anyone with reduced hearing, but they never restore perfect hearing.

Digital aids: Digitally process the sound. Usually digital aids are supplied to children. Advantages over analogue aids include:

- Filtering out of background noise
- Less whistling than analogue aids
- Can be customized to an individual's pattern of hearing loss
- Can be programmed with different settings for different sound environments e.g. classroom, outdoors, TV at home etc.

Behind-the-ear hearing aids: The hearing aid rests behind the ear and is connected to an earmould within the ear by a plastic tube. This is the most common type of hearing aid provided by the NHS.

Body-worn hearing aids: The hearing aid is a small box that is clipped to the clothes or put in a pocket and connected by a lead to an earphone and earmould. These are the most powerful hearing aids available so are used for the most profoundly deaf, and can be easier to use for patients with sight problems and/or problems using their hands.

Bone conduction hearing aids: For those with conductive hearing loss or for people who are unable to wear conventional hearing aids because of previous ear surgery or ear malformation.

CROS/BiCROS hearing aids: For those with unilateral complete deafness. CROS hearing aids pick up sound from the side with no hearing and feed it to the better ear. BiCROS aids amplify sound from both sides and feed it into the ear that has some hearing.

Cochlear implants: May benefit children with profound bilateral sensorineural hearing loss. They have 2 components.

- *The external component:* Is worn behind the ear. It consists of a microphone, processor which filters and simplifies sound and a transmitter which sends the resulting signal to the inner component.
- *The internal component:* Contains a decoder and complex band of electrodes. This is surgically inserted into the inner ear (the cochlea). When the signal from the outer component is received it is translated into a series of electrical impulses which directly stimulate nerve fibres in the cochlear.

Advice for patients: Information and support for deaf children and their parents

National Deaf Children's Society ☎ 0808 800 8880
🖳 www.ndcs.org.uk
Royal National Institute for the Deaf ☎ 0808 808 0123 *Text phone*
☎ 0808 808 9000 🖳 www.rnid.org.uk
Hearing Concern ☎ 0845 074 4600 🖳 www.hearingconcern.com
ENT UK Information about deafness and hearing aids
🖳 www.entuk.org

Otitis media

Inflammation of the middle ear.

Acute suppurative otitis media: Caused by viral or bacterial infections, or bacterial infection complicating a viral illness (e.g. URTI, measles) – clinically indistinguishable.

Presentation:
- *Symptoms:* Ear pain – usually unilateral and often accompanied by fever and systemic upset. There may also be ear discharge associated with relief of pain if there is a spontaneous perforation of the drum.
- *Signs:* Red, bulging drum (Figure 8.21). If perforation has occurred the external canal may be filled with pus, obscuring the drum.

🛈 If you can't see the drum, review the patient after treatment.

Acute management:
- In 80% patients, symptoms resolve in ≤3d. without treatment. Advise fluids + paracetamol and/or ibuprofen for analgesia and fever control.
- Symptoms resolve 24h. earlier with antibiotics but antibiotics carry the risk of side effects and their use ↑ community antibiotic resistance. Many GPs are now using a 'delayed' approach–prescribing if symptoms are no better in 3d.
- Most GPs prescribe antibiotics (e.g. amoxicillin tds for 5–7d.) at presentation if a perforation is present.
- If recurrent attacks (>4 episodes in 6mo.) or if acute perforation does not heal in <1mo., refer to ENT.

Prevention: Parental smoking ↑ children's risk of otitis media. Encourage parents to stop smoking.

Mastoiditis: Rare complication. The result of extension of acute otitis media into the mastoid. Symptoms include: fever, persistent headache, profuse creamy ear discharge and increasing conductive deafness. On examination there is tenderness ± swelling over the mastoid and the ear may stick out (pinna pushed down and forwards). The eardrum should be red and bulging or perforated – if it is normal it is not mastoiditis. If suspected, admit to ENT for IV antibiotics.

Chronic suppurative otitis media: Persistent drainage (>1mo.) from the ear associated with tympanic membrane perforation and some degree of conductive hearing loss. Not usually painful. (⚠ Earache or headache suggest the possibility of an intracranial complication – refer urgently to ENT). Management depends on the site of the perforation.

Central perforation: 'Safe disease'. Treat as for otitis externa (📖 p.282) to dry the discharge and encourage drum healing[C]. Refer to ENT if there is persistent discharge, deafness, vertigo or earache. Surgery to close the drum may help.

Attic or marginal perforation: 'Unsafe disease'. May indicate *cholesteatoma* development in the pars flaccida of the eardrum. Refer to ENT for further assessment.

Figure 8.21 The normal eardrum and eardrum in acute otitis media

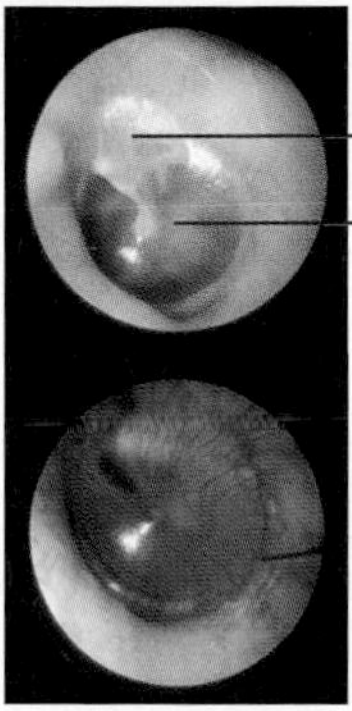

Normal tympanic membrane

Pars flaccida (attic)

Pars tensa

Otitis media

GP Notes: Otitis media

Frequently asked questions about treatment of otitis media:

In acute otitis media, are there certain groups I should routinely prescribe antibiotics for?

There is some evidence antibiotics have a greater benefit in:

- The very young (<2y. old)
- Those with severe ear signs – very inflamed and bulging drum
- Those with systemic symptoms – high temperature or vomiting.
- Those with bilateral acute otitis media.

Can antibiotic ear drops be used when the eardrum is perforated?

Advice varies regarding the use of topical aminoglycoside and polymyxin antibiotics in the presence of a perforated eardrum. There is good evidence they help in chronic secretory otitis media, but they do have a potentially ototoxic effect. Most ENT surgeons prescribe them. A pragmatic position for GPs is to only prescribe for short periods before seeking the advice of an ENT specialist.

Advice for parents of children with acute otitis media:

- Earache is common.
- Most earaches settle without treatment within 3 days.
- Most people do not need antibiotics to get better and antibiotics can cause side effects.
- Use paracetamol and/or ibuprofen regularly to help ease the pain.
- If your symptoms are not improving in 3–4 days, see your doctor.

285

Further information

SIGN Diagnosis and management of childhood acute otitis media in primary care (2003) 🖳 www.sign.ac.uk

Photographs are reproduced with permission from the Hawke Library of Ear Disease 🖳 www.earphotos.com

Cholesteatoma: Skin or stratified squamous epithelium growing in the middle ear. Thought to result from formation of a *retraction pocket* in the pars flaccida of the eardrum.

Presentation: Smelly discharge from the ear and conductive hearing loss. Other symptoms depend on which other structures are affected and can include headache, facial nerve palsy and symptoms of intracranial abscess formation. Examination reveals perforation of the pars flaccida of the tympanic membrane with pearly white debris within it (Figure 8.22).

Management: Refer to ENT. Treatment is either with suction to clear out the cholesteatoma and/or surgery. Following surgery, the ear should be dry and trouble free; if not, refer back to ENT. Lifelong follow-up is required as cholesteatomas recur.

Serous/secretory otitis media (glue ear): Non-infected fluid accumulation in the middle ear. Commonest cause of hearing loss amongst children. Fluid accumulates behind the eardrum due to dysfunction or obstruction of the eustachian tube e.g. due to throat or ear infections, or tonsillar hyperplasia. More common in children with Down's syndrome or cleft lip/palate.

Presentation:
- *Symptoms:* Deafness ± earache, difficulties with speech and language, behavioural problems.
- *Signs:* Dull, concave drum with visible peripheral vessels (Figure 8.23). Behind the drum there may be a fluid level or air bubbles.

Management in children[CE]: In children, glue ear is an age-related condition that resolves as the child grows older – any treatment is aimed at reducing the impact of symptoms until natural resolution occurs. 75% of children with glue ear have no remaining symptoms or signs within 3mo. However, bilateral hearing loss persisting >12mo. affects 5%.

If not resolving after 3mo. or accompanied by frequent otitis media, refer to the community audiology service or ENT depening on local arrangements – especially important if there is speech or language delay. Treatment options include:
- *Watchful waiting:* Can be used in asymptomatic or mild cases.
- *Medical:*
  - Long-term antibiotics (e.g. amoxicillin for 2–6wk.) and mucolytics may confer short-term benefit but evidence for their use is limited
  - Autoinflation with a nasal balloon may benefit older motivated children. It works by increasing intranasal pressure and opening the eustachian tube. It is not available on prescription
- *Surgical:* Grommets ± adenoidectomy give temporary benefit (6–24mo.).

Grommets: Air-conducting tubes inserted through the eardrum to drain the middle ear (Figure 8.23). Most are extruded spontaneously <9mo. after insertion and may need reinsertion if deafness recurs. Discharge from the ear occurs in some children with grommets – treat with antibiotic/steroid ear drops ± aural toilet (see otitis externa, 📖 p.282). Children with grommets can swim and bathe but should avoid diving.

Tympanosclerosis: Thickening and calcification of the tympanic membrane as a result of scarring from recurrent ear infections or after grommet insertion. Usually asymptomatic. No action is needed.

Figure 8.22 Cholesteatoma: perforation of the pars flaccida with pearly white debris within it

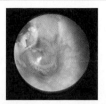

Figure 8.23 Glue ear and after treatment with grommet *in situ*

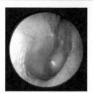 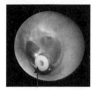

Serous/secretory otitis media ('glue ear')   Grommet *in situ*

Advice to give parents of children with glue ear

- Glue ear is common.
- Fluid behind the eardrum causes the hearing loss.
- It often starts after an ear infection, sore throat or cold.
- In most cases it will settle in 3 months without treatment.
- If it persists children are referred for consideration of grommets – speech and language problems can develop due to the hearing loss and grommets temporarily relieve the glue ear until the child grows out of it. Hearing loss can also lead to frustration and behaviour problems.
- Speak clearly, loudly and face to face to your child. Avoid background noise (e.g. TV) when talking to your child.
- Discuss the problem with your child's school teacher – minor changes may be needed, for example moving to the front of the classroom.
- Passive smoking can make glue ear worse. If you smoke – stop.

Further information for parents
Patient UK Information leaflet on glue ear 🖳 www.patient.co.uk

Figures 8.22 and 8.23 permission sought from the Hawke Library of Ear Disease
🖳 www.earphotos.com

Chapter 9

Diagnosis and management of common childhood mental health problems

Common childhood behaviour problems

There is no right or wrong way to deal with these problems and the approach outlined here is usually just one way to tackle these problems.

Sleep problems: 📖 p.296

School refusal and truancy: 📖 p.300

Toilet training problems: 📖 p.294

Feeding problems: 📖 p.68

Recurrent functional pains in children:
- Recurrent abdominal pain – 📖 p.170
- Recurrent headache – 📖 p.214
- Recurrent limb pains – 📖 p.206

Fears and phobias:

Fears:
- Fears of the dark, monsters and spiders are common in 3–4y. olds.
- Fears of injury and death are more common in older children.
- Statements made by the parents in anger or jest may be taken literally by pre-school children and can be disturbing.
- Frightening stories, films or TV programmes may be upsetting and intensify fears.

Phobias: Phobias cause persistent, unrealistic, yet intense anxiety in reaction to external situations or stimuli.

Management: Normal developmental stage-related fears must be differentiated from true phobias and anxiety states. If the phobia or fear is intense and interferes with the child's activity or if the child does not respond to simple reassurance, refer to child psychiatry.

Tics: Sudden, repetitive coordinated movements of no apparent purpose. Commonly involve facial grimacing, head movements or shoulder movements. Average age of onset ≈2y. Tics are present at some point in ~4% of children. Often a family history is present. The majority are precipitated by stress and disappear spontaneously, though some persist into adulthood.

Gilles de la Tourette syndrome: ♂:♀≈3:1. Characterized by multiple motor tics and irrepressible verbal outbursts – sometimes obscene. There may also be repetitive blinking, nodding, gesturing, echoing of speech and/or stuttering. Usually begins in childhood. Associated with obsessive–compulsive disorder and ADHD. Probable genetic aetiology.

Management: Refer for confirmation of diagnosis and specialist management. Spontaneous remissions do occur. Haloperidol or clonidine may help those severely affected with tics. Treat any associated obsessive–compulsive disorder or ADHD (📖 p.302).

GP Notes: Simple behaviour management techniques

For simple problems, parental education, reassurance and a few specific suggestions tailored to the problem are often sufficient. Follow-up is important to ensure that the problem is resolving. If simple measures are not succeeding within 3–4mo., consider referral to other agencies e.g. health visitor, school nurse, child psychiatrist etc. Specific behavioural techniques include:

Behaviour modification: Behaviour modification is a learning process that requires care-givers to set consistent rules and limits. Parents should try to minimize anger when enforcing rules and increases positive contact with the child.

Discipline: Ineffective discipline may result in inappropriate behaviour. Scolding or physical punishment may briefly control a child's behaviour if used sparingly, but may reduce the child's sense of security and self-esteem. Threats to leave or send the child away are damaging. *Options:*
- *Positive reinforcement for appropriate behaviour:* This is a powerful tool for controlling a child's behaviour with no adverse effects.
- *Time-out procedure:* The child must sit alone in a dull place for a brief period. Time-outs are a learning process for the child and are best used for controlling a single inappropriate behaviour or a few at one time.

Breaking vicious circle patterns: The child's behaviour (be it normal for that developmental stage or abnormal) evokes a response in the parent or carer which provokes the child to behave in that manner further – thus generating another response from the parent. Try to identify vicious circle patterns and suggest alternative parental responses which make the behaviour futile.

Conduct disorders: Poor behaviour e.g. aggression, destructive tendencies and antisocial behaviour are common complaints. Tolerance varies from family to family. Try simple strategies such as rewarding good behaviour and ignoring poor behaviour ± 'time-out' strategies (📖 p.xxx). If not succeeding, refer to child psychiatry.

Rhythmic behaviour: Head rocking or banging, thumb sucking, self-stimulation, baby behaviour and many other variants all occur during normal development. They usually appear if the child is tired, uncertain or anxious. Reassure parents. Most resolve spontaneously.

Excessive crying in babies: Babies vary in the amount they cry and ease with which they are soothed. Likewise parents vary in their ability to tolerate a crying baby. Babies cry for many reasons – discomfort, hunger, loneliness, separation, boredom etc. If crying excessively:
- Take a history from the parent(s) – when does the baby cry? Can he be consoled? What do the parents do when the baby cries?
- Examine fully from head to toe to exclude causes of discomfort e.g. nappy rash, otitis media, eczema etc.
- Check the baby is growing along his centile line.
- Consider family stress (including postnatal depression) as a reason why the parents can't tolerate the crying.
- Treat any underlying cause found and support the family. Information about behavioural techniques used to manage babies that cry excessively is available from Cry-sis ☎ 0845 1228 669 🖥 www.cry-sis.org.uk

Childhood depression: Response to childhood stress. Distinguish from depressive symptoms occurring as part of other emotional or conduct disorders. Most common in adolescence (♀>♂).

Diagnosis: Difficult, especially among adolescents. Teenage unhappiness is common (~½ 14y. olds feel miserable; ¼ are self-depreciatory; 8% have suicidal thoughts) and does not necessarily indicate depression. But adolescents often don't communicate well with their parents and have little contact with health professionals, resulting in late diagnosis.

Presenting features:
- Unhappiness and/or tearfulness, apathy, boredom, ↓ ability to enjoy life
- Antisocial behaviour – ♂>♀ – especially after bereavement
- ↓ school performance – may admit to poor concentration
- Separation anxiety reappearing in adolescence
- Frequent unexplained illness or undue worries about health
- Self-harm
- Bipolar depressive disorder is not seen before puberty

Management: Unless a mild episode, related to a single precipitating event and no other risk factors for depression, refer for specialist advice. Specialist treatment includes counselling, family therapy, CBT and drug therapy. ❶ With the exception of fluoxetine, risks of treatment with SSRIs outweigh benefits in children.

Further information:
NICE Depression in children and young people (2005) 🖥 www.nice.org.uk

Advice for patients: Crying baby? Guide to coping

Is baby hungry or thirsty? Offer breast-feed, bottle-feed or drink from spoon or bottle.

Is baby uncomfortable, in pain or generally cranky?
- Check for illness or nappy/clothing rashes – check with GP or health visitor if unsure.
- Talk to your baby and play with him/her.
- Change baby's nappy – let baby kick nappy free.
- Check baby's temperature by feeling tummy – adjust clothing.
- Offer breast, bottle or dummy.
- Offer cool boiled water, an infant colic remedy e.g. Infacol.
- Try gentle massaging of baby's tummy or a warm bath.
- Try changing baby's position, picking baby up and walking about with him/her, gently rocking up and down or making a soothing noise. Baby slings, rockers and bouncers can help – always follow manufacturer's instructions on use.
- Take baby out in the pram or car. Consider visiting a friend.

Is baby tired but fighting sleep?
- Offer breast, bottle or dummy.
- Try rocking baby horizontally in your arms or in the pram/pushchair, or take the baby for a car ride or pram walk.
- Try a quieter room, softer light or darker room.
- Leave baby to cry for a short time.
- Use a baby soother cassette or sing to your baby; some very quiet background noises may soothe baby e.g. ticking clocks, or make cassettes of vacuum cleaners, hairdryer noises etc.
- Check baby is comfortable and that he/she is not too hot or cold – check tummy to gauge temperature.
- Let baby sleep in fresh air.
- Try a warm bath.

Sensitive baby?
- Handle and talk to baby gently and quietly but don't overwhelm with stimulation.
- Try a quieter environment.
- Try to keep to a routine and limit the number of visitors.

Still crying?
- Put baby down, shut door, walk out of room for a break.
- Give baby to someone else for a few hours if possible. Use any time away from baby to look after yourself, eat well and unwind.
- Go out with baby.
- Phone a friend or relative, the Cry-sis helpline, health visitor or GP if unable to cope or worried.
- Alternative therapies e.g. homeopathy or cranial osteopathy may be helpful in some cases but always go to a registered and insured practitioner.

Crying baby? Guide to coping reproduced with permission from the Cry-sis website.
www.cry-sis.org.uk

Toilet training problems

Most children can do without nappies by day from 2–3y. and by night from 2–5y.

Nocturnal enuresis or bed wetting: Affects 30% of children aged 4y.; 10% at 6y.; 3% at 12y. and 1% at 18y. ♂>♀. Tends to run in families.

Causes and management:

Physical abnormality:
- 1–2% presenting with enuresis have an underlying physical abnormality – usually UTI.
- Rare causes – congenital anomalies, sacral nerve disorders, DM, diabetes insipidus, pelvic mass.
- In all children presenting with enuresis, exclude physical causes with history, examination and urinalysis for glucose, protein and M,C&S.
- If a physical cause is found, treat the cause.

Delay in maturation:
- By far the most common cause of bed wetting.
- Management:
  - <6y. – no need for treatment – most will resolve spontaneously
  - ≥ 6y. – refer to the school nurse who can provide equipment and training to control bed wetting. Techniques used – Table 9.1.

Emotional distress:
- Enuresis is occasionally caused by emotional distress.
- The child may have been dry then start wetting the bed at night again.
- If suspected, ask gently about any problems the child is having and manage those problems before treating the enuresis *per se*.

> ⓘ Don't forget diabetes as a possible diagnosis if a child starts wetting the bed again after being dry at night – always check urine for glucose.

Encopresis: Most children are continent of faeces by 2½ –3y. Faecal soiling after this age usually occurs during the day.

If:
- The child has bowel control but passes stool in unacceptable places, cause is usually emotional. Expert help from child psychiatry is needed – refer.
- Firm stool is passed occasionally in the toilet but usually in the pants, developmental delay (mental or social) is likely. Try a firm, consistent training programme similar to motivational counselling for enuresis (Table 9.1).
- Soft stool oozes out causing the child to constantly soil himself and smell of faeces – consider overflow incontinence to chronic constipation. Treat constipation. Refer to paediatrics if not settling.

Table 9.1 Methods of enuresis control

Method	Features
Motivational counselling	Child avoids drinks for 2–3h. before bed; urinates before going to bed; records wet and dry nights and changes clothing and bedding when wet. Rewards (e.g. star chart) are given for dry nights. The child is reassured throughout that the problem is not his fault and just a developmental problem likely to resolve in time.
Enuresis alarms	An alarm is triggered when the child starts to pass urine. In the first few weeks the child wakes after complete emptying of the bladder; in the next few weeks partial inhibition usually occurs; eventually the child wakes up in response to bladder contractions before he wets the bed. ~70% effective. Relapse occurs in 10–15%. The alarm should be used for at least 3wk. after the last bed-wetting episode.
Desmopressin	Synthetic version of antidiuretic hormone. Taken at night. Adverse effects include headache, nausea, nasal congestion, nosebleed, sore throat, cough, flushing and mild abdominal cramps. Effective in the short term (for 4–6wk.) e.g. to cover holidays.

Advice for parents: General rules for toilet training

- *Wait until your child is ready* – this usually means when he can indicate to you that he is going to the toilet and has shown an interest in using the toilet/potty. It is helpful to have a potty or child's toilet seat to put on the normal toilet for him to become familiar with before starting toilet training.
- *Pick a good time* when your child can have a few days at home without nappies in an environment where accidents don't matter. Make sure plenty of spare clothes are available.
- *Keep the potty handy or stay within easy reach of the toilet.* When your child says he wishes to go, sit him immediately on the toilet. Reward any result with praise and don't punish your child for any accidents – ask him to help clear up any mess and reinforce that it would be better to use the potty/toilet next time.
- *Until both you and your child are confident in your child's ability to use the toilet, continue using nappies when out and at night.* Take your child to the toilet at night before bedtime. When dry nappies are consistently noted in the mornings, try without nappies at night – a plastic sheet on the mattress is a good idea. Even when your child has been dry day and night for some time, accidents are common if your child is tired, unwell or unsettled – whether excited or unhappy.
- If your child does not succeed within a few days, either try training pants or revert to nappies and try again at a later date.

Information for parents of children with enuresis

ERIC (enuresis resource and information) ☎ 0845 370 8008
🖥 www.eric.org.uk

Childhood sleep problems

Sleeping patterns and habits of children vary considerably and should only be regarded as problems when they are presented as such by the family. First take a careful history. Ask about:

- *Medical problems* e.g. night cough related to asthma, itching from eczema, obstructive sleep apnoea. Treat appropriately
- *Physical problems* e.g. hunger or cold
- *Night terrors* (📖 p.298)
- *The sleep pattern* – usually ≥1 of:
  - Difficulty settling
  - Waking during the night
  - Waking early in the morning
- *The amount of daytime sleep.*

General advice: In all cases it is helpful to recommend a regular calming bedtime routine (e.g. bath, story, cuddle, bed) and minimal fuss when a child does wake at night e.g. try to settle back to sleep without taking out of cot, not rewarding waking with games, snacks etc.

Resistance to going to bed: The baby/child who cries incessantly when put to bed is a common problem with a peak age of 1–2y. The child cries when left alone or climbs out of bed and seeks the parents. *Causes include:*

- Separation anxiety
- Increasing attempts by the child to control his environment
- Long naps late in the afternoon
- Rough, overstimulating play before bedtime
- A disturbed parent – child relationship and/or tension in the home

Management: Letting the child stay up, staying in the room and comforting the child or punishing the child are all ineffective. Options include:

- *Leaving the child to cry:* This often does work and the crying diminishes after a few nights but it is very hard for parents to do and can be impossible if they are in shared accommodation.
- *Controlled crying:* The child is left to cry for a set length of time e.g. 2–10min. before the parent returns to settle him again with minimum fuss and then leaves. Length of time before returning is gradually ↑. Easier for parents than leaving the child to cry and still effective.
- *Staying with the child until he sleeps but gradually withdrawing proximity:* e.g. sit on bed with child, after a few nights sit next to bed, then nearer door etc. until child learns to go to sleep alone. This method is gentler than the above but may take longer.

Advice for patients: Checklist for settling babies (0–6 months)

- Try to put baby down awake, allowing him to settle down himself. Do not go back at the first whimper. It is worth noting that young babies often need to cry for a period to get themselves to sleep.
- Young babies will often wake for a night feed; this is natural. However, try to keep feeds as low-key as possible (no eye contact, no loud noises, subdued lighting). This will help baby distinguish between day and night and will hopefully prevent night feeds from becoming a comfortable habit as s/he gets older.
- Make sure that baby is comfortable (check nappy), well fed and not thirsty.
- Is baby cold or in a draught?
- Is baby too hot? It is very important not to allow baby to get overheated.
- Some babies like dark, others a soft night-light.
- Some babies like background noise. Various soother tapes are widely available and may help baby to fall asleep. Try the static noise from the radio which can have a soothing effect. Ordinary household appliances often work in this way too (vacuum cleaner, hairdryer etc.). Sudden noises should be avoided.
- Music can often help babies to settle; try a mobile or musical cot toy.
- Rhythmic movement often calms babies. The motion of a pram or motorized crib or a swinging seat can have an hypnotic effect. Baby slings provide continual movement with the additional comfort of closeness with mum or dad.
- Playthings on the cot can prevent boredom and make the cot a more enjoyable place to be, especially as baby gets to 3 months or older. Soft toys in the cot can act as insulation – avoid overheating baby.

Checklist for settling older babies and young children (7 months – 3 years): 📖 p.299

Information and support for parents

Parentline ☎ 0808 800 2222 🖳 www.parentlineplus.org.uk
Cry-sis Support for families with crying and sleepless babies
☎ 0845 1228 669 🖳 www.cry-sis.org.uk

Waking during the night: Occurs in ½ children aged 6–12mo. and is related to separation anxiety. In older children, episodes often follow a stressful event (e.g. moving, illness).

Management: Allowing the child to sleep with the parents, playing, feeding or punishing the child usually prolongs the problem.

- Try the methods used for resistance to going to bed (opposite), but advise parents to always check to see that the child is not ill/needing a clean nappy etc before being left to cry.
- Scheduled waking where a child is woken 15–60min. before the time he usually wakes and then resettled has also been shown to improve night waking.
- If a child wakes early, another strategy is to make toys or books accessible. The child may then amuse himself for a period of time without disturbing his parents. Some 2–3y. olds wander around without waking the parents – fitting a stair gate across the child's bedroom door prevents the child coming to any harm doing this.
- Use of sedatives e.g. alimemazine (for children >2y.) is often discouraged but can be useful, particularly when parents feel desperate. Only use as a short-term measure.

Nightmares: Occur during rapid eye movement (REM) sleep. Nightmares can be caused by frightening experiences (e.g. scary stories, television violence), particularly in 3–4y. olds. The child usually becomes fully awake and can vividly recall the details of the nightmare. An occasional nightmare is normal, but persistent or frequent nightmares warrant evaluation by an expert.

Sleepwalking (somnambulism): Involves walking clumsily, usually avoiding objects. The child appears confused but not frightened. 15% of children aged 5–12y. have sleepwalked ≥1 time. It is most common amongst school-aged boys and may be triggered by stressful events.

- Advise parents/carers not to try to wake the child.
- If the child is in danger, gently steer him away from any harm.
- If the child sleepwalks frequently, consider taking action to prevent the child coming to any harm whilst sleepwalking e.g. stair gate across bedroom door.
- If the sleepwalks occur repeatedly at the same time, waking the child ~15min. before the predicted time can break the cycle.

Night terror: Sudden awakening with inconsolable panic and screaming. Usually in the first 1–3h. of sleep. Episodes last seconds to minutes.
Features:
- Blank or confused stares
- Incomplete arousal with poor responsiveness to people
- Amnesia for the episode

Most common in children aged 3–8y. and require no treatment apart from simple reassurance. Advise parents not to wake the child as this ↑ disturbance. If frequent, consider waking the child before episodes occur and keeping the child awake for a few minutes to break the cycle. If the terrors persist beyond 8y., consider a diagnosis of temporal lobe epilepsy.

Advice for patients: Checking routine for older babies and young children (7 months – 3 years)

1. Ensure both parents and baby are well. Give yourself 2 clear weeks when you are not going out in the evening or going away.
2. Babies and children need a routine, especially at bedtime. Set a bedtime and stick to it. Make sure there is a good 'winding down' period: quiet games, stories and a relaxing bath.
3. Put baby to bed, tuck him in, say 'good night' and leave. Make sure he has any comfort objects with him before you go.
4. When he cries, leave him for a set time (5–10 minutes) then go back, 'check' him, tuck him in and leave. Do not pick him up. Do this until he goes to sleep; some parents leave the period of time between checking a little longer each time.
5. If your child gets up return him gently but firmly to bed. Ensure he knows you mean business and that you are not going to give in. It may help to use the same repetitive phrase and tone of voice each time you go in to your child.
6. Do not give drinks (unless it is exceptionally hot), cuddles or stories as this can be interpreted as a 'reward' for not going to sleep.
7. Be determined. If you give in now he will try much harder the next time; he knows you will give in in the end.
8. If baby wakes in the night do exactly the same as before. Go back as many times as is necessary to 'check'. In this way you and your baby know everything is OK.
9. Be consistent. If you have the support of a partner, make sure you work together.
10. Be prepared for a battle of wills. Baby will not give in without a fight. Tell your neighbours what you are going to do and discuss it with your health visitor.

The gradual retreat method: This method is probably easier on the nerves (less crying) but will take longer than the checking routine. Like the checking routine you will still need a routine but, instead of leaving, you stay and sit by the cot or bed until baby falls asleep–stroking him as necessary. Over the next few nights gradually sit further away from him until he will go to sleep with you outside the bedroom door.

Checklist for settling babies (0–6 months): 📖 p.297

Information and support for parents

Parentline ☎ 0808 800 2222 🖥 www.parentlineplus.org.uk
Cry-sis Support for families with crying and sleepless babies
☎ 0845 1228 669 🖥 www.cry-sis.org.uk

Checking routine for older babies reproduced with permission from Cry-sis website.
🖥 www.cry-sis.org.uk

Poor progress at school

~20% of school-age children require special educational services at some point in their schooling. ♂:♀≈5:1.

Severe learning difficulty: 📖 p.306

Autistic spectrum disorder: 📖 p.304

Attention deficit hyperactivity disorder (ADHD): 📖 p.302

Specific learning disorders:

Speech and language delay: May be a learning disorder, or due to deafness or neurological problems. Usually detected during routine paediatric developmental screening. Refer for hearing assessment and speech and language assessment promptly.

Dyslexia: Affects 3–5% to varying degrees. ♂>♀. Sufferers have difficulties with reading, writing and spelling in their native language. There is considerable overlap with other learning difficulties e.g. dyscalculia and dyspraxia. IQ is often normal/high and the child appears bright and alert. There may be a FH. If suspected liaise with the child's school via the teacher. Formal testing by an educational psychologist confirms diagnosis.

Dyscalculia: Rarer than dyslexia but contains many of the same features. The core problem is a difficulty handling numbers and mathematical concepts. Management is the same as for dyslexia.

Dyspraxia: Affects 2% of the population in varying degrees – 70% ♂. IQ is often normal or high. As with dyslexia, children have varying features. Common features include:

- Clumsiness
- Poor posture
- Awkward gait
- Difficulty holding a pen or pencil properly
- Poor short-term memory
- Poor body awareness

- Reading and writing difficulties
- Confusion about which hand to use
- Difficulties throwing/catching balls
- Poor sense of direction
- Difficulty hopping, skipping and/or riding a bike
- Slow to learn to dress and feed

Management is as for dyslexia.

School refusal and truancy:

Children <10y.: Younger children may refuse to go to school or recurrently complain of symptoms (e.g. abdominal pain) that justify staying home. Usually school refusal is a form of separation anxiety, though occasionally it is due to a problem at school e.g. bullying. Advise parents to consult the school – a star chart with a star from the teacher for each morning the child goes to school without a fuss may help. Relapses can occur if the child is absent or after holidays.

Older children: School refusal is a more difficult problem. Speak to parents and child together and separately. Try to ascertain if there is a genuine reason why the child avoids school. Liaise with the school. If not succeeding, refer to child psychiatry.

GP Notes: Questions to ask if a child presents with poor progress at school

- Does the child have a physical illness affecting his school work e.g. asthma, eczema?
- Is the child on any drugs that might affect his academic performance (e.g. anticonvulsants)?
- Is the family stable or is there family upset?
- Does another member of the family have a chronic or life-threatening illness?
- Is the child's home environment conducive to doing his school work?
- Is this school refusal?
- Is the child happy at school?
- Is there a problem with vision or hearing?
- Is the child of normal intelligence?
- Does the child interact socially with adults and other children?
- Have developmental milestones been met?
- Does the child have specific difficulty with certain aspects of his school work e.g. mathematics, reading, writing?

Advice for patients: Information and support for parents

British Dyslexia Association ☎ 0118 966 8271
🖳 www.bdadyslexia.org.uk
Dyspraxia Foundation ☎ 01462 454 986
🖳 www.dyspraxiafoundation.org.uk
Children of high intelligence ☎ 0208 347 8927
🖳 www.chi-charity.org.uk
Independent panel for Special Education Advice (IPSEA)
☎ 0800 018 4016 🖳 www.ipsea.org.uk

Hyperactivity

Not easily defined because claims a child is hyperactive often reflect the tolerance level of the person complaining. More active children with shorter-than-average attention spans create management problems. Hyperactivity may have an underlying cause (e.g. an emotional disorder, CNS dysfunction, a genetic component) or may be an exaggeration of normal temperament. Often it is stage-related – support until that stage has passed. Simple behaviour management techniques (📖 p.291) may also help. If persistent and associated with learning difficulty or developmental delay, refer to child psychiatry.

Attention deficit hyperactivity disorder (ADHD):

- Common neurodevelopmental disorder which interferes with normal social function, learning and development.
- Aetiology is probably multifactorial with overstimulation, family environment and genetic factors all contributing.
- Affects 0.5–1% of the school-age population in the UK; rare <7y.; ♂:♀≈6:1.
- ~50% also have disruptive behaviour/conduct disorders, 20–30% a learning disorder and 25–40% an anxiety disorder. Emotional problems, low self-esteem, nocturnal enuresis, depression, family and relationship problems are also common.
- Long-term ADHD is associated with low academic achievement, substance misuse, unemployment and antisocial tendencies.

Diagnosis: ❶ Many of these behaviours are seen in normal children.
- *Inattention:* Poor attention to detail and organization of tasks; appears not to listen; easily distracted; forgetful; lack of concentration on tasks
- *Impulsivity:* Lack of social awareness; shouts out answers to questions; difficulty waiting (unable to take turns or wait in a queue); excessive talking – interrupts others; lack of social awareness
- *Hyperactivity:* Fidgets; inappropriate running, climbing or leaving seat

Diagnosis depends on several symptoms being present for ≥6mo. in >1 setting (e.g. school and home) and exclusion of other diagnoses causing similar behavioural pictures.

Differential diagnosis:
- Learning disorder
- Hearing problems
- Epilepsy
- Autistic disorder
- Thyroid disease
- Drug ingestion
- Psychological problems (depression, emotional trauma e.g. divorce)

Management: If suspected refer to community paediatrics or child psychiatry. Specialist treatment includes behavioural therapy, dietary manipulation (though evidence is slim) and drug therapy (e.g. ritalin – controlled drug, multiple side effects, growth must be monitored). Self-help and local support groups can be helpful.

GP Notes: Before referral

Ask the parents to obtain a report from the child's school before referral. This:
- Shows whether the problem occurs in more than one place
- Provides additional information for referral and
- Tests motivation – if the parents don't get a report (or provide a good reason why they haven't got a report), will they keep a child psychiatry appointment?

Advice for patients:

Information and support for parents:

Green & Chee *Understanding ADHD* (1997) Vermilion ISBN 0091817005

National Attention Deficit Disorder Information and Support Service (ADDISS) ☎ 020 8952 2800 ▯ www.addiss.co.uk *e-mail:* info@addiss.co.uk

Parentline ☎ 0808 800 2222 ▯ www.parentlineplus.org.uk

Independent Panel for Special Education Advice (IPSEA) ☎ 0800 018 4016 ▯ www.ipsea.org.uk

Information and support for children

National Attention Deficit Disorder Information and Support Service (ADDISS) ☎ 020 8952 2800 ▯ www.addiss.co.uk *e-mail:* info@addiss.co.uk

Childline 24h. confidential counselling service ☎ 0800 1111 ▯ www.childline.org

Further information

NICE Attention deficit hyperactivity disorder: pharmacological and psychological interventions in children, young people and adults (due to publish in April 2008) ▯ www.nice.org.uk

Autism and Asperger's syndrome

Autism: A developmental disorder of unknown cause affecting 2/10,000 children, though autistic spectrum disorders are much commoner (9/1000). $\male{:}\female{\approx}4:1$. Autism is a severely disabling condition for both child and family which requires a great deal of support from the community services, including the GP.

Diagnosis: Not apparent at birth. Usually detected from 18mo.–3y. when failure of social interaction and lack of speech becomes apparent. GPs play a vital role in detection and diagnosis.

Screening: Consider using a screening tool such as the Checklist for Autism in Toddlers (CHAT) for all toddlers with problems with social interaction or speech and language delay at the 18mo. check (opposite). If the 5 key items (shaded) are answered 'NO', the child has a high risk of developing autism. Children failing items A7 and Biv have a medium risk of developing autism.

Features of autism: Triad of:
- Impaired reciprocal social interaction (A symptoms)
- Impaired imagination associated with abnormal verbal and non-verbal communication (B symptoms)
- Restricted repertoires of activities and interests (C symptoms).

Management: There is no proven treatment though behaviour therapy is sometimes tried. Be approachable, willing to listen and prepared to be an advocate for the family if they have any problems. Having a child or living with an adult with autism is very hard. *Advise families:*
- To set unwavering rules for behaviour
- To reward and give more attention to good behaviour
- To contact self-help and support organizations
- To ensure they receive all benefits payable (e.g. carer's allowance, disability living allowance).

Prognosis:
- 70% remain severely handicapped – special schooling is often needed
- 50% develop useful speech
- 20% develop fits in adolescence
- 15% lead an independent life

Asperger's syndrome (autistic psychopathy): A variety of autism in which a child, from the age of ~2y., shows obsessive preoccupation with routines and stereotyped behaviour with distress if the environment is altered. Social isolation and linguistic difficulties are absent. Better prognosis than autism.

Advice for patients: Information and support for parents and patients

National Autistic Society of the UK (NAS) ☎ 0845 070 4004
🖥 www.nas.org.uk

Table 9.2

The Checklist for Autism in Toddlers (CHAT):

To be used by GPs or health visitors during the 18mo. developmental check-up.

Section A: Ask Parent:

1	Does your child enjoy being swung, bounced on your knee etc.?	yes/no
2	Does your child take an interest in other children?	yes/no
3	Does your child like climbing on things, such as up stairs?	yes/no
4	Does your child enjoy playing peek-a-boo/hide-and-seek?	yes/no
5	Does your child ever PRETEND, for example to make a cup of tea using a toy cup and teapot, or pretend other things?	yes/no
6	Does your child ever use his/her index finger to point, to ASK for something?	yes/no
7	Does your child ever use his/her index finger to point, to indicate INTEREST in something?	yes/no
8	Can your child play properly with small toys (e.g. cars or bricks) without just mouthing, fiddling or dropping them?	yes/no
9	Does your child ever bring objects over to you (parent) to SHOW you something?	yes/no

Section B: GP or HV Observation:

i	During the appointment, has the child made eye contact with you?	yes/no
ii	Get child's attention, then point across the room at an interesting object and say 'Oh look! There's a [name of toy]!' Watch child's face. Does the child look across to see what you are pointing at?	yes/no*
iii	Get the child's attention, then give child a miniature toy cup and teapot and say 'Can you make a cup of tea?' Does the child pretend to pour out tea, drink it etc.?	yes/no**
iv	Say to the child 'Where's the light?' or 'Show me the light'. Does the child point with his/her index finger at the light?	yes/no***
v	Can the child build a tower of bricks? (If so, how many? Number of bricks:............)	yes/no

* To record YES on this item, ensure the child has not simply looked at your hand but has actually looked at the object you are pointing at.

** If you can elicit an example of pretending in some other game, score a YES on this item.

*** Repeat this with 'Where's the teddy?' or some other unreachable object, if child does not understand the word 'light'. To record YES on this item, the child must have looked up at your face around the time of pointing.

GMS contract

Learning disability 1	The practice can produce a register of patients diagnosed with learning disability (see 📖 p.307 for the definition of learning disability used for the purpose of the QoF).	4 points

CHAT is reproduced with permission from the National Autistic Society UK (NAS)
🖥 www.nas.org.uk

Severe learning difficulty (mental handicap)

Arrested or incomplete development of the mind characterized by subnormality of intelligence. May exist alone or with other disabilities. Often noted by a parent first – take any concerns seriously.

Causes: Varied – many are rare. Divide into:

Congenital:
- Genetic e.g. Down's syndrome
- Metabolic e.g. congenital hypothyroidism
- Others e.g. prenatal rubella

Acquired: e.g. trauma, meningitis, birth injury

Management: Refer to paediatrics/genetics to ensure no treatable cause is missed. *Then:*

Communicate with carers:
- Explain referrals, test results and their implications, the local system and who is responsible for what.
- Find out about the condition (as far as possible) and tell the carers where to get more information.
- Ensure carers receive information about benefits and housing/schooling options available.

Refer to other community services e.g. paediatrician; district handicap team. Ensure follow-up happens and assist with assessment of special needs for schooling, housing and employment purposes. Continue prescription of medication started by other team members.

Manage medical problems not related to disability e.g. sore throats.

Promote compliance with long-term therapy ± education or rehabilitation programmes.

Offer family planning, preconceptual counselling and/or antenatal diagnosis for parents of children with severe learning disability and patients with severe learning difficulty reaching reproductive age.

Prognosis:
- *IQ 50–70:* 80% of people with learning disability. Most lead an independent life and require just special attention to their schooling.
- *IQ 35–49:* Special schooling, or extra support within mainstream schooling, and supervision may be needed.
- *IQ <35:* Severe learning difficulty. Limited social activity and speech may be impaired. Special schooling and medical services are needed. Support and counselling for families involved are important.

Advice for patients: Information and support for parents

MENCAP ☎ 0808 808 1111 ⌨ www.mencap.org.uk
Independent Panel for Special Education Advice (IPSEA)
☎ 0800 018 4016 (Scotland – 0131 454 0096/0144;
Northern Ireland – 0232 705654) ⌨ www.ipsea.org.uk

GMS contract

Learning disability 1	The practice can produce a register of patients diagnosed with learning disability*	4 points

*Learning disability is defined as presence of:
- Significantly reduced ability to understand new or complex information to learn new skills (impaired intelligence), with:
- Reduced ability to cope independently (impaired social functioning)
- Which started aged <18y., with a lasting effect on development.

Mental health problems in adolescence

Changes of adolescence start gradually – from ~11y. for girls and ~13y. for boys – and are complete by the age of ~17y. Adolescence is characterized by rapid physical development and emotional change. Adjusting to these changes causes problems:

- **Concerns about appearance:** Some become very concerned about their appearance. They need reassurance, especially if not growing or maturing as quickly as their friends
- **Clothes/style** are important to express solidarity with friends and declare independence
- **Hormonal changes** result in body shape, voice, hair and skin changes, body hair growth and menstruation. All can be hard to adjust to
- **Acne** may need treatment, especially if scarring (📖 p.250)
- **Dieting and consumption of junk food** are common. Rarely eating disorders develop.

Emotional problems: In the course of their adolescence, >1:5 children think so little of themselves that life does not seem worth living. Emotional disorders are often not recognized, even by family and friends. Overeating, excessive sleepiness, promiscuity and a persistent over-concern with appearance may be signs of emotional distress. More obviously, phobias and panic attacks appear.

School problems:
- **School refusal:** 📖 p.300
- **Truancy:** Usually children who are unhappy at home and frustrated at school. They spend their days with others who feel the same.
- **Poor school work:** Emotional problems e.g. worry about problems at home often affect school work and make it difficult to concentrate; pressure to do well/pass exams may be counter-productive. Exams are important, but advise parents not to let them dominate life or cause unhappiness.

Abuse: Physical, emotional or sexual abuse may occur in adolescence.

Behaviour problems: It is normal for teenagers and their parents to complain about each other's behaviour and disagree frequently. Parents often feel they have lost control over their child. Adolescents resent parental restrictions on their freedom, but still want parental guidance. Advise parents to lay down sensible ground rules and stick to them. Evidence suggests children are at greater risk of getting into trouble if their parents don't know where they are – advise teenagers to let their parents know where they are going and parents to ask.

Trouble with the law: ♂>♀. Most young people do not break the law – when they do, it usually only happens once. Repeated offending may reflect family culture or may result from unhappiness – always ask about emotional feelings when an adolescent is repeatedly getting into trouble.

Drugs, solvents and alcohol: Most teenagers never use drugs or inhale solvents, and of those that do, most never get beyond the experimenting stage. Alcohol is the most common drug causing problems for adolescents but consider the possibility of any form of drug use when parents notice serious, sudden changes in behaviour.

Cannabis: Is the most common drug of misuse. 30–50% of 16–17y. olds have tried it. Many perceive it as harmless (particularly when compared with tobacco). However, it does have adverse effects including:
• Cognitive impairment
• ↑ rates of respiratory infection, chronic bronchitis and possibly lung cancer
• ↑ risk of psychosis.

Solvent abuse: It is estimated that ~5% of teenagers abuse solvents.
• Solvents are easily obtained and cheap.
• Initial effects of inhalation are euphoria, incoordination, blurred vision and slurring of speech.
• Rarely the solvent may cause bronchoconstriction or arrhythmia.
• Deaths, when they occur, are usually due to hypoxia, VF or accidents whilst intoxicated.

Symptoms to look for in the surgery are changes in behaviour (e.g. drop in school performance or attendance, irritability, mood swings) and local changes due to inhalation e.g. cough, headaches, conjunctivitis. If detected, refer to the youth support agencies.

Psychiatric illness: Rarely, changes in behaviour and mood can mark the beginning of more serious psychiatric disorders. Manic depression and schizophrenia, as well as commoner disorders such as anxiety and depression, may emerge during adolescent years. Refer for psychiatric assessment if concerned.

Eating disorders: 📖 p.312

GP Notes: Distinguishing normal adolescent behaviour from mental illness

Teenage behavioural problems may be signs of mental illness if:
• They go on for more than a few weeks
• They don't vary e.g. persistently low mood in all circumstances
• They are severe e.g. self-harming behaviour, violence
• There is a significant impact on relationships, school performance and/or usual activities.

Advice for patients:

Information and support for parents
Parentline ☎ 0808 800 2222 🖳 www.parentlineplus.org.uk

Information and support for teenagers
Childline 24h. confidential counselling service
☎ 0800 1111 🖳 www.childline.org
Solvent abuse ☎ 01785 810762 🖳 www.re-solv.org

Acute panic attack

Features: Common, especially amongst teenage girls. Fear, terror and feeling of impending doom accompanied by some or all of the following:
- Palpitations
- Shortness of breath
- Choking sensation
- Dizziness
- Paraesthesiae
- Chest pain/discomfort
- Sweating
- Carpopedal spasm.

Differential diagnosis:
- Dysrhythmia
- Asthma
- Anaphylaxis
- Thyrotoxicosis
- Temporal lobe epilepsy
- Hypoglycaemia
- Phaeochromocytoma (very rare)

Action:

Talking down: Explain the nature of the symptoms to the patient:
- Racing of the heart is due to adrenaline produced by the panic
- Paraesthesiae and feelings of dizziness are due to overbreathing due to panic
- Count breaths in and out, gently slowing breathing rate.

Rebreathing techniques:
- Place a paper bag over the patient's mouth and ask him to breath in and out through the mouth.
- A connected but not switched on O_2 mask or nebulizer mask is an alternative in the surgery.
- This raises the partial pressure of CO_2 in the blood and symptoms due to low CO_2 (e.g. tetany, paraesthesiae, dizziness) resolve. This demonstrates the link between hyperventilation and the symptoms too.

Propranolol: 10–20mg stat for a teenager may be helpful – DON'T USE for asthmatics, younger patients or patients on verapamil.

Advice for patients: Self-help

One way of tackling panic attacks is to look at the way you talk to yourself, especially during times of stress and pressure. Panic attacks often begin or escalate when you tell yourself scary things, like 'I feel light-headed...I'm about to faint!' or 'I'm trapped in this lift and something terrible is going to happen!' or 'If I go outside, I'll freak out.' These are called "negative predictions" and they have a strong influence on the way your body feels. If you're mentally predicting a disaster, your body's alarm response goes off and the 'fight–flight response' kicks in.

To combat this, try to focus on calming, positive thoughts, like 'I'm learning to deal with panicky feelings and I know that people over-come panic all the time' or 'This will pass quickly, and I can help myself by concentrating on my breathing and imagining a relaxing place' or 'These feelings are uncomfortable, but they won't last forever.'

Remind yourself of these FACTS about panic attacks:
• A panic attack cannot cause heart failure or a heart attack.
• A panic attack cannot cause you to stop breathing.
• A panic attack cannot cause you to faint.
• A panic attack cannot cause you to 'go crazy'.
• A panic attack cannot cause you to lose control of yourself.

If it's too hard to think calming thoughts when you're having a panic attack, find ways to distract yourself. Some people do this by talking to other people when they feel the panic coming on. Others prefer to exercise or work on a detailed project or hobby. Changing scen-ery can sometimes be helpful, too, but it's important not to get into a pattern of avoiding necessary daily tasks. If you notice that you're regularly avoiding things like driving, going shopping, going to work or taking public transport, it's probably time to get some profes-sional help.

Slow, abdominal breathing (6 breaths per minute) has been shown to stop panic attacks. Learning slow abdominal breathing can be quite difficult and people who have panic attacks are almost always chest breathers. Practice abdominal breathing (moving upper part of tummy to breathe rather than chest wall) when relaxed at home. If you can learn to breathe slowly with your diaphragm, you will not panic!

Cut down on alcohol and caffeine – these can make panic attacks worse. Try relaxation techniques (such as yoga) and exercise regu-larly – both can help reduce the number of panic attacks people have.

Information and support for patients
Royal College of Psychiatrists Patient information sheets
⌨ www.rcpsych.ac.uk
No more panic ⌨ www.nomorepanic.co.uk

Eating disorders

⚠ Patients who are pregnant or have DM are particularly at risk of complications if they have co-morbid eating disorders. Refer early for specialist support and ensure everyone involved in care is aware of the eating disorder.

Anorexia nervosa: Prevalence 0.02–0.04%. ♀>>♂. Usually begins in adolescence. Peak prevalence at 16–17y. *Features:*

- Refusal to maintain body weight >85% of that expected (BMI <17.5kg/m^2).
- Intense fear of gaining weight, though underweight.
- Disturbed experience of body weight or shape or undue influence of shape on self-image.
- Amenorrhoea in women for ≥3 mo. and ↓ sexual interest.

Patients tend to have a set daily calorific intake e.g. 600–1000 calories and may employ strategies e.g. bingeing and vomiting, purging or excessive exercise to try to lose weight. Depression and social withdrawal are common as are symptoms 2° to starvation (see opposite).

Management[N]:

- Give ongoing support and information.
- Check electrolytes.
- Refer to a specialist eating disorders clinic (if available) or psychiatry. Treatment involves family therapy for adolescents, psychotherapy and possible admission for refeeding.

Follow-up: Patients with enduring anorexia nervosa not under 2° care follow-up should be offered an annual physical and mental health check.

⚠ Many patients with anorexia nervosa have compromised cardiac function. Avoid prescribing drugs which adversely affect cardiac function (e.g. antipsychotics, TCAs, macrolide antibiotics, some antihistamines). If prescribing is essential then follow up with ECG monitoring.

Bulimia nervosa: Prevalence 1–2%. Mainly ♀ aged 16–40y. *Features:*

- Recurrent episodes of binge eating, far beyond normally accepted amounts of food.
- Inappropriate compensatory behaviour to prevent weight ↑ e.g. vomiting, use of laxatives, diuretics and/or appetite suppressants. Bulimics can be subdivided into those that purge and those that just use fasting and exercise to control their weight.
- Self-image unduly influenced by body shape (see anorexia above).
- Normal menses & normal weight. If low BMI classified as anorexia.

Management:

- Give ongoing support and information.
- Check electrolytes.
- First-line treatment: evidence-based self-help programme e.g. Overcoming bulimia – CD-ROM available from Calipso

🖳 www.calipso.co.uk; telephone-based self-help programme run by the Eating Disorders Association – details below, cost ~£200.

- If unsuccessful, refer to a specialist eating disorders clinic (if available) or psychiatry. CBT and drug treatment with fluoxetine may help.

GP Notes: Identification of and screening for eating disorders

Target groups for screening include:
- Young women/teenagers with low BMI compared with age norms
- Patients consulting with weight concerns who are not overweight
- Women with menstrual disturbances or amenorrhoea
- Patients with GI symptoms
- Patients with symptoms/signs of starvation – sensitivity to cold, delayed gastric emptying, constipation, ↓ BP, bradycardia, hypothermia
- Patients with physical signs of repeated vomiting – pitted teeth ± dental caries, general weakness, cardiac arrhythmias, renal damage, ↑ risk of UTI, epileptic fits, ↓ K⁺
- Children with poor growth
- Young people with type 1 DM and poor treatment adherence

Screen target populations with simple screening questions:
- Do you worry excessively about your weight?
- Do you think you have an eating problem?

Advice for patients: Advice for patients purging

- *Vomiting:* Advise patients to avoid brushing their teeth after vomiting, rinse with a non-acid mouthwash after vomiting, and decrease acid oral environment (e.g. by limiting acid foods).
- *Laxatives:* Where laxative abuse is present, advise patients to gradually decrease laxative intake. Laxative abuse does not significantly ↓ calorie absorption.

Information and support for patient and parents
Eating Disorders Association (EDA) ☎ 0845 634 1414 (adults) 0845 634 7650 (youths) 🖳 www.b-eat.co.uk

Futher information
NICE Core interventions in the treatment and management of anorexia nervosa, bulimia nervosa and related eating disorders (2004) 🖳 www.nice.org

Threatened suicide and deliberate self-harm (DSH)

GPs are frequently called to patients who have deliberately self-harmed themselves, are threatening suicide or if relatives are worried about suicide risk.
- Assessment algorithm – Figure 9.1
- Management algorithm – Figure 9.2

Figure 9.1 Assessment of threatened suicide or deliberate self-harm

If any self-harm: Assess the situation and admit to A&E as needed.

⬇

Ask about suicidal ideas and plans in a sensitive but probing way. It is a common misconception that asking about suicide can plant the idea into a patient's head and make suicide more likely. Evidence is to the contrary.

⬇

Ask about present circumstances:
What problems are making the patient feel this way?
Does s/he still feel like this?
Would the act of suicide be aimed to hurt someone in particular?
What kind of support does the patient have from friends and relatives and formal services (e.g. CPN)?

⬇

Assess suicidal risk: Ask patient and any relatives/friends present.
Risk factors:
♂>♀
Admission or recent discharge from psychiatric hospital.
Social isolation
History of deliberate self-harm (100x ↑risk)
Depression
Alcohol or substance abuse
Personality disorder
Schizophrenia
Serious medical illness (e.g. cancer).

⬇

Assess psychiatric state: Features associated with ↑ suicide risk are:
Presence of suicidal ideation
Hopelessness–good predictor of subsequent and immediate risk
Depression
Agitation
Early schizophrenia with retained insight–especially young patients who see their ambitions restricted
Presence of delusions of control, poverty and/or guilt.

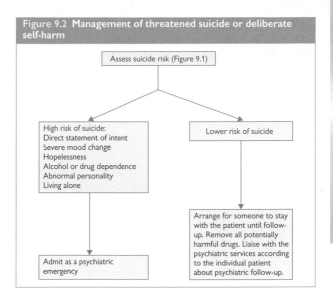

Figure 9.2 Management of threatened suicide or deliberate self-harm

Assess suicide risk (Figure 9.1)

High risk of suicide:
Direct statement of intent
Severe mood change
Hopelessness
Alcohol or drug dependence
Abnormal personality
Living alone

Lower risk of suicide

Admit as a psychiatric emergency

Arrange for someone to stay with the patient until follow-up. Remove all potentially harmful drugs. Liaise with the psychiatric services according to the individual patient about psychiatric follow-up.

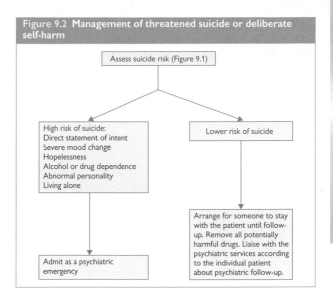 People who have self-harmed should be treated with the same care, respect and privacy as any other patient.

Deliberate self-harm (DSH): Deliberate non-fatal act committed in the knowledge that it was potentially harmful and, in the case of drug overdose, that the amount taken was excessive. 90% DSH is due to self-poisoning. Paracetamol or aspirin are the most common drugs used (📖 p.52). Self-harm is often aimed at changing a situation (e.g. to get a boyfriend back), a communication of distress ('cry for help'), a sign of emotional distress or may be a failed genuine suicide attempt.

Advice of patients: Information and support for patients and relatives

Self Injury and Related Issues (SIARI) 🖥 www.siari.co.uk
Samaritans 24h. emotional support via telephone ☎ 08457 909090
Survivors of bereavement by suicide ☎ 0870 241 3337
🖥 www.uk-sobs.org.uk

Further information

NICE Self-harm: the short-term physical and psychological management and secondary prevention of self-harm in primary and secondary care (2004) 🖥 www.nice.org.uk
DoH National Suicide Prevention Strategy for England (2002)
🖥 www.dh.gov.uk

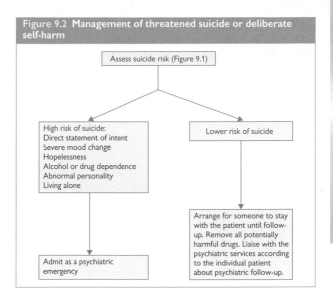

Chapter 10

Miscellaneous topics

Prescribing for children

> ⚠ Keep all medicines out of the reach of children (and preferably in a locked cupboard).

Children differ from adults in their response to drugs and the doses they require. Particular care is needed in first 30d. of life. Consult the *BNF, BNF for Children* or *Paediatric Vade Mecum* before prescribing unfamiliar drugs and always check drug doses carefully.

Prescriptions for children:

- Prescriptions for children <12y. must include age or date of birth (recommended for older children as well).
- All children <16y. (and those <18y. in full-time education) are entitled to free prescriptions.

Licensing of drugs: In the UK, the Medicines Act (1968) makes it essential for anyone who manufactures or markets a drug for which therapeutic claims are made to hold a licence. Although doctors usually prescribe according to the licensed indications, they are not obliged to.

Prescribing outside licence: Many drugs are not licensed for use with children but children sometimes need these drugs and there may not be a licensed alternative. In these circumstances, drugs are often prescribed 'off-licence'. Don't prescribe unlicensed drugs unless you have experience of and can justify their use (e.g. there is an evidence base for their use or established drug texts like the *BNF* advocate use). If in doubt refer for a specialist opinion.

> ⚠ Before prescribing any medication (whether within or outside the licence), weigh risks against benefits. The more dangerous the medicine, and the flimsier the evidence base for treatment, the more difficult it is to justify the decision to prescribe.

When prescribing licensed drugs for unlicensed indications:

- Inform patients and carers of what you are doing and why and obtain consent for the drug's use in that way.
- Explain that the patient information leaflet (PIL) will not have information about the use of the drug in these circumstances.
- Record in the patient's notes your reasons for prescribing outside the licensed indications for the drug.

❗ The person signing the prescription is legally responsible.

Prescribing paediatric suspensions:

- Paediatric suspensions often contain sugar.
- For long-term use or children having frequent prescriptions consider sugar-free versions.
- Don't advise adding medicines to infant feeding bottles – drugs may interact with milk and the dose is ↓ if not all the contents are drunk.
- Oral syringes are supplied by pharmacies where dose is <5ml. They are also useful for administering larger doses to reluctant children.

Suspected adverse reactions: To any therapeutic agent (whether OTC, herbal/alternative medication or prescribed by a doctor) should be reported to the Medicines and Healthcare Products Regulatory Agency (MHRA – CSM Freepost, London SW8 5BR). Forms ('yellow cards') are available from that address or in the back of the *BNF*. Alternatively report online at 🖥 www.mhra.gov.uk

- *For new drugs* (marked ▼ in *BNF*): Doctors are asked to report all reactions whether or not causality is clear.
- *For established drugs:* Doctors are asked to report all reactions in children.

GP Notes: Tips on prescribing for children

- If a child needs medication in more than one place (e.g. school and home, separated parents), prescribe sufficient so they can keep a supply at both.
- Intramuscular injections are painful – avoid giving them to children wherever possible.

Further information

Information on drugs used to treat rare paediatric conditions: Alder Hey Children's Hospital (☎ 0151 252 5381) or Great Ormond Street Hospital (☎ 020 7405 9200)

BNF 🖥 www.bnf.org

BNF for Children 🖥 www.bnfc.org

DTB Prescribing unlicensed drugs or using drugs for unlicensed applications (1992) 30 pp.97–9

Consent and confidentiality

Definition of competence A competent child is able to understand the nature, purpose and possible consequences of a proposed procedure, as well as the consequences of not undergoing that procedure. This is termed 'Frazer competence' (previously 'Gillick competence').

Consent: Implies willingness of a patient to undergo examination, investigation or treatment (collectively termed 'procedure' on this page). It may be expressed (i.e. specifically says yes or no/signs a consent form) or implied (i.e. complies with the procedure without ever specifically agreeing to it – use with care).

For consent to be valid: The person giving consent must:
- Be competent to make the decision
- Have received sufficient information to take it and
- Not be acting under duress.

In the case of children (<16y.): Consent can only be given by:
- A parent, other individual or local authority with parental responsibility
- The child if he or she is judged to be competent
- A court.

🔵 A competent child may consent to treatment. However, if treatment is refused, a parent or court may authorize procedures in the child's best interests.* If in doubt, seek legal advice.

> ⚠ **Emergencies:** When consent cannot be obtained, you may provide medical treatment, provided it is limited to what is immediately necessary to save life or avoid significant deterioration in the patient's health. Respect the terms of any advance statement/living will you are aware of.

Confidentiality: The Human Rights Act (1998) and Data Protection Act (1998) are the main pieces of legislation preserving confidentiality of health records. But respect for confidentiality is also an essential requirement for the preservation of trust between patient and doctor. Failure to comply with standards can lead to disciplinary proceedings and even restriction/cessation of practice.

With regard to children:
Young people judged to be competent:
- Have a right to refuse parental access to their health record
- Can make their own decisions regarding disclosure
- Can apply for access to their own records

For other children:
- Disclosure can be authorized by a person with parental responsibility.
- Any person with parental responsibility may apply for access to records of a child (<18y. or <16y. in Scotland). Where >1 person has parental responsibility, each may apply independently without consent of the other parent.

---

* In Scotland, parents do not have this power to overrule a competent child's decision.

Breaching confidentiality: Only breach confidentiality in exceptional cases and with justification. This includes discussing a patient with another health professional not involved currently with that patient's care.

Situations where breach of confidentiality may be justified:
- *Child abuse:* The welfare of the child is paramount – 📖 p.322
- *Emergencies:* Where necessary to prevent or lessen a serious and imminent threat to life or health e.g. teenager with suicidal intent
- *Statutory requirement:* e.g. social services may request information under section 47 of the Children's Act when investigating possible child abuse. Ask under which legislation disclosure is sought – if unfamiliar with the legislation check details before giving information
- *The public interest:* The BMA has produced guidance
- *Public health:* Reporting notifiable diseases (statutory duty – 📖 p.89)
- *Required by court or tribunal*
- *Adverse drug reactions:* Routine reporting to the Medicines and Healthcare Products Regulatory Agency
- *Complaints:* As part of the complaints procedures involving doctors

> **GP Notes: Frequently asked questions about competence to consent**
>
> *Who determines whether a child is competent?*
> It is the responsilbility of the treating doctor to decide whether a child is competent to consent.
>
> *How can I decide if a child is competent to consent to treatment?*
> A competent child should be able to understand in simple terms:
> - What the treatment involves
> - Why it needs to be done
> - What its benefits and risks are and the effect of not having treatment.
>
> In addition, children must:
> - Believe the information applies to them
> - Retain information long enough to make a choice
> - Make the choice without pressure.
>
> *If a child is deemed competent once, is that child always competent?*
> No – competence varies according to what the treatment proposed is. For example, a teenager may be competent to decide to take contraception but not to consent to major surgery.

Further information
DoH guidance 🖥 www.dh.gov.uk
BMA 🖥 www.bma.org.uk
- Consent toolkit
- Confidentiality and people under 16
- Access to health records by patients
Gilbert & Tripp *Consent, rights and choices in healthcare for children and young people* (2001) BMJ Books ISBN: 0727912283
GMC 🖥 www.gmc-uk.org
- Seeking patients' consent: the ethical considerations
- Guidance on good practice: confidentiality

Child abuse and neglect

Defined as depriving children of their human rights. These are:

- **Being healthy:** Enjoying good physical and mental health and living a healthy lifestyle
- **Staying safe:** Being protected from harm and neglect
- **Enjoying and achieving:** Developing broad skills for adulthood
- **Making a positive contribution:** To the community and society
- **Economic well-being:** Overcoming disadvantages to achieve their full potential.

Statistics: ~3/100 children are abused each year in the UK; there were 4109 reported offences of cruelty or neglect of children in England and Wales in 2002/3, and every year ~30,000 children's names are added to the child protection register in England alone.

Presentation: *Always* have a high index of suspicion. *Suspect abuse if:*

- The child discloses it
- The story is inconsistent with injuries found
- There is late presentation after an injury or lack of concern about the injury by the parent(s)
- Presentation to an unknown doctor
- Accompanying adult is not the parent or guardian
- Sibling has been a victim of abuse
- Reluctance to allow the child to be examined
- Characteristic injuries – look for marks consistent with cigarette burns; scalds (especially if symmetrical or doughnut shaped on buttocks); finger mark or bite mark bruises; perineal bruising or anogenital injury; linear marks consistent with whipping; buckle or belt marks
- Multiple injuries or old injuries coexistent with new
- Unlikely sites for injuries e.g. mouth, ears, genitalia, eyes
- Behaviour of the child is suggestive e.g. withdrawn, 'frozen watchfulness', sexually precocious behaviour, abnormal interaction between child and parents, unwilling to speak about the injury etc.
- Vaginal discharge, sexually transmitted disease or recurrent UTI in any child <14y.
- Failure to thrive, developmental delay and/or behavioural problems: neglect and/or emotional abuse are included in the differential diagnosis of failure to thrive and developmental delay. Any type of abuse may result in behavioural problems

---

Risk factors for child abuse:

Parent/carer factors:

- Mental illness
- Substance/alcohol abuse
- Being abused themselves as children or adults
- Ongoing physical illness
- Learning disabilities
- Unemployment/impoverished living conditions

Child factors:

- History of sibling abuse
- Learning, behaviour or physical problems
- Unplanned pregnancy/premature birth
- Poor attachment to parents/carers
- Environment high in criticism
- 'Looked after' children

Table 10.1 Classification of child abuse	
PHYSICAL	**EMOTIONAL**
Hitting, shaking, throwing, burning, suffocating, poisoning, including factitious or induced illness	The child is made to feel worthless, afraid, unloved or inadequate (e.g. if developmentally inappropriate expectations are imposed)
NEGLECT	**SEXUAL**
Failure to meet the child's basic needs, allowing the child to be exposed to danger	Forcing/enticing a child to take part in sexual activities – may involve physical contact, or production of pornographic material

ⓘ In practice there is often overlap and >1 type of abuse may co-occur.

GP Notes: How to safeguard children with confidence

- Make sure you are familiar with the practice and local child protection procedures.
- Make sure you attend child protection training regularly.
- Share your concerns with colleagues and try to use shared documentation and computer templates as much as possible.

GMS Contract

Management 1	Individual health care professionals have access to information on local procedures relating to child protection	1 point

Immediate action:

⚠ Welfare of the child is *paramount*. Not to report abuse is to collude with the abuser. Do *not* perform a forensic-type examination unless you are trained to do so and be careful not to ask leading questions which might contaminate the evidence.
- Wherever possible, arrange for another health professional to be present during the consultation.
- Take a history from any accompanying adult. If possible also take a history from the child alone too.
- Examine the child. Ask for an explanation for any injuries noted.
- Keep thorough notes, recording dates and times, history given, injuries noted and any explanation of those injuries.

Further action: Depends on nature of the suspected abuse, suspected abuser (e.g. if someone outside the home is suspected, the child is safe to return home), nature of the injuries and response of the parents. Be familiar with and follow local guidelines and practice policy. *Options are:*

- Hospital admission – protects the child and allows full assessment.
- Liaison with social services child protection team (on call 24h./d.).
- If admission is refused, contact social services to arrange a Place of Safety Order, or the police to take the child into police protection.
- Contact social services if your observations and discussions lead you to feel that this is a child protection issue and follow up the referral in 48h. with a written referral – you should receive confirmation of your referral within 1 but certainly within 3 working days.
- You can also refer directly to the police, particularly if you feel emergency action may be required to protect the child.

Difficult issues for safeguarding children:

- Confidentiality of medical information
- Sharing information with parents and carers
- Fear of damaging future relationships with the family
- Fear of causing family disruption
- Fear of dealing with other agencies e.g. police and social services
- Fear of being mistaken in one's suspicions
- Fear of missing abuse
- Fear of attending court
- Fear of negative peer review

Refugee children: Have special problems and needs. *Consider:*

- Language barriers – consider the use of professional interpreters even if the child is with an English speaking carer.
- Cultural and religious issues – if in doubt, ask
- Physical needs – health needs are diverse depending on country of origin and previous level of health care. Consider immunization status.
- Psychological needs – many children refugees have traumatic backgrounds. Approach children with sensitivity and consider involving specialist child psychiatric services and specialist refugee support services early.
- Family – some children will have left family members behind. The Red Cross or Red Crescent can help with tracing (⌨ www.redcross.org.uk)

Further information

The refugee council ⌨ www.refugeecouncil.org.uk

⚠ **Special circumstances to watch out for:**
- *Circumcision of female infants*
- *Forced marriage of minors (<16y.)*

Both these practices are illegal in the UK but it is not uncommon for children to be taken abroad to be circumcised/married. If you suspect this might be going to happen to any patient of yours, inform social services and/or the police immediately.

Figure 10.1 The 4-step approach to managing child abuse

Step 1

Recognition

Health professionals either identify or suspect a situation where a child may be at risk of abuse or neglect.

Step 2

Reporting

Suspicions are reported or discussed with social services, police and/or child protection agencies.

Concerns regarding a family become 'public'—this is often the threshold at which those in primary care hesitate and step back from the brink.

Step 3

Enquiry and assessment of risk

Concerns and allegations are explored, information is gathered and risk to children determined.

A multi-agency approach is usually employed.

Step 4

Intervention

Consists of supportive and rehabilitation measures in order to enable child development.

GP Notes: Determining child abuse

⚠ This guidance appears simple – and *is* when abuse is overt – but often it is *difficult* to decide if a child is being abused. If you have worries but cannot justify them sufficiently to invoke child protection procedures:
- Check via social services whether the child is on the 'at risk' register
- Check notes of siblings and other family members to see if there has been any suggestion of abuse in the family before
- Discuss your worries with the health visitor and/or other involved members of the primary health care team.

If any of these sources ↑ your suspicion, you may be justified in investigating further or invoking child protection measures at that point.

If you are still unsure what to do, record your worries and the reasons for them in the child's notes and alert all other involved members of the practice team. Review whenever that child is seen again in the practice.

Further information

DoH 🖥 www.dh.gov.uk
- Working together to safeguard children (1998)
- What to do if you're worried a child is being abused (2003)

RCGP *Carter & Bannon* The role of primary care in the protection of children from abuse and neglect (2003) 🖥 www.rcgp.org.uk

Department for Education and Skills Every child matters (2004) 🖥 www.everychildmatters.gov.uk

The chronically disabled child

Chronic disability due to a wide variety of causes affects ~10% of children in the UK.

Effects on the child: Vary from child to child dependent on the nature of the disability, personality of the child and support the child has at home and in the community. Common problems include:

- Physical discomfort – both due to the disability and to painful or embarrassing treatments
- Alterations in the normal pattern of growth and development and/or physical differences may lead to social isolation and ↓ motivation
- Frequent hospitalizations and outpatient visits prevent the child integrating into school or ongoing community activities
- Dependence – the disability may prevent the child reaching his own goals and achieving his own independence. Many children also realize the additional burden they cause their parents and carers.

Effects on the family: Vary from family to family depending on financial and/or social support, relationship between parents and other siblings and many other factors. Stress may cause family break-up, especially when other marital and intra-family problems exist. Common problems:

- Grieving for the loss of the 'ideal child' – conditions that affect the appearance of the child particularly affect attachment between parents and child. The grief might take the form of shock, denial, anger, sadness, depression, guilt or anxiety and may occur any time in the child's development
- Neglected siblings
- Inconsistent discipline – due to demands placed on the family and sympathy for the child – resulting in behaviour problems
- Marginalization of 1 parent – 1 parent tends to take on the bulk of the caring activities. There is a danger the other parent starts to feel inadequate and isolated with respect to the care of the child
- Major expense and time commitment – frequently 1 parent has to give up work to look after a disabled child, resulting not only in loss of income but loss of that parent's independence and opportunities for the future
- Social isolation
- Confusion over the health, benefits and social services available.

Care coordination: Inconsistent policies and funding, inadequate access to facilities (including physical barriers to access) and poor communication and coordination between the health care, educational and community support systems → misery for children with disability and their families. Without coordination of services, care is crisis oriented.

Care coordination requires knowledge about the child's condition, the family and the community in which they function. In all cases *someone* should be designated responsible for coordinating care – the best person to do that will vary according to circumstances. Regardless of who assists in coordination of services, the family and child must be partners in the process.

Role of the GP:

- The GP of any patient with a chronic illness in the community is a team member and may be the key worker who coordinates care.
- Maintain an open door policy and encourage children and carers to seek help for problems early.
- Try to become familiar with a child's disease, even if it is rare. It is impossible to plan care without knowledge of course and prognosis and an easy way to lose a child's confidence if you appear ignorant of their condition.
- If progress is slower than expected, or stalls, consider other medical problems (e.g. anaemia, infection), behavioural problems and communication problems (e.g. poor vision/hearing).
- Information alone can improve outcome.

Advice for patients: Parents' experiences of having a child with chronic disability

'She was our baby. She was our first. To us, whether there was something wrong or not, she was still a baby. She still needed us, and so we just got on with it.'

'For me, the beginnings of bringing up a child with learning difficulties (I prefer this more inspiring label to "handicapped") were not so easy. Although my books on baby play helped, I still had to feel my way through, especially as my daughter was my first child.'

'When our little girl was born with Down's syndrome, it was a terrible shock and we were very sad. Our parents and friends were very supportive, which helped enormously. One of the most helpful things was being introduced, through the local Down's Syndrome Association group, to a family with a nine-month-old daughter with Down's syndrome. Meeting them showed us that we would be able to cope because they had.'

'Please do not misunderstand me. A child like X who has special needs, no matter how complex their condition, I think brings such joy to their family. Their achievements, which so often cost so much to themselves and their family, mean so much.'

'I find that I have to try very hard not to dwell on what problems may occur as they might not, and it is enough for anyone to deal with what problems actually arise. Looking too far into the future is not a useful occupation either.'

Information and support for parents and children

Department of Work and Pensions (DWP) Information on benefits for disabled children and their carers ☎ 0800 88 22 00 🖳 www.direct.gov.uk

Contact a Family Support and information for families with disabled children (any disability) ☎ 0808 808 3555 🖳 www.cafamily.org.uk

Whizz-Kidz Mobility for non-mobile disabled children ☎ 020 7233 6600 🖳 www.whizz-kidz.org.uk

Holiday Care Holidays for families with a disabled child ☎ 0845 124 9971 🖳 www.holidaycare.org.uk

Children with cancer: Once the diagnosis of cancer is made, most children embark on an intensive regime of treatment which may involve surgery, chemotherapy and/or radiotherapy. They are usually referred to specialist paediatric oncology units who share care with local hospitals, and have direct access to advice and admission via those units. Outreach nurses provide support in the community (e.g. administration of IV drugs via Hickman lines) with the aim of maintaining as normal a lifestyle as possible.

The GP's role: The role of the GP is important in management of children with cancer even if it is peripheral:
- Keep in touch with the family and up to date with what is going on
- Provide support to the child and other family members
- Give advice on any benefits or local services the family might find of assistance
- Ensure prescriptions requested by specialist services are supplied promptly.

Palliative care: Sadly, despite treatment, some children progress to the terminal stages of their illnesses. General principles of palliative care apply but the emotional traumas are often much greater. If possible engage specialist palliative care services early. Try to maintain continuity of care with as few professionals involved as possible. Provide ongoing support to family members after the child has died.

Bereaved children: Children understand what death is by 8y. and even children of 2–3y. have some understanding of death. Exclusion makes children isolated and often makes the death of someone they have known more, not less, painful. Prepare children for a death if possible and give them a chance to have their questions answered. If a child has problems, seek specialist help.

Further information

DoH Children's NSF (2004) ▢ www.dh.gov.uk
HM Government Carers and Disabled Children Act (2000)
▢ www.hmso.gov.uk/acts/acts2000/20000016.htm
Audit Commission Services for disabled children (2003)
▢ www.audit-commission.gov.uk/disabledchildren

Advice for patients: Parent experiences of having a child with a terminal disease

'That stab of pain in the heart, that feeling of having your insides ripped out when you find out that your child has a disease that is incurable, with symptoms that can only get worse, that pain never goes away, or hasn't yet…. When I first heard the news I felt that my life had effectively come to an end. I had dreams for my family. I had high hopes, you know, the ones involving famous football players, rugby players, airline pilots, whatever. None of them included someone disabled and wheelchair bound.'

'Sometimes it felt as if I was being punished. But someone else shouldn't be paying for my faults; that just wasn't fair. Or maybe it was. After all, seeing someone you love from the depths of your heart degenerate before your very eyes is pretty effective punishment. Or maybe there is no such thing as fairness. Fairness is a human concept and nothing about this made sense.'

Information and advice for children and parents

Help Adolescents With Cancer (HAWC) ☎ 0161 688 6244
🖥 www.hawc-co-uk.com
Association for Children's palliative care (ACT) ☎ 0845 108 2201
🖥 www.act.org.uk
Association of Children's Hospices (ACH) ☎ 0117 989 7820
🖥 www.childhospice.org.uk
Winston's Wish (support for children and young people following death of a sibling or parent) ☎ 0845 2030 405
🖥 www.winstonswish.org.uk
Cruse Bereavement Care Young Persons' Helpline
☎ 0808 808 1677 🖥 www.crusebereavementcare.org.uk
Child Bereavement Trust ☎ 0845 357 1000
🖥 www.childbereavement.org.uk
Child Death Helpline ☎ 0800 282 986
🖥 www.childdeathhelpline.org.uk

GP Notes: Checklist of areas to cover when looking after children with chronic disability or terminal conditions

- Can physical symptoms be improved?
- Can psychological symptoms be improved (including self-esteem)?
- Can functioning within the home be improved? (aids and adaptations within the home, extra help)
- Can functioning in the community be improved? (mobility outside the home, school, social activities)
- Can the family's financial state be improved? (benefits)
- Does the carer need more support? (voluntary and self-help organizations, social services)

Benefits

> ⚠ Information in this section is up to date at the time of going to press but benefits issues change rapidly.

Millions of pounds of benefits go unclaimed every year. This section is a rough guide to the benefits available to enable GPs to point their patients in the right direction. It is not intended as a comprehensive reference.

Table 10.2 Guide to agencies involved in delivering benefits			
Agency	**Function**	**Website: www. + suffix**	**Telephone**
Department of Work and Pensions (DWP)	Administers all benefits *except:* Tax credits (Inland Revenue) Statutory Sick Pay (employer) Housing Benefit (local authority) Council Tax Benefit (local authorities)	dwp.gov.uk *or* direct.gov.uk *or* jobcentreplus.gov.uk	*Benefits enquiry line* – 0800 882200 *Help with form completion* – 0800 441144 *Information for employers and the self-employed* – 0845 7143143
HM Revenues and Customs (HMRC)	Administers tax credits	hmrc.gov.uk	*Tax credit enquiry line* – 0845 300 3900
Appeals Service	Provides an independent tribunal body for hearing appeals	appeals-service.gov.uk	N/A

🛈 0800 numbers are free; 0845 numbers are charged at local rate.

> ⚠ Benefit fraud: The DWP provides a freefone number which members of the public can telephone in confidence to give information about benefit fraud. ☎ 0800 85 44 40

Further information for health professionals
Department of Work and Pensions (DWP) ▢ www.dwp.gov.uk

Further information for patients and carers
Government information and services ▢ www.direct.gov.uk
Citizens' Advice Bureau ▢ www.adviceguide.org.uk
Counsel and Care ☎ 0845 300 7585 ▢ www.counselandcare.org.uk

Table 10.3 Benefits for mothers and children

	Eligibility	How to apply	Benefits gained
Child benefit	Anyone responsible for the upbringing of a child aged <16y.	Application form from local social security office or ▣ www.direct.gov.uk	Oldest child – £18.10/wk. Other children – £12.10/wk.
Statutory Maternity Pay (SMP)*	• Worked for the same employer for 26wk. into the 15th week before the baby is due • Pregnant at (or have had the baby by) the 11th week before the baby is due • Earning ≥ NI lower earnings limit in the relevant period	• Inform employer at least 28d. before starting leave • Mat B1 form	Paid for up to 26wk. (Maternity Pay Period – MPP)– can start any time from 11th week before the baby is due until the week of birth. • 1st 6wk. – 90% usual average earnings • 6–26wks. – 90% of usual earnings or £112.75/wk. – whichever is lower.
Maternity Allowance (MA)*	• Employed/self-employed for ≥26wk. in the 66wk. preceding the baby's due date (test period). • Average weekly earnings of ≥ £30/wk. for at least 13wk. of the test period • Do not qualify for SMP (e.g. changed jobs, become unemployed, self-employed).	Apply > 26/40 and within 3mo. of date MA due to start. Need: • Form MA1 (available from social security offices, employer or DWP ▣ www.direct.gov.uk • MATB1; and, if employed, • Form SMP1 from employer.	Paid for 26wk. ìMaternity Allowance Period – MAP)– can start any time from 11th week before the baby until the day after birth. 90% of usual earnings or £112.75/wk. – whichever is lower.

* Incapacity benefit and income support may be available for women unable to claim SMP or MA

Table 10.3 Contd.

	Eligibility	How to apply	Benefits gained
Sure start Maternity Grant	• From 11wk. before baby is due to <3mo. after birth/adoption • Claiming IS or income based JSA; Child Tax Credit at a higher rate than the maximum family element or Working Tax Credit with a disability or severe disability element	Form SF100 from social security offices.	£500 payment

⬤ Free prescriptions/dentistry are available to all children <16y., mothers while pregnant and <1y. after birth, and families with low income

Table 10.4 Benefits for disabled children and their carers

	Eligibility	How to apply	Amount
Disability Living Allowance (DLA)▽	Disability >3mo. and expected to last >6mo. more*. *Mobility Component:* Help needed to get about outdoors ● *Higher rate* – unable/virtually unable to walk (age >3y.) ● *Lower rate* – help to find way in unfamiliar places (age >5y.) *Care Component:* Help needed with personal care ● *Lower rate* – attention/supervision needed for a significant proportion of the day or unable to prepare a cooked meal. ● *Middle rate* – attention/supervision throughout the day or repeated prolonged attention or watching over at night. ● *Higher rate* – 24 hours attention/supervision day or terminal illness*	☎ 0800 882200 (0800 220674 in Northern Ireland) or Leaflet DS704 available from Post Offices or Using claim packs available at CAB and social security offices or 🖥 www.direct.gov.uk	**Mobility Component:** *Higher rate* – £45.00/wk. *Lower rate* – £17.10/wk. **Care Component:** *Higher rate* – £64.50/wk. *Middle rate* – £43.15/wk. *Lower rate* – £17.10/wk. ● If a child receives DLA, families may be able to claim additional child tax credit
Community Care Grant	Receiving Income Support or income-based Jobseeker's allowance and: ● want to re-establish or help the applicant or a family member stay in the community ● ease exceptional pressure on the applicant or a family member. ● to help with certain travel costs	Form SF300 from local social security offices or 🖥 www.direct.gov.uk	Minimum payment £30. No maximum amount.

▽ No need to receive help to apply. Not means tested.

* Terminal illness (not expected to live >6mo.) – claim under Special Rules. Claims are processed much faster and the highest care rate is automatically awarded. GP or hospital specialist fills in form DS1500 to provide clinical information to support application (fee can be claimed).

Table 10.4 Contd.

	Eligibility	How to apply	Amount
Disabled facilities grant	For work essential to help a disabled person live an independent life. Means tested.	Apply via local housing department.	Any reasonable application for funds is considered.
Carer's allowance	• Aged ≥16y; and • Spends ≥35h/wk. caring for a person with a disability who is getting constant attendance allowance or middle or higher rate care component of DLA; and • Earning ≤ £87.00/wk. after allowable expenses • Not in full time education	Complete form in leaflet DS700 available from local security offices or ⧉ www.direct.gov.uk	£48.65/wk. Plus additions for dependants. (ⓘ no new claims for dependent children have been accepted since April 2003)
Home responsibilities protection (HRP)	Scheme which protects Basic State Pension for people who don't work or have low income and are caring for a child.	Further information is available at: ⧉ www.thepensionservice.gov.uk	
Vaccine damage payment	Payable if the claimant is >80% impaired by a vaccination given within the NHS.	Apply via the vaccine damage payments unit, Palatine House, Lancaster Road, Preston PR1 1HB ☎ 01772 899944 ⧉ www.direct.gov.uk	Recipients receive a lump sum

Table 10.5 Benefits for families with low income

	Eligibility	How to Apply	Benefits gained
Income Support (IS)	• ≥18y, (16y, in some circumstances) and <60y. • Low income, <£8000 in savings (£16000 if in residential care) and not in receipt of JSA. • <16h paid work/wk. (and partner <24h/wk.)	Form A1 from local Jobcentre plus office.	**Money** – depends on circumstances **Other benefits** – housing benefit, community tax benefit, health benefits and social fund payments. Children >5y. – and pregnant women – free milk and vitamins (free fruit soon to be introduced). Children >5y. free school meals and, in some areas, uniform grants. **Christmas bonus** – annual one-off payment
JobSeekers Allowance (JSA)	• ≥19y. (women) or <65y. (men). • Unemployed or working <16h/wk. • Capable of and available for work • Have a JobSeekers agreement that contracts the recipient to actively seek work.	Apply by visiting local JobCentre.	**Contributions-based JobSeekers allowance** – can claim for up to 26wk. Age-dependent fixed weekly payment. **Income-based JobSeekers allowance** – allowance dependent on circumstances. Entitles claimants to same benefits as income support (see above). **Hardship payments** – available to people is disallowed JSA.
Council Tax Benefit and Second Adult rebate	• **Council tax benefit:** Low income. Exclusions as for housing benefit. • **Second adult rebate:** Payable if someone who lives with you is aged >18y. does not pay rent or council tax and has low income. • **Council tax reduction:** if single occupier or disabled. • **Disregarded occupants:** Certain people including students, carers and children, are not counted in calculating the number of people living at a property.	Via local authority	**Council tax benefit:** pays council tax. **Council tax reductions:** • all disregarded occupants – 50% • disabled – reduction to next lowest council tax band. • single occupier – 25% discount

Table 10.5 (Contd.)

	Eligibility	How to apply	Benefits gained
Working Tax Credit (WTC)	• Age ≥16y, working ≥16h./wk. and responsible for a child (<16y. or 16–19y. in full time education)	Apply to HMRC ☎ 0845 300 3900 🖥 www.hmrc.gov.uk	**Tax credits** – amount depends on individual circumstances ⊕ Childcare – up to 70% childcare costs can be reclaimed
Children's Tax Credit (CTC)	• Age ≥16y. and • Responsible for ≥1 child (<16y. or 16–19y. in full time education). • Family income < £50,000 pa.	Apply to HMRC ☎ 0845 300 3900 🖥 www.hmrc.gov.uk	**Tax credits:** • Family element – credit for any family eligible – ↑ if there is a child <1y. old in the family. • Child element – credit for each individual child in the family – ↑ if the child is disabled/severely disabled.
Housing Benefit	Low income, living in rented housing	Via local authority	Pays rent for up to 60wk. Then need to reapply.
The 6 social Fund payments	• **Crisis loan** • **Budgeting loan** – for a large purchases. Must receive IS, pension credit or income-based JSA. • **Funeral Payments** – Must receive low income benefit and be responsible for the funeral. • **Cold weather payments** – average temperature <0°C for ≥7d. Must receive IS, pension credit or income-based JSA and live with a pensioner, child <5y. or disabled person. • **Maternity grant** • **Community care grant** – 🕮 p.333	Cold weather payments – should be automatic. All others claim via local job-centre plus office or 🖥 www.jobcentreplus.gov.uk	• **Crisis loan** – up to £1000 – interest free loan repayable when crisis finished over 78wk. • **Budgeting loan** – as crisis loan • **Funeral expenses** – sum towards cost of funeral – usually does not cover full expenses. • **Cold weather payments** – £8.50/wk.

Table 10.6 Mobility for disabled children			● Local public transport schemes also exist
	Eligibility	How to apply	Benefits gained
Blue Badge Scheme	Age >2y. and ≥1 of the following: ● Higher rate of the mobility component of DLA ● Motor vehicle supplied by a Government Health department ● Registered blind ● Permanent and substantial difficulty walking	Apply through local social services department. ● The badge should not be used if the disabled person is not in the car. Further information: 🖳 www.dft.gov.uk	Entitles holder to park: ● in specified disabled spaces: ● free of charge or time limit at parking meters or other places where waiting is limited ● on single yellow lines for up to 3h (no time limit in Scotland)
Motability Scheme	Higher rate mobility component of DLA	Contact motability. Application guide available at 🖳 www.motability.co.uk or ☎ 0845 456 4566	Registered Charity. Mobility payments can be used to lease or hire-purchase a car, powered scooter or wheelchair. Grants may also be available for advance payments, adaptations or driving lessons.
Road Tax Exemption	● Higher rate mobility component of DLA or ● Person nominated as someone who regularly drives for a disabled person	Usually received automatically. If not and claiming DLA ☎ 0845 7123456	Exemption from Road Tax.

Table 10.7 Adaptations and equipment for disabled children   ❶ All purchases related to disability are VAT exempt

	Eligibility	Applying	Benefits received
Occupational Therapy (OT) Assessment	All disabled people	Request needs assessment by occupational therapist via local social services department.	Enables provision of equipment and adaptations necessary to maintain an independent lifestyle.
Disabled Living Centres/Disabled Living Foundation	All disabled people	49 **Disabled Living Centres** in the UK – list available at 🖥 www.assist-uk.org/centres/centres **Disabled Living Foundation:** ☎ 0845 130 9177 🖥 www.dlf.org.uk	**Disabled Living Centres** – Look at and try out equipment with OTs on hand to advise. **Disabled Living Foundation:** Information on aids and adaptations.

Chapter 11

Useful information and contacts for GPs and patients

Useful information and contacts for GPs

General information

DoH Children's National Service Framework (2004) 🖥 www.dh.gov.uk
DIPEx patient experience database 🖥 www.dipex.org
NICE Referral guidelines for suspected cancer – quick reference guide (2005) 🖥 www.nice.org.uk
National Library for Health 🖥 www.library.nhs.uk

Acne

BMJ Webster GF Acne vulgaris (2002) 325 pp.475–9 🖥 www.bmj.com

Addiction and dependence

DoH Drug misuse and dependence – guidelines on clinical management (1999) 🖥 www.dh.gov.uk

Adolescents

NICE Preventing sexually transmitted infections and reducing under 18 conceptions (2007) 🖥 www.nice.org.uk
BMJ McPherson Adolescents in primary care (2005) 330 pp.465–7 🖥 www.bmj.com

Allergy/anaphylaxis

British Society for Allergy and Clinical Immunology (BSACI) 🖥 www.bsaci.org
Resuscitation Council UK Emergency medical treatment of anaphylactic reactions for first medical responders (2005) 🖥 www.resus.org.uk

Amblyopia

Royal College of Ophthalmologists Guidelines for the management of strabismus and amblyopia (2000) 🖥 www.rcophth.ac.uk

Anaemia

British Committee for Standards in Haematology 🖥 www.bcshguidelines.com
● Diagnosis and management of acquired aplastic anaemia (2003)
● Diagnosis and management of hereditary spherocytosis (2004)

Artificial eyes

National Artificial Eye Service ☎ 0845 6050561 🖥 www.naes.nhs.uk

Asthma

British Thoracic Society 🖥 www.brit-thoracic.org.uk
British Thoracic Society/SIGN British guideline on the management of asthma (revised 2005) 🖥 www.sign.ac.uk
Peak flow 🖥 www.peakflow.com
Cochrane: Accessed via 🖥 www.library.nhs.uk
● Abramson *et al* Allergen immunotherapy for asthma (2003)
● Bhogal *et al* Written action plans for asthma in children (2005)
● Dennis & Cates Alexander technique for chronic asthma (2000)
● Gøtzsche *et al* House dust mite control measures for asthma (2004)

- Holloway & Ram Breathing exercises for asthma (2004)
- Hondras *et al* Manual therapy for asthma (2005)
- Kilburn *et al* Pet allergen control measures for allergic asthma in children and adults (2001)
- McCarney *et al* Acupuncture for chronic asthma (2003)
- McCarney *et al* Homeopathy for chronic asthma (2004)
- Ram *et al* Physical training for asthma (2005)
- Thien *et al* Dietary marine fatty acids (fish oil) for asthma (2002)
- York & Shuldham Family therapy for chronic asthma in children (2005)

Thorax
- Huntley & Ernst Herbal medicines for asthma: a systematic review (2000) 55(11) pp.925–9
- Huntley *et al* Relaxation therapies for asthma: a systematic review (2002) 57(2) pp.127–31

Clinical evidence: Accessed via 🖥 www.library.nhs.uk
- Dennis *et al* Asthma (2004)
- Keeley & McKean Asthma and other wheezing disorders in children (2004)

BMJ Learning Childhood asthma: diagnosis and treatment
🖥 www.bmjlearning.com

Attention deficit hyperactivity disorder (ADHD)

NICE Attention deficit hyperactivity disorder: pharmacological and psychological interventions in children, young people and adults (due to publish in April 2008) 🖥 www.nice.org.uk

Benefits – see disability and benefits
Child abuse
DoH 🖥 www.dh.gov.uk
- Working together to safeguard children (1998)
- What to do if you're worried a child is being abused (2003)

RCGP Carter & Bannon. The role of primary care in the protection of children from abuse and neglect (2003) 🖥 www.rcgp.org.uk
Department for Education and Skills Every child matters (2004) 🖥 www.everychildmatters.gov.uk

Child surveillance
Hall, Hill & Elliman *The child surveillance handbook* (1994) Radcliffe Medical Press ISBN: 1870905245
UK Newborn Screening Programme Centre
🖥 www.newbornscreening-bloodspot.org.uk
NHS Newborn hearing screening programme 🖥 www.nhsp.info

Coeliac disease
British Society of Gastroenterology Interim guidelines for the management of patients with coeliac disease (2002) 🖥 www.bsg.org.uk

Confidentiality and consent
DoH guidance 🖥 www.dh.gov.uk
BMA 🖥 www.bma.org.uk
- Consent toolkit
- Confidentiality and people under 16
- Access to health records by patients

Gilbert & Tripp *Consent, rights and choices in healthcare for children and young people* (2001) BMJ Books ISBN: 0727912283

GMC ⊞ www.gmc-uk.org
- Seeking patients' consent: the ethical considerations
- Guidance on good practice: confidentiality

Congenital heart disease (see also heart disease)

Journal of the Royal College of Physicians of London Hunter S Congenital heart disease in adolescence (2000) 34(2) pp.150–2

NEJM Brickner *et al* Congenital heart disease in adults (2000) 342(4) pp.256–63

Congenital infection

RCOG ⊞ www.rcog.org.uk
- Chickenpox in pregnancy (2001)
- Management of genital herpes in pregnancy (2002)
- Prevention of early-onset neonatal group B streptococcal disease (2003)
- Management of HIV in pregnancy (2004)

British HIV Association Management of HIV in pregnant women and the prevention of mother-to-child transmission of HIV (2005) ⊞ www.bhiva.org

DTB Chickenpox, pregnancy and the newborn (2005) 45(9) pp.69–72 ⊞ www.dtb.org.uk

Conjunctivitis

Lancet Rose PW *et al* Chloramphenicol treatment for acute infective conjunctivitis in children in primary care: a randomised double-blind placebo-controlled trial (2005) 366(9479) pp.6–7

BMJ Everitt, Little & Smith A randomised controlled trial of management strategies for acute infective conjunctivitis in general practice (2006) **333**: 468

Constipation

NEJM Iacono *et al* Intolerance of cow's milk and chronic constipation in children (1998) 339(16) pp. 1100–4

Cot death

Foundation for the Study of Infant Deaths (FSID) Guidelines for general practitioners when a baby dies suddenly and unexpectedly (2003); information; support; administration of the CONI scheme ⊞ www.sids.org.uk

Cystic fibrosis

CF Trust Standards for the clinical care of children and adults with CF in the UK (2001) ⊞ www.cftrust.org.uk

UK Newborn Screening Programme Centre CF screening programme and leaflets about CF screening for parents ⊞ www.newbornscreening-bloodspot.org.uk

Deafness

NHS Newborn hearing screening programme ⊞ www.nhsp.info

Depression

NICE Depression in children and young people (2005) ⊞ www.nice.org.uk

Diabetes

WHO Definition, diagnosis and classification of diabetes mellitus and its complications (2000) ⌨ www.diabetes.org.uk

NICE Diagnosis and management of type 1 diabetes in children and young people (2004) ⌨ www.nice.org.uk

Diet and feeding

DoH Infant feeding recommendation ⌨ www.dh.gov.uk
Drugs in Lactation Advisory Service ⌨ www.ukmicentral.nhs.uk
UNICEF Baby Friendly Initiative ⌨ www.babyfriendly.org.uk

Diploma in child health

Royal College of Paediatrics and Child Health ⌨ www.rcpch.ac.uk

Disability and benefits

HM Government Carers and Disabled Children Act (2000) ⌨ www.hmso.gov.uk/acts/acts2000/20000016.htm
Audit Commission Services for disabled children (2003) ⌨ www.audit-commission.gov.uk/disabledchildren
Department of Work and Pensions (DWP) ⌨ www.dwp.gov.uk
Disability Discrimination Act ⌨ www.direct.gov.uk

Drug abuse

DoH Drug misuse and dependence guidelines on clinical management (1999) ⌨ www.dh.gov.uk

Drugs

BNF ⌨ www.bnf.org
BNF for children ⌨ www.bnfc.org
Information on drugs used to treat rare paediatric conditions: Alder Hey Children's Hospital (☎ 0151 252 5381) or Great Ormond Street Hospital (☎ 020 7405 9200)
DTB Prescribing unlicensed drugs or using drugs for unlicensed applications (1992) 30 pp.97–9
Obtaining steroid cards:
● England and Wales: Department of Health ☎ 08701 555455
● Scotland: Banner Business Supplies ☎ 01506 448440
Medicines and Healthcare Products Regulatory Agency (MHRA – formerly MCA) ⌨ www.mhra.gov.uk
UK National Poisons Information Service ☎ 0870 600 6266
TOXBASE poisons database ⌨ www.toxbase.org
Drugs in Lactation Advisory Service ⌨ www.ukmicentral.nhs.uk

Eating disorders

NICE Core interventions in the treatment and management of anorexia nervosa, bulimia nervosa and related eating disorders (2004) ⌨ www.nice.org

Eczema

NICE Atopic eczema in children: Management of atopic eczema in children from birth up to the age of 12 years (due to publish in December 2007) ⌨ www.nice.org.uk
BMJ ⌨ www.bmj.com
● Barnetson & Rogers Childhood atopic eczema (2002) 324 pp.1376–9
● Santer *et al* Childhood eczema (2005) 331 p.497

British Association of Dermatologists Guidelines for the management of contact dermatitis (2001) ▦ www.bad.org.uk

ENT problems

ENT UK British Association of Otorhinolaryngologists – Head & Neck Surgeons (BAO – HNS) ▦ www.entuk.org
British Association of Oral and Maxillofacial Surgeons ▦ www.baoms.org.uk
ENT Specialist Library ▦ www.library.nhs.uk/ent
Hawke Library of Ear Disease ▦ www.earphotos.com

Epilepsy

NICE ▦ www.nice.org.uk
- The epilepsies: the diagnosis and management of the epilepsies in adults and children in primary and secondary care (2004)
- Newer drugs for epilepsy in children (2004)

Eye problems

Royal College of Ophthalmologists ▦ www.rcopth.ac.uk
Eye Atlas – excellent photographs of many conditions ▦ www.eyeatlas.com
Eye examination tips ▦ http://eyelearn.med.utoronto.ca

Glue ear – see otitis media

GP contract

DoH The GMS Contract ▦ www.dh.gov.uk
BMA ▦ www.bma.org.uk
- The GMS Contract and supporting documents
- Quality and outcomes framework guidance
- Read codes

Hayfever – see rhinitis

Headache

British Association for the Study of Headache Guidelines for all doctors in the diagnosis and management of migraine and tension-type headache (2nd edition – 2003) ▦ www.bash.org.uk
DTB Managing migraine in children (2004) 42 pp.25–8

Head injury

NICE Triage, assessment investigation and early management of head injury in infants, children and adults (2003) ▦ www.nice.org.uk

Heart disease

British Heart Foundation ☎ 0845 708070 ▦ www.bhf.org.uk
British Heart Foundation Factfiles:
- Infective endocarditis (12/2003 & 01/2004)
- Palpitations: their significance and investigation (04/2004)
DoH National Service Framework: Coronary Heart Disease (2005) ▦ www.dh.gov.uk
BMJ *ABC of clinical electrocardiography* (2002) ▦ www.bmj.com

HIV

Medical Foundation for AIDS and Sexual Health HIV in primary care (2004 and revision 2005) 🖥 www.medfash.org.uk
British HIV Association 🖥 www.bhiva.org
• HIV Treatment Guidelines (2006)
• Management of HIV infection in pregnant women and the prevention of mother-to-child transmission of HIV (2005)
RCOG Management of HIV in pregnancy (2004) 🖥 www.rcog.org.uk

Immunization

DoH The Green Book: immunization against infectious disease 🖥 www.dh.gov.uk
Immunisation 🖥 www.immunisation.org.uk
NHS 🖥 www.mmrthefacts.nhs.uk
Health Protection Agency (HPA) 🖥 www.hpa.org.uk
• Topics A–Z
• Information on vaccines and vaccination schedules

Infection – see also: congenital infection, HIV

Hyposplenism/asplenism: Patient cards and information sheets are available from Department of Health, PO Box 410, Wetherby, LS23 7LL.
DoH Winning ways: reducing healthcare-associated infection in England (2004) 🖥 www.dh.gov.uk
NICE 🖥 www.nice.org.uk
• Infection control, prevention of health care associated infection in primary and community care (2003)
• Feverish illness in children: Assessment and initial management in children up to 5 years (due to publish in May 2007)
• Acute diarrhoea and vomiting in children: diagnosis and management (due to publish in February 2009)
Health Protection Agency (HPA) 🖥 www.hpa.org.uk
• Topics A–Z
• Guidance on management of communicable diseases in schools and nurseries
• Information on notification of infectious diseases
British Association of Dermatologists Guidelines for the management of cutaneous warts (2001) 🖥 www.bad.org.uk
BMJ Fuller *et al* Diagnosis and management of scalp ringworm (2003) 326 p. 539 🖥 www.bmj.com

Influenza

NICE Guidance on the use of zanamivir, oseltamivir and amantadine for the treatment of influenza (2003) 🖥 www.nice.org.uk
Health Protection Agency (HPA) Topics A–Z: Influenza 🖥 www.hpa.org.uk
DoH (Chief Medical Officer) Explaining pandemic flu (2005) Available from 🖥 www.dh.gov.uk

ITP

British Committee for standards in Haematology Guidelines for investigation and Management of ITP (2003) 🖥 www.bcshguidelines.com

345

Neonatal screening – see child surveillance

Obesity

NICE Obesity: the prevention, identification, assessment and management of overweight and obesity in adults and children (2006) ⌨ www.nice.org.uk

Children's BMI Charts ⌨ www.healthforallchildren.co.uk

Otitis externa

Clinical Evidence Hajioff D. Otitis externa (2005) ⌨ www.clinicalevidence.com

Journal of the Royal College of General Practitioners Lambert IJ A comparison of the treatment of otitis externa with otosporin and aluminium acetate: a report from a services practice in Cyprus (1981) 31 pp.291–294

Otitis media

SIGN Diagnosis and management of childhood acute otitis media in primary care (2003) ⌨ www.sign.ac.uk

Clinical Evidence Williamson I. Otitis media with effusion (2004) ⌨ www.clinicalevidence.com

Overdose – see drugs

Pneumonia

British Thoracic Society Guidelines for the management of community-acquired pneumonia in children (2002) ⌨ www.brit-thoracic.org.uk

Poisoning – see drugs

Psoriasis

British Association of Dermatologists Recommendations for the initial management of psoriasis (2003) ⌨ www.bad.org.uk

Refugee children:

The Refugee Council ⌨ www.refugeecouncil.org.uk

Asylum Aid ☎ 0207 247 8741 ⌨ www.asylumaid.org.uk

Health for asylum seekers and refugees ⌨ www.harpweb.org.uk

Red Cross Family tracing ⌨ www.redcross.org.uk

Resuscitation

Resuscitation Council (UK) ⌨ www.resus.org.uk
- Resuscitation guidelines (2005)
- Emergency medical treatment of anaphylactic reactions for first medical responders (2005)

Rhinitis

British Society for Allergy and Clinical Immunology (BSACI) (2000) Rhinitis management guidelines ⌨ www.bsaci.org

Sinusitis

Cochrane Williams J. *et al* Antibiotics for acute maxillary sinusitis (2000)

Sore throat

SIGN Management of sore throat and indications for tonsillectomy (1999) ⌨ www.sign.ac.uk

Sports medicine
British Association of Sport and Exercise Medicine
🖥 www.basem.co.uk
ABC of sports medicine (1999) BMJ Publishing ISBN: 072 791 3662

Squint
Royal College of Ophthalmologists Guidelines for the management of strabismus and amblyopia (2000) 🖥 www.rcophth.ac.uk
Squint/strabismus 🖥 http://eyelearn.med.utoronto.ca/
Lectures04-05/Paediatric/03Strabismus.htm#strab

Suicide and self-harm
DoH National Suicide Prevention Strategy for England (2002)
🖥 www.dh.gov.uk
NICE Self-harm: the short-term physical and psychological management and secondary prevention of self-harm in primary and secondary care (2004) 🖥 www.nice.org.uk

Travel
DoH Health advice for travellers 🖥 www.dh.gov.uk
National Travel Health Network and Centre (funded by DoH) Information for travellers and health professionals including yellow fever vaccination centres. Advice line for health professionals
☎ 0845 602 6712 🖥 www.nathnac.org
Fit for Travel NHS (Scotland) travel site ☎ 09068 44 45 46 (premium rate) 🖥 www.fitfortravel.scot.nhs.uk
Medical Advisory Service for Travellers Abroad (MASTA)
☎ 0113 283 7500 🖥 www.masta.org

Tuberculosis
NICE Tuberculosis: Clinical diagnosis and management of tuberculosis, and measures for its prevention and control (2006) 🖥 www.nice.org.uk
British Thoracic Society 🖥 www.brit-thoracic.org.uk
- *Thorax* Chemotherapy and management of tuberculosis in the UK (1998) 53(7) pp.536–48
- *Thorax* Control and prevention of tuberculosis in the UK: code of practice (2000) 55 pp.887–901
Health Protection Agency (HPA) Topics A–Z: Tuberculosis
🖥 www.hpa.org.uk
DoH Stopping tuberculosis in England: an action plan from the Chief Medical Officer (2004) 🖥 www.dh.gov.uk

Urinary tract infection
NICE Urinary tract infection: diagnosis, treatment and long-term management of urinary tract infection in children (due to publish in June 2007) 🖥 www.nice.org.uk

Urticaria
British Association of Dermatologists Guidelines for the management of urticaria and angio-oedema (2001) 🖥 www.bad.org.uk

Information and contacts for children, parents and carers

General information and support
Parentline ☎ 0808 800 2222 ▯ www.parentlineplus.org.uk
Childline 24h. confidential counselling service ☎ 0800 1111
▯ www.childline.org
Patient UK Patient information on a range of topics
▯ www.patient.co.uk
DIPEx patient experience database ▯ www.dipex.org

Accidents
Royal Society for the Prevention of Accidents ▯ www.rospa.co.uk

Acne
Acne support group ☎ 0870 870 2263 ▯ www.stopspots.org

Addiction and dependence
ADFAM Support for families of addicts ☎ 020 7553 7640
▯ www.adfam.org.uk
Solvent abuse ☎ 01785 810 762 ▯ www.re-solv.org
'Talk to FRANK' (England and Wales) Government-run information,
advice and referral service. ☎ (24h.) 0800 77 66 00
▯ www.talktofrank.com

Attention deficit hyperactivity disorder (ADHD)
Green & Chee *Understanding ADHD* (1997) Vermilion ISBN: 0091817005
National Attention Deficit Disorder Information and Support Service
(ADDISS) ☎ 020 8952 2800 ▯ www.addiss.co.uk

Adolescence
Teenage Health Freak ▯ www.teenagehealthfreak.org

Allergy/anaphylaxis
Allergy UK ☎ 01322 619 898 ▯ www.allergyuk.org
Anaphylaxis Campaign ☎ 01252 542029 ▯ www.anaphylaxis.org.uk
Medic-Alert Foundation Supply Medic-Alert bracelets ☎ 0800 581420
▯ www.medicalert.co.uk
BBC pollen index ▯ www.bbc.co.uk/weather/pollen

Anaemia
Aplastic Anaemia Trust ☎ 0870 487 0099 ▯ www.theaat.org.uk

Arthritis
Arthritis Research Campaign (ARC) ☎ 0870 850 5000
▯ www.arc.org.uk
Arthritis Care ☎ 0808 800 4050 ▯ www.arthritiscare.org.uk.
Arthritis Foundation ▯ www.arthritis.org

Asthma
Asthma UK ☎ 08457 01 02 03 ▯ www.asthma.org.uk

Ataxia

Ataxia UK ☎ 0845 644 0606 🖳 www.ataxia.org.uk

Autism

National Autistic Society of the UK (NAS) ☎ 0845 070 4004
🖳 www.nas.org.uk

Behaviour problems

Cry-sis Support for families with crying and sleepless babies
☎ 0845 1228 669 🖳 www.cry-sis.org.uk
Green *Beyond toddlerdom: every parent's guide to the 5–10s* (2000)
Vermilion ISBN: 0091816246
Green *Toddler taming: a parent's guide to the first four years* (2000)
Vermilion ISBN: 0091875285

Benefits

Benefit fraud line ☎ 0800 85 44 40
Citizens' Advice Bureau 🖳 www.adviceguide.org.uk
Department of Work and Pensions 🖳 www.dwp.gov.uk
☎ *Benefits Enquiry Line* — 0800 882200; 0800 243355 (minicom facility);
0800 441144 (for help with form completion)
Government information and services 🖳 www.direct.gov.uk
HM Customs & Revenue (HMCR) 🖳 www.hmcr.gov.uk *Tax credit
enquiry line* ☎ 0845 300 3900
Jobcentre Plus 🖳 www.jobcentreplus.gov.uk

Bereavement

Winston's Wish (support for children and young people following
death of a sibling or parent) ☎ 0845 2030 405
🖳 www.winstonswish.org.uk
Cruse Bereavement Care Young Persons' Helpline ☎ 0808 808 1677
🖳 www.crusebereavementcare.org.uk
Child Bereavement Trust ☎ 0845 357 1000
🖳 www.childbereavement.org.uk
Child Death Helpline ☎ 0800 282 986
🖳 www.childdeathhelpline.org.uk
Survivors of Bereavement by Suicide ☎ 0870 241 3337
🖳 www.uk-sobs.org.uk

Blindness

LOOK Support for families of blind or visually impaired children
☎ 0121 428 5038 🖳 www.look-uk.org
Royal National Institute for the Blind Information and talking book
service ☎ 0845 766 9999 🖳 www.rnib.org.uk
Action for Blind People ☎ 0800 915 4666 🖳 www.afbp.org
Deafblind UK ☎ 0800 132 320 🖳 www.deafblind.org.uk
National Association of Local Societies for Visually Impaired People
☎ 01302 571888 🖳 www.nalsvi.org
Guidedogs for the Blind Association ☎ 0118 983 5555
🖳 www.guidedogs.org.uk
British Blind Sport ☎ 01926 424 247 🖳 www.britishblindsport.org.uk
National Library for the blind ☎ 0161 355 2000 🖳 www.nlb-online.org
Calibre cassette library ☎ 01296 432 339 🖳 www.calibre.org.uk
ClearVision UK Postal lending library of children's books with added
braille ☎ 020 8789 9575 🖳 www.clearvisionproject.org

Talking Newspaper Association of the UK ☎ 01435 866102
📖 www.tnauk.org.uk

Brain tumour

Brain Tumour UK ☎ 0845 450 0386 📖 www.braintumouruk.org.uk
Brain and Spine Foundation ☎ 0808 808 1000
📖 www.brainandspine.org.uk
Brain Tumour Action (mainly Scotland) ☎ 01506 436 164
📖 www.braintumouraction.org.uk

Breast-feeding – see feeding and weaning

Cancer and terminal illness

Cancer Research UK (Cancer Help UK) Information sheets on many
different types of cancer ☎ 0800 226 237 📖 www.cancerhelp.org.uk
CancerBACUP ☎ 0808 800 1234 📖 www.cancerbacup.org.uk
Help Adolescents With Cancer (HAWC) ☎ 0161 688 6244
📖 www.hawc-co-uk.com
Association for children's palliative care (ACT) ☎ 0845 108 2201
📖 www.act.org.uk
Association of Children's Hospices (ACH) ☎ 0117 989 7820
📖 www.childhospice.org.uk

Cardiomyopathy

Cardiomyopathy Association ☎ 0800 018 1024
📖 www.cardiomyopathy.org
Cardiac Risk in the Young (Cry) ☎ 01737 363 222
📖 www.c-r-y.org.uk

Carers

Carers UK ☎ 0808 808 7777 📖 www.carersonline.org.uk
Counsel and Care ☎ 0845 300 7585 📖 www.counselandcare.org.uk
Princess Royal Trust for Carers ☎ 020 7480 7788 📖 www.carers.org
Disability and Carers' service 📖 www.direct.gov.uk

Cerebral palsy

SCOPE (cerebral palsy) ☎ 0808 800 3333 📖 www.scope.org.uk

Cleft lip and palate

Cleft Lip and Palate Association (CLAPA) ☎ 020 7833 4883
📖 www.clapa.com

Coeliac disease

Coeliac UK ☎ 0870 444 8804 📖 www.coeliac.co.uk

Congenital heart disease – see heart disease

Contraception – see sexual health

Crohn's disease and ulcerative colitis

National Association for Colitis and Crohn's disease (NACC)
☎ 0845 130 2233 (info); 0845 130 3344 (support) 📖 www.nacc.org.uk

Cystic fibrosis

Cystic Fibrosis Trust ☎ 0845 859 1000 ▣ www.cftrust.org.uk
UK Newborn Screening Programme Centre Leaflets about CF screening for parents ▣ www.newbornscreening-bloodspot.org.uk

Deafness

National Deaf Children's Society ☎ 0808 800 8880
▣ www.ndcs.org.uk
Royal National Institute for the Deaf (RNID) ☎ 0808 808 0123
▣ www.rnid.org.uk
Sign Community (British Deaf Association) ▣ www.bda.org.uk
Hearing Concern ☎ 0845 074 4600 ▣ www.hearingconcern.org.uk
Deafblind UK ☎ 0800 132 320 ▣ www.deafblind.org.uk
Hearing dogs for deaf people ▣ www.hearing-dogs.co.uk
UK Deaf Sport ▣ www.ukdeafsport.org.uk
RNID Typetalk ▣ www.typetalk.org

Diabetes

Diabetes UK ☎ 0845 120 2960 ▣ www.diabetes.org.uk

Disability

Department of Work and Pensions (DWP) Information on benefits for disabled children and their carers ☎ 0800 88 22 00
▣ www.direct.gov.uk
Contact a Family Support and information for families with disabled children (any disability) ☎ 0808 808 3555 ▣ www.cafamily.org.uk
Citizens' Advice Bureau ▣ www.adviceguide.org.uk
Royal Association for Disability and Rehabilitation (RADAR)
▣ www.radar.org.uk
Disablement Information and Advice Line (DIAL) ▣ www.dialuk.info
Disabled Living Foundation ☎ 0845 130 9177 ▣ www.dlf.org.uk
Forum of Mobility Centres (advice on use of motor vehicles for disabled people) ☎ 0800 559 3636 ▣ www.mobility-centres.org.uk
Motability ☎ 0845 456 4566 ▣ www.motability.co.uk
Whizz-Kidz Mobility for non-mobile disabled children
☎ 020 7233 6600 ▣ www.whizz-kidz.org.uk
Holiday Care Holidays for families with a disabled child
☎ 0845 124 9971 ▣ www.holidaycare.org.uk

Down's syndrome

Down's Syndrome Association ☎ 0845 230 0372
▣ www.downs-syndrome.org.uk

Drug abuse

Talk to Frank (England & Wales) Government run information, advice and referral service ☎ (24h.) 0800 77 6600 ▣ www.talktofrank.com
Know the Score (Scotland) ☎ 0800 587 5879
▣ www.knowthescore.info
Drugscope ▣ www.drugscope.org.uk
Drug-info Information about drug abuse for families of addicts
▣ www.drugs-info.co.uk

Dyslexia

British Dyslexia Association ☎ 0118 966 8271
▣ www.bdadyslexia.org.uk

Dyspraxia
Dyspraxia Foundation ☎ 01462 454 986
🖳 www.dyspraxiafoundation.org.uk

Dystonia
Dystonia Society ☎ 0845 458 6322 🖳 www.dystonia.org.uk

Ear, nose and throat problems
ENT UK Information on a range of ENT topics 🖳 www.entuk.org

Eating disorders
Eating Disorders Association (EDA) ☎ 0845 634 7650 (youths)
🖳 www.b-eat.co.uk

Eczema
National Eczema Society ☎ 0870 241 3604 🖳 www.eczema.org

Enuresis
ERIC Enuresis resources and information ☎ 0845 370 8008
🖳 www.eric.org.uk

Epilepsy
Epilepsy Action ☎ 0808 800 5050. 🖳 www.epilepsy.org.uk
Epilepsy Scotland ☎ 0808 800 2200 🖳 www.epilepsyscotland.org.uk
Joint Epilepsy Council of the UK and Ireland
🖳 www.jointepilepsycouncil.org.uk
West's Syndrome Support Group 🖳 www.wssg.org.uk

Eye problems
Royal College of Ophthalmologists 🖳 www.rcopth.ac.uk
Royal National Institute for the Blind Information and talking book
service ☎ 0845 766 9999 🖳 www.rnib.org.uk
Moorfields Eye Hospital Patient information sheets
🖳 www.moorfields.org.uk
Good Hope NHS Hospital Trust Patient information sheets and lots
of useful weblinks 🖳 www.goodhope.org.uk/departments/eyedept
Eye Care Trust Information on a range of eye problems and eye care
☎ 0845 129 5001 🖳 www.eye-care.org.uk
Specific eye conditions (SPECS) Information about support organizations for specific eye conditions 🖳 www.eyeconditions.org.uk

Feeding and weaning
National Childbirth Trust ☎ 0870 444 8708
🖳 www.nctpregnancyandbabycare.com
La Leche League ☎ 0845 120 2918 🖳 www.laleche.org.uk
Baby Café 🖳 www.thebabycafe.co.uk
Association of Breast-feeding Mothers ☎ 0870 4017711
🖳 www.abm.me.uk
Breast-feeding Network ☎ 0870 9000 8787
🖳 www.breastfeedingnetwork.org.uk

Weaning information leaflet available from 🖥 www.dh.gov.uk

Lewis S Practical parenting: weaning and first foods – which foods to introduce and when (2003) Hamlyn ISBN: 0600605647

Fragile X
Fragile X Society ☎ 01371 875100 🖥 www.fragilex.org.uk

Genetic disorders
Genetics Interests Group ☎ 020 7704 3141 🖥 www.gig.org.uk
Unique Rare Chromosome Disorder Support Group
☎ 01883 330766 🖥 www.rarechromo.org
Contact a Family ☎ 0808 808 3555 🖥 www.cafamily.org.uk

Glycogen storage diseases
Association for Glycogen Storage Disease (UK) 🖥 www.agsd.org.uk

Growth problems
Height Matters 🖥 www.heightmatters.org.uk

Haemophilia
Haemophilia Society ☎ 0800 018 6068 🖥 www.haemophilia.org.uk

Hayfever
BBC pollen index 🖥 www.bbc.co.uk/weather/pollen
Allergy UK ☎ 01322 619898 🖥 www.allergyuk.org

Headache
Migraine Action Association ☎ 0870 050 5898 🖥 www.migraine.org.uk
The Migraine Trust ☎ 020 7436 1336 🖥 www.migrainetrust.org

Heart disease
British Heart Foundation ☎ 0845 0708 070 🖥 www.bhf.org.uk
Children's Heart Federation ☎ 0808 808 5000 🖥 www.childrens-heart-fed.org.uk
Cardiac Risk in the Young (Cry) ☎ 0173 7363 222 🖥 www.c-r-y.org.uk
Heartline Association ☎ 01276 707636 🖥 www.heartline.org.uk
Children's Heart Association ☎ 01706 221988 🖥 www.heartchild.info

Heart transplant
Transplant Support Network ☎ 0800 027 4490/1
🖥 www.transplantsupportnetwork.org.uk

Hepatitis B
Department of Health Hepatitis B: how to protect your baby. Available from 🖥 www.dh.gov.uk

HIV
NAM Aidsmap ☎ 0207 840 0050 🖥 www.aidsmap.com
National AIDS Helpline ☎ 0800 567 123 (24h. helpline)
Terrence Higgins Trust ☎ 0845 1221 200 🖥 www.tht.org.uk
Children with AIDS Charity (CWAC) ☎ 020 7033 8620
🖥 www.cwac.org

Hydrocephalus – see spina bifida

Hypermobility
Hypermobility Syndrome Association (HMSA) ☎ 0845 345 4465
🖥 www.hypermobility.org

Ichthyosis
Ichthyosis Support Group ☎ 0845 602 9202 🖥 www.ichthyosis.co.uk

Idiopathic thrombocytopenic purpura – see ITP

Immune deficiency
Immune Deficiency Foundation 🖥 www.primaryimmune.org

Immunization
Immunization NHS website for patients 🖥 www.immunisation.org.uk

Infection
Health Protection Agency (HPA) Topics A–Z 🖥 www.hpa.org.uk

ITP
ITP Support Association 🖥 www.itpsupport.org.uk

Kawasaki disease
Kawasaki Support Group ☎ 0247 661 2178

Kidney disease
UK National Kidney Federation ☎ 0845 601 0209
🖥 www.kidney.org.uk
Kidney Patient Guide 🖥 www.kidneypatientguide.org.uk

Leukaemia
Children with Leukaemia ☎ 020 7404 0808 🖥 www.leukaemia.org.uk
Leukaemia Research Fund ☎ 020 7405 0101 🖥 www.lrf.org.uk
Leukaemia Care 🖥 www.leukaemiacare.org
CLIC and Sargent ☎ 0800 197 0068 🖥 www.clicsargent.org.uk

Lower limb problems
Steps Support for patients with lower limb conditions and their families
☎ 0871 717 0044 🖥 www.steps-charity.org.uk
Arthritis Research Campaign (ARC) ☎ 0870 850 5000
🖥 www.arc.org.uk

Lymphoma
Lymphoma Association ☎ 0808 808 5555 🖥 www.lymphoma.org.uk

Meningitis
Meningitis Research Foundation ☎ 080 8800 3344
🖥 www.meningitis.org.uk
Meningitis Trust ☎ 0800 028 18 28 🖥 www.meningitis-trust.org

Mental health problems
National Association for Mental Health (MIND) ☎ 0845 766 0163
🖥 www.mind.org.uk
Royal College of Psychiatrists Patient information sheets
🖥 www.rcpsych.ac.uk

Microphthalmia

Micro- and Anophthalmic Children's Society (MACS)
☎ 0800 169 8088 🖥 www.macs.org.uk

Migraine – see headache

MMR vaccination
Immunization 🖳 www.immunisation.org.uk
NHS 🖳 www.mmrthefacts.nhs.uk
Health Protection Agency (HPA) MMR information sheet and weblinks
🖳 www.hpa.org.uk

Muscular dystrophy
Muscular Dystrophy Campaign ☎ 020 7720 8055
🖳 www.muscular-dystrophy.org

Myaesthenia gravis
Myaesthenia Gravis Association ☎ 0800 919 922 🖳 www.mgauk.org

Neurofibromatosis
Neurofibromatosis Association UK ☎ 020 8439 1234 🖳 www.nfauk.org

Osteogenesis imperfecta
Brittle Bone Society ☎ 0800 0282 459 🖳 www.brittlebone.org

Osteopetrosis
Osteopetrosis Support Trust 🖳 www.osteopetrosis.org.uk

Panic attacks
No More Panic 🖳 www.nomorepanic.co.uk

Phenylketonuria
National Society for Phenylketonuria (NSPKU) ☎ 020 8364 3010
🖳 www.nspku.org

Premature babies
Bliss support line ☎ 0500 618 140 🖳 www.bliss.org.uk
Premature Babies website 🖳 www.premature-babies.co.uk

Psoriasis
Psoriasis Association ☎ 0845 676 0076
🖳 www.psoriasis-association.org.uk

Retinitis pigmentosa
British Retinitis Pigmentosa Society ☎ 0845 123 2354
🖳 www.brps.org.uk

Retinoblastoma
Childhood Eye Cancer Trust (CHECT) ☎ 0121 708 0583
🖳 www.chect.org.uk

Rhinitis
BBC pollen index 🖳 www.bbc.co.uk/weather/pollen
Allergy UK ☎ 01322 619898 🖳 www.allergyuk.org

Scoliosis
Scoliosis Association (UK) ☎ 020 8964 1166 🖳 www.sauk.org.uk
Arthritis Research Campaign (ARC) ☎ 0870 850 5000
🖳 www.arc.org.uk

Self-harm – see suicide

Severe learning difficulty
MENCAP ☎ 020 7454 0454 🖳 www.mencap.org.uk

Sexual health

Brook Advisory Service Contraceptive advice and counselling for teenagers ☎ 0800 0185 023 ▢ www.brook.org.uk
Family Planning Association ▢ www.fpa org.uk
Sexwise For under 19s ☎ 0800 28 29 30

Sickle cell anaemia

Sickle Cell Society ☎ 0800 001 5660 ▢ www.sicklecellsociety.org
UK Newborn Screening Programme Centre Leaflets about neonatal bloodspot screening for parents
▢ www.newbornscreening-bloodspot.org.uk

Special education

Independent Panel for Special Education Advice (IPSEA) ☎ 0800 018 4016 ▢ www.ipsea.org.uk
Children of High Intelligence ☎ 020 8347 8927
▢ www.chi-charity.org.uk

Spina bifida and hydrocephalus

Association for Spina Bifida and Hydrocephalus (ASBAH)
☎ 0845 450 7755 ▢ www.asbah.org.uk

Sturge-Weber syndrome

Sturge-Weber Foundation UK ☎ 01392 464675
▢ www.sturgeweber.org.uk

Suicide and self-harm

Self-injury and related issues (SIARI) ▢ www.siari.co.uk
Samaritans 24h. emotional support via telephone ☎ 08457 909 090
Survivors of Bereavement by Suicide ☎ 0870 241 3337
▢ www.uk-sobs.org.uk

Terminal illness – see cancer

Thalassaemia

UK Thalassaemia Society ▢ www.ukts.org

Tuberous sclerosis

Tuberous Sclerosis Association ☎ 0121 445 6970
▢ www.tuberous-sclerosis.org

Turner's syndrome

Turner's Syndrome Support Society ☎ 0845 230 7520
▢ www.tss.org.uk

Ulcerative colitis - see Crohn's disease and ulcerative colitis

Index